Adolescents and AIDS

Dedication

For my family—Mom, Dad, Uncle Mike, Aunt Lily, Margaret, Mike, John, Rebecca, Michelle, Tom, Jennifer, Jason, Casper, and Sebastian for your love and support.

For C. Terry Hendrix, C. Deborah Laughton, Diane S. Foster, and all the staff at Sage for their invaluable support and their incomparable expertise.

For everyone working tirelessly to create a safer and healthier world for adolescents.

Adolescents and AIDS

A Generation in Jeopardy

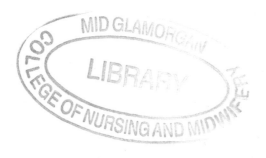

EDITED BY
RALPH J. DiCLEMENTE

SAGE Publications
International Educational and Professional Publisher
Newbury Park   London   New Delhi

For information address:

SAGE Publications, Inc.
2455 Teller Road
Newbury Park, California 91320

SAGE Publications Ltd.
6 Bonhill Street
London EC2A 4PU
United Kingdom

SAGE Publications India Pvt. Ltd.
M-32 Market
Greater Kailash I
New Delhi 110 048 India

Printed in the United States of America

Library of Congress Cataloging-in-Publication Data

Main entry under title:

Adolescents and AIDS: a generation in jeopardy / Ralph J. DiClemente, editor.
      p.   cm.
    Includes bibliographical references and index.
    ISBN 0-8039-4181-1 (cl).—ISBN 0-8039-4182-X (pb)
    1. AIDS (Disease) in adolescence—United States. 2. AIDS (Disease) in adolescence—United States—Prevention. 3. AIDS (Disease) in adolescence—Government policy—United States.
    [DNLM: 1. Acquired Immunodeficiency Syndrome—epidemiology—United States. 2. Acquired Immunodeficiency Syndrome—in adolescence. 3. Acquired Immunodeficiency Syndrome—prevention & control—United States. 4. Public Policy—United States. WD 308 A239]
RJ387.A25A36   1992   92-19402
362.1'969792'00835—dc20   CIP

93 94 15 14 13 12 11 10 9 8 7 6 5 4 3 2

Sage Production Editor: Diane S. Foster

13.1.9k

Contents

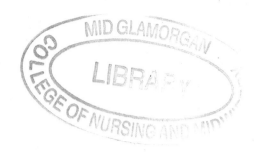

Foreword

THOMAS J. COATES

AIDS has taken its toll in the United States and will continue to do so, especially among those who do not have the knowledge, skills, or resources to protect themselves against its slow march. AIDS is especially unfortunate because it attacks those who are at, or just beginning, the prime of their lives. It is now the second leading cause of death among males and the fifth leading cause of death among females aged 25 to 44. Even more discouraging are the rampant growth rates in Africa, Latin America, and Asia. The young and productive population is vulnerable; the losses to individuals, families, and society are inestimable.

The next generation—those who are now adolescents—will not be spared the scourge unless we, in all of the societies in the world, can gather the courage to develop and disseminate effective prevention programs aimed at youth in all segments of society: those in school, out of school, in trouble, who have run away, who are experimenting with sexuality and sexual orientation, who have to sell sex in order to survive, who become involved in drug use, who have childhoods that cause them to grow up in a hurry, who are in the military, and who are incarcerated.

This book, and the research underlying it, lay the foundations for understanding the problems and what to do about them. Prevention programs that will have any chance of success, first need good data about the prevalence and incidence of AIDS, of HIV infection, and of sexual practices among adolescents. The second requirement is a thoroughgoing understanding of the determinants of high risk behaviors and the consequent diseases in these populations. The full range of determinants—economic, social, psychological, policy— need to be explored. The third requirement is good sound data on the impact of preventive programs on behavior and disease spread in this vulnerable population.

It has not been easy to collect this information. The United States and many other countries around the world are fearful that the collection of such data, or the implementation of prevention programs, will cause adolescents to become more sexual or will provide a social environment that promotes sexual activity in opposition to the norms or values of influential segments of these societies. Legal and policy impediments have interferred with the collection of basic epidemiological data and have made it difficult to find sites to evaluate programs which, based on sound theory, might have a chance of influencing adolescents to protect themselves sexually.

This is discouraging because AIDS is not the first sexually transmitted problem to affect teenagers in this country and other countries. The United States is experiencing a phenomenal growth in the birth rate among teenagers. In 1988, 488,981 teenagers gave birth, and this accounted for 12.5% of all births. The sharpest increase in the birth rate occurred among teens, ages 15 to 17 years. The pregnancy rate among teens is twice that of England, France, and Canada, and more than six times that of the Netherlands.[1] Every year, about 2.5 million U.S. teenagers are infected with sexually transmitted diseases.[2]

Thus, in addition to good information, we need policies that will recognize that teens are sexual, and that this activity will cause problems for them and society unless it is addressed directly and courageously. How will we resolve the deep differences in our society about whether or not this information should be collected and what kinds of programs should be implemented to address the problems that are revealed? More information will provide one of the answers. If we are concerned that data and programs will have untoward side effects, then we should design studies to reveal whether or not teens gain or lose control over their sexuality when these data and programs are available. The information in this book shows that the problems have not gone away because we as a society are reluctant to address adolescent sexuality directly. Quite the opposite. The book shows that information can be collected, that programs can be evaluated, and that they may have impact acceptable to many segments of society. Let us hope that more of this kind of work can be done.

Notes

1. U. S. Government Printing Office. (1992). Statement of the Center for Population Options, Hearing before the Select Committee on Children, Youth, and Families, House of Respresentatives, June 18, 1991. Washington, DC: Author.

2. U.S. Government Printing Office. (1992). Statement of Dr. Lloyd Kolbe, Centers for Disease Control, Hearing before the Select Committee on Children, Youth, and Families, House of Representatives, June 17, 1991. Washington, DC: Author.

Preface

Acquired immunodeficiency syndrome (AIDS) is a complex and multidimensional biological, social, and psychological phenomenon that rapidly has become a major public health crisis. The specter of AIDS has deeply affected many lives not only in the United States but on every continent of the world. While our understanding of the virology, immunology, and epidemiology of AIDS has increased substantially in a relatively brief period of time, at present no cure is known, and an effective vaccine is not anticipated in the foreseeable future. Thus prevention of HIV infection is the only means of stemming the tide of morbidity and mortality associated with this disease.

It is important to differentiate the biological roots of the disease from the roots of the epidemic. While the virus, human immunodeficiency virus (HIV), is the etiologic agent associated with AIDS, clearly the epidemic is driven by behavior. Transmission depends to a large extent on individuals engaging in risk behaviors that allow for exposure to the virus. From this perspective, the epidemic is as much a psychosocial phenomenon as it is a biological phenomenon in which protection from infection requires the adoption and maintenance of HIV-preventive behaviors.

Adolescents only recently have been recognized as being at risk for HIV infection. Adolescence is a time of growth and experimentation, a period marked by establishing autonomy and confronting new challenges. It is also a period in which many adolescents will initiate sexual and drug-related risk behaviors that increase the probability of HIV infection.

Adolescents and AIDS: A Generation in Jeopardy is an attempt to understand the threat the HIV epidemic poses for our youth and to propose strategies for curtailing this threat. To accomplish this goal, a multidisciplinary group of researchers, clinicians, and policy analysts offers a variety of perspectives with direct relevance, implications, and practical strategies for promoting the health and well-being of our adolescents. Specifically the book serves to highlight the epidemiologic data demonstrating adolescents' risk behavior, to help us understand the factors that motivate their behavior, to examine psychosocial models relevant for enhancing the adoption and maintenance of HIV-preventive behavior, to evaluate the effectiveness of current intervention strategies and consider new and innovative approaches, and to consider the impact of health and public policy with respect to adolescents' exposure to prevention activities and treatment.

Part I "Epidemiology: The Scope of the Problem" includes five chapters that focus on describing adolescents' behavior. Chapter 1, "Adolescents at Risk for HIV Infection," by Karen Hein, provides an overview of the AIDS epidemic among adolescents in the United States. In Chapter 2, "Monitoring Adolescents' Response to the AIDS Epidemic: Changes in Knowledge, Attitudes, Beliefs, and Behaviors," Ralph Hingson and Lee Strunin describe changes in these psychosocial and behavioral indicators over the course of the epidemic. In Chapter 3, "Psychosocial Determinants of Condom Use Among Adolescents," Ralph J. DiClemente focuses on identifying and understanding the role of psychosocial and behavioral factors associated with HIV-preventive sexual behavior (i.e., consistent condom use). Chapter 4, "Incarcerated Youth at Risk for HIV Infection," by Robert E. Morris, Charles J. Baker, and Susan Huscroft, and Chapter 5, "HIV Infection and Disease Among

Homeless Adolescents," by Diane L. Sondheimer, provide a more in-depth examination of the prevalence of HIV, sexually transmitted diseases, and HIV-related risk behaviors among such high-risk adolescent populations as incarcerated and homeless adolescents and suggest specific intervention and health care strategies for these youth.

Part II "Prevention: Theory, Design, and Evaluation" includes seven chapters that deal directly with the development, implementation, and evaluation of intervention strategies for promoting the adoption and maintenance of HIV-preventive behaviors. Chapter 6, "A Social Cognitive Approach to the Exercise of Control Over AIDS Infection," by Albert Bandura, provides an insightful presentation of the utility of self-regulation and self-efficacy theory for behavior change. Chapter 7, "Impact of Perceived Social Norms on Adolescents' AIDS-Risk Behavior and Prevention," by Jeffrey D. Fisher, Stephen J. Misovich, and William A. Fisher, offers a psychosocial model for understanding how perceived normative influences motivate adolescents' behavior and how this model can be useful in developing prevention programs. In Chapter 8, "Using Mass Media for Prevention of HIV Infection Among Adolescents," Daniel Romer and Robert C. Hornick focus on the use of social marketing strategies delivered by mass media approaches for implementing HIV-prevention efforts on a communitywide level. Chapter 9, "School-Based Prevention Programs: Design, Evaluation, and Effectiveness," by Douglas Kirby, specifically assesses the development and impact of school-based HIV-prevention programs and proposes recommendations for designing more effective programs. In Chapter 10, "Innovative Approaches to Interpersonal Skills Training for Minority Adolescents," Steven P. Schinke and Adam N. Gordon propose new strategies for reaching minority adolescent populations. Chapter 11, "Community-Based HIV-Prevention Programs for Adolescents" by Benjamin P. Bowser and Gina M. Wingood, addresses the issue of prevention from a community perspective in which existing community-based organizations can be utilized as social change agents. In Chapter 12, "Developmentally Tailoring Prevention Programs: Matching Strategies to Adolescents' Serostatus," Mary Jane Rotheram-Borus, Cheryl Koopman, and Margaret Rosario describe the need to adapt our primary models and strategies for promoting behavior change among HIV-infected adolescents.

Part III "Policy and Legal Perspectives" includes three chapters that describe the role of health and public policy as it affects adolescents in the context of the AIDS epidemic. Chapter 13, "Public Policy Perspectives on HIV Education," by James A. Wells, offers an analysis of the public policy that impacts the development and implementation of school-based HIV education programs, including condom-availability programs. Chapter 14, "Public Policy, HIV Disease, and Adolescents," by Lawrence J. D'Angelo, redirects our attention to the broader health policy issues at the national level and how they affect adolescents' access to health care. In Chapter 15, "Expanding Access to HIV Services for Adolescents: Legal and Ethical Issues," Abigail English focuses on the legal issues involved in adolescents seeking health care and participation in clinical trails.

The academic focus of *Adolescents and AIDS: A Generation in Jeopardy* is purposefully multidisciplinary in order to bring to bear the many professional perspectives necessary to begin to understand the enormity of the threat HIV poses for our adolescent population and the complex social forces that affect adolescents' behavior. Additionally the book is intended to bridge the chasm between epidemiology, behavior change theory, prevention research, and policy. Because the HIV epidemic is a multifaceted and complex social problem, the solutions for protecting our nation's youth will not be unidimensional or simplistic. I trust this book will be of value to a broad spectrum of individuals concerned with the health of adolescents: behavioral and medical researchers, counselors, and practitioners, as well as policy analysts, program administrators, planners, and others.

The gauntlet is down. HIV poses a direct challenge to the health and well-being of adolescents. If we cannot accept the challenge and rise to the occasion by marshalling our fiscal resources and collective intellectual energy to protect our nation's most valuable resource—its youth—then a generation will be in dire jeopardy. I trust we will vigorously accept and meet this challenge. The future depends on it.

RALPH J. DICLEMENTE

PART I

Epidemiology:
The Scope of the Problem

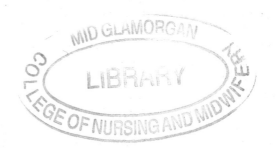

1

Adolescents at Risk for HIV Infection

KAREN HEIN

Introduction

A healthy, productive generation of adolescents in the 1990s will ensure that America has the healthy generation of adults needed to support the growing elderly population in the 21st century. The AIDS epidemic threatens the viability, perhaps the very existence, of this next generation. The social and economic well-being of this first "AIDS generation" may well predict the future well-being of this nation as a whole in the next century.

As of mid-1989, it is estimated that between 1-1.5 million Americans and 4.5-10 million people worldwide are infected with HIV (Mann, 1989). As more people of all ages are identified as being HIV-positive, requirements for counseling, early care, and interventions will accelerate (Arno, 1989). Given the current estimates of latency of 11 years from the time of infection to development of disease, the majority of people infected as teenagers will remain asymptomatic until they reach their 20s (Gayle, Manoff, & Rogers, 1989).

Changing Demographics
in the Next 50 Years

By the year 2000, there will be 20% fewer 15- to 24-year-olds than in 1980 (Hevesi, 1989). The generation of cohorts born between 1964 and 1977 is particularly small (Novello, Wright, & Sondheimer, 1989). These cohorts, now ages 11-24, comprise the current adolescent population. There are 16% fewer adolescents ages 16-19 today than 10 years ago.

AIDS as a Cause of Death
in Adolescence

Unheard of before 1981, AIDS is rising rapidly in the ranks of the leading causes of death among children. It is already the ninth leading cause of death among children 1-4 years of age, and the sixth in young people between ages 15-24. In the latter age group, AIDS deaths have increased 100-fold between 1981 and 1987. If current trends continue, AIDS could well be among the top five causes of death for young people ages 15-24 in the next few years.

Patterns of Premature Death

From 1975 to 1982, premature mortality decreased in New York City. This trend, however, reversed in 1982 until the present due to increased mortality from AIDS. AIDS has become the leading cause of premature mortality in both men and women in New York City. In 1985, AIDS was the leading cause of years of potential life lost in males ages 15-64, surpassing suicide and homicide. Similarly in 1982, AIDS became the leader in the cause-specific mortality in narcotic-related deaths in New York City.

Factors Affecting the Rate
of HIV Infection Among Adolescents

The number of HIV-infected youth in the United States is unknown. In considering the degree of penetration of HIV infection into the adolescent age group, three major factors must be weighed, as shown in Figure 1.1. The first is the number of susceptible teenagers, the second is the number of infected contacts of these

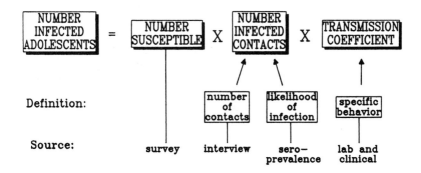

Figure 1.1. Key Factors to Be Considered in Estimating the Potential Number of HIV-Infected Adolescents

SOURCE: From "AIDS in Adolescence: The Next Wave of the HIV Epidemic?" by K. Hein, 1989, *Journal of Pediatrics*, 114. Reprinted by permission.

adolescents, and the third is a transmission coefficient that is specific for each type of behavior.

Surveys of sexual and drug use practices among youth will help determine the number of susceptible adolescents. Examples include the national surveys conducted in the 1960s, 1970s, and mid-1980s, which obtained information about the age of first intercourse, patterns of sexual behavior, number of partners, and contraceptive use patterns.

Estimation of the number of infected contacts is based on two components: the number of contacts (e.g., the number of sexual partners), and the likelihood of infection. Behavioral interventions are being instituted now to try to delay the age of first intercourse and either to limit the number of partners or to encourage abstinence or monogamy. Will these measures be sufficient to avoid widespread HIV infection in adolescents? A key factor is the likelihood of a partner's being infected. In areas of high viral prevalence, having only one or two partners may result in HIV infection because the chances of having an infected partner are much greater. Therefore both the geographic differences in seroprevalence rates and any increase in seroprevalence rates over time are critical factors in rapidity of HIV spread to and among adolescents.

The degree of risk also depends on the specific behavior being discussed. Anal intercourse has a higher transmission coefficient than vaginal intercourse, which in turn is a more efficient means of spread than oral intercourse. Little is known about the frequency of these behaviors in adolescents. Recent data reveal that anal intercourse was practiced by 26% of teenagers attending an adolescent outpatient clinic in New York City. Of those who reported anal intercourse, however, 70% never used condoms (Jaffe, Sheehaus, Wagner, & Leadbeater, 1988). Condoms were less likely to be used during anal as compared to vaginal intercourse. In another study of San Francisco teenage girls, 21% of sexually experienced patients attending a clinic reported anal intercourse (Kegeles, Adler, & Irwin, 1988). The incidence of oral-genital contact among adolescents appears to be increasing (Newcomer & Udry, 1985). Although apparently less risky than vaginal or anal intercourse, oral intercourse has been implicated in HIV transmission (Spitzer & Weiner, 1989). National data show that male partners of heterosexual female adolescents tend to be 2-3 years older (Sorenson, 1973), but for homosexual male adolescents who have had intercourse, the average age of their partners is 7 years older (Ramefedi, 1988).

HIV Seroprevalence Studies in Adolescents

Few studies of seroprevalence have included adolescents. Recent data from seroprevalence studies among 69,233 Job Corps entrants 16-21 years of age revealed a seroprevalence rate of 3.9/ 1,000, roughly three times higher than the rate reported in the military (St. Louis, Hayman, & Miller, 1989). In a center serving runaway and homeless youth in New York City, 6% of these disenfranchised youth were HIV-positive. The rates increased with age, so that seropositivity was present in 15% of those who were 18-20 years of age (Kennedy, 1988). Most of these young people were well at the time of the survey. Anonymous serologic surveys of 13,810 specimens on 13 college campuses from students attending health services revealed HIV-positive rates of 1/500 (Gayle,

Keeling, & Garcia-Tonon, 1989). Positive results were identified in 5 college campuses in different parts of the United States out of the total of 13 campuses sampled.

Since October 1985, the U.S. Department of Defense has routinely tested civilian applicants for military service for serologic evidence of infection with HIV type 1 (HIV-1). From October 1984 through March 1988, 1,525,869 recruit applicants were tested; presence of HIV-1 antibody was confirmed by enzyme immunoassay and Western blot in 2,152 (1.4 per 1,000) (Burke et al., 1990). The male-to-female ratio for teenagers under 20 years of age was 0.5 (Brundage et al., 1988).

HIV seroprevalence rates among all clinic patients attending a sexually transmitted disease clinic in Baltimore increased steadily with age, from 2.2% in those 15-19 years old to 9.9% in those 30 years old or older (Quinn et al., 1988).

The prevalence of human immunodeficiency virus (HIV) infection was determined in women at the time of childbirth throughout New York State between November 30, 1987, and November 30, 1988. Rates for newborns whose mothers were ages 20-29 years (1.30%) and 30-39 years (1.35%) were significantly higher than rates for those with mothers younger than age 20 years (0.72%) (Novick et al., 1989). Recent data, however, point to a changing pattern, with only 10 HIV-positive babies born to mothers under age 20 years up until April 1988, but 88 such babies born in the 13 months between April 1988 and May 1989. Of all HIV-positive babies born in New York State, the rate was 1/1,000 for HIV-positive babies born to 15-year-old mothers and 1/100 for babies born to 19-year-old mothers (Novick, Glebatis, Stricof, & Berns, 1989).

Using standard criteria for identifying at-risk adolescents, 62% of HIV-positive teenagers were missed in a seroprevalence study in Washington, DC (D'Angelo, Geston, Luban, & Gayle, 1991).

Only a tiny percentage of at-risk adolescents have been part of any type of seroprevalence study whether anonymous or confidential. Yet the number of sexually experienced adolescents exceeds half of the total American adolescent population by the age of 19. The number of reported cases of AIDS in 13- to 21-year-olds is doubling every 14 months, but the incidence and prevalence of HIV-infected youth are largely unknown.

Differences in Transmission Category Profiles
of Children, Adolescents, and Adults

Adolescents should be separated from younger children and adults for four reasons.

1. Adolescence is the period in the life cycle when the risk-related sexual and drug activities begin (Hein, 1987).
2. Evidence exists that HIV infection has entered the adolescent population (Hein, 1989). From previous experience with other sexually transmitted diseases, once introduced, HIV is likely to spread quickly but silently among American youth (Bell & Hein, 1984).
3. The vast majority of infected youth are unaware of their HIV status and, based on studies of sexual behavior during adolescence (Hein, 1991a), they are likely to unwittingly continue to transmit the virus to other partners.
4. The notion of *risk groups* may not be a useful concept in adolescence.

The majority of United States teenagers have had sexual intercourse by the age of 19 years (Hofferth, Kahn, & Baldwin, 1987). Although some teenagers are clearly at increased risk compared with others, risk status currently may be more a reflection of geography (i.e., prevalence of HIV in a given area) than being a member of a "risk group." By adulthood, the majority of adolescents will be at risk for acquiring HIV because most will have had several partners. Risk-related behaviors cross over from traditional risk groups to all adolescents who are sexually experienced. For example, many teenage boys who identify as being homosexual have not had intercourse (Ramefedi, 1987). Alternatively, unprotected receptive anal intercourse is reported by more than 20% of teenage females in some surveys of heterosexual adolescents attending clinics in New York and San Francisco (Moscicki, Millstein, Broering, & Irwin, 1988). Despite the fact that most teenagers were well aware of the AIDS epidemic by the mid-1980s, an accelerated increase occurred in the proportion having premarital sex from 1986 to 1988 (Centers for Disease Control, 1991).

Briefly stated, the differences between affected children and affected adolescents are (a) the route of infection, which in young children is usually vertical from an infected mother; (b) the shorter mean survival time in young children; and (c) the need for day care and foster care for preschool children.

Some of the differences between adolescents and adults are as follows: (a) More teenage cases are acquired by heterosexual transmission; (b) a higher percentage of teenaged patients are asymptomatic (but will become symptomatic during adulthood); (c) a higher percentage of patients are black or Hispanic; (d) a special set of ethical and legal issues exists regarding testing and informing partners and parents of adolescents under the age of majority (Hein, 1991b); (e) there are cognitive differences, which affect the processing of information, and differences in coping styles; and (f) special medical, economic, and social implications arise when teenaged mothers deliver HIV-infected babies. Additional differences include the lack of a unified support community (such as the adult homosexual community); the sexual behavior patterns in the teenage population, which has a higher percentage of "sexual adventurers" (with less use and availability of contraceptives); and the lack of availability of services that are convenient, appropriate, and attractive to youth. Specific biologic, behavioral, and social attributes of adolescents point to the need for a different approach to organizing educational interventions and health services for teenagers.

Characteristics of Adolescent AIDS Cases

As of January 19, 1988, 605 (1.2%) of 51,334 reported AIDS cases in the United States were in 13- to 21-year-olds, 518 male and 87 female (Vermund, Hein, Gayle, Cary, & Thomas, 1989). While only 3% of the nation's 13- to 21-year-olds live in New York City, 20% of all reported United States AIDS cases in this age range live there. Thus New York City accounted for 16% of total AIDS cases reported in United States male adolescents and 32% of reported United States female adolescents (Figure 1.2). Frequency of AIDS in the adolescent age group rises markedly with increasing age. Half of the cases in the 13- to 21-year-old category are seen in 20- to 21-year-old persons, who would be expected to represent only about 22% of the 13- to 21-year age group ($p<0.001$). The adolescent ratio of male-to-female cases is 3:1 in New York City and 7:1

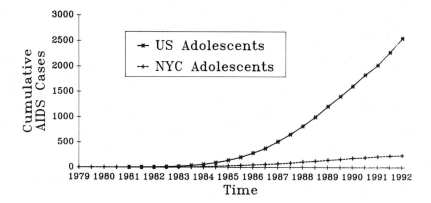

Figure 1.2. Reported Cases of AIDS in New York City (NYC) and in the United States (US) Excluding NYC

SOURCE: Adapted from "AIDS Among Adolescents in NYC: Case Surveillance Profiles Compared With the Rest of the US" by S. V. Vermund, K. Hein, H. Gayle, J. Cary, and P. Thomas, 1989, *American Journal of Disease in Children, 143*. Reprinted by permission.

in the United States excluding New York City, while the adult ratio is 7:1 in New York City and 15:1 in the United States excluding New York City.

The rate of growth in the cumulative incidence of AIDS in the United States is rapid in the first 9 years of the AIDS epidemic (Figure 1.3). The reported onset of the epidemic in adults and children, as documented from surveillance reports, preceded the recognition of AIDS among adolescents, who were first diagnosed in 1981.

Adolescents Compared to Adults

Proportional frequencies of risk behavior associated with AIDS are different in adolescents and adult cases. Both in New York City and in the United States excluding New York City, adolescents with AIDS are proportionately less likely than adults with AIDS to have acquired infection by male homosexual activities or IV drug use (Figure 1.4). Adolescents with AIDS are comparatively more likely to have acquired infection from transfusion of blood

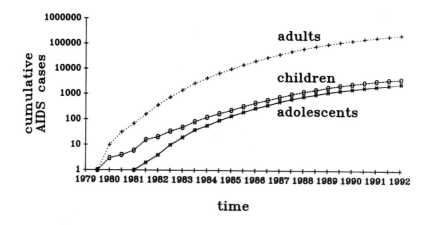

Figure 1.3. Cumulative Prevalence of AIDS Cases Reported to the CDC as of January 1988 by 6-Month Periods From 1979-1987 for the United States. Adults Are Over 21 Years of Age, Adolescents Are 13-21 Years, and Children Are Under 13 Years of Age

SOURCE: From "AIDS Among Adolescents in NYC: Case Surveillance Profiles Compared With the Rest of the US" by S. V. Vermund, K. Hein, H. Gayle, J. Cary, and P. Thomas, 1989, *American Journal of Disease in Children, 143.* Reprinted by permission.

products (20% among all adolescent cases, compared to 3% among all adult cases) or from heterosexual transmission (9% among all adolescent cases, compared to 4% among all adults) ($p<0.0001$). The preponderance of transfusion/blood products-acquired AIDS is largely among males, because of the many AIDS cases with hemophilia. The heterosexual proportional differences can be attributed to differences among female cases; 47% of AIDS cases in female adolescents and 29% of AIDS cases in female adults are reportedly due to heterosexual spread, while the comparable figure among males is 2% for both adolescents and adults.

Adolescents in New York City Compared With Adolescents in the Rest of the United States

Among males, a history of IV drug use, with or without a history of homosexual activity, is reported in 16% of New York City

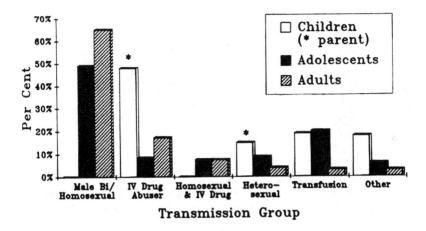

Figure 1.4. Transmission Profiles of AIDS Cases Reported for Adults (Over 21 Years), Adolescents (13-21 Years), and Children (Under 13 Years) for the United States

SOURCE: Adapted from "AIDS Among Adolescents in NYC: Case Surveillance Profiles Compared With the Rest of the US" by S. V. Vermund, K. Hein, H. Gayle, J. Cary, and P. Thomas, 1989, *American Journal of Disease in Children, 143.* Reprinted by permission.

adolescent AIDS cases, compared with 4% of adolescent AIDS cases from the rest of the United States. Adolescent cases in New York City and the United States show a similar proportion of cases in males reporting homosexual/bisexual activity, from 55% to 57% of all adolescent AIDS cases (Figure 1.5). Transfusion-related cases are proportionately more common outside New York City. Comparing all proportional differences between New York City male cases and those from the rest of the United States, significant differences are evident ($p<0.0001$).

Proportionately more female adolescent AIDS cases are IV drug use related and heterosexually acquired in New York City reports than in those from elsewhere in the United States ($p = 0.4$) (Figure 1.6). As with males, few transfusion-related cases are noted in female New York City adolescents with AIDS, compared with those from elsewhere in the United States. Overall differences between AIDS cases in female adolescents in New York City and in the rest of the United States are not significant, but the number of reported cases for female adolescents is small.

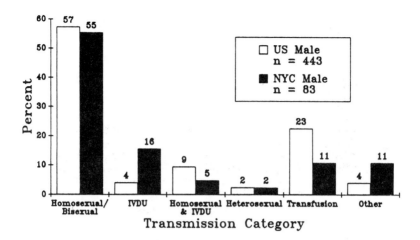

Figure 1.5. Transmission Profiles for Male Adolescents Ages 13-21 Years With AIDS in New York City and the United States Excluding NYC

SOURCE: From "AIDS Among Adolescents in NYC: Case Surveillance Profiles Compared With the Rest of the US" by S. V. Vermund, K. Hein, H. Gayle, J. Cary, and P. Thomas, 1989, *American Journal of Disease in Children, 143.* Reprinted by permission.

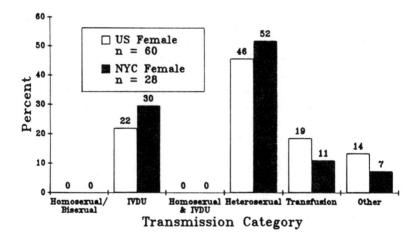

Figure 1.6. Transmission Profiles for Female Adolescents Ages 13-21 Years With AIDS in New York City and the United States Excluding NYC

SOURCE: From "AIDS Among Adolescents in NYC: Case Surveillance Profiles Compared With the Rest of the US" by S. V. Vermund, K. Hein, H. Gayle, J. Cary, and P. Thomas, 1989, *American Journal of Disease in Children, 143.* Reprinted by permission.

The Importance of Filling Gaps
in Knowledge Quickly

The United States in the next few decades will rely on a productive work force that has the shape of an inverted pyramid. The shrinking size of the pool of potential workers due to the aging out of the "baby boomers" and the corresponding increase in the proportion of elderly citizens will put new pressures on young adults in the 21st century.

As demonstrated by reported cases of AIDS and HIV seroprevalence studies, the virus clearly has entered some segments of the adolescent population already. Currently some of the adolescents at highest risk are also the most disenfranchised youth. Therefore more flexible, innovative, age-specific primary and secondary prevention services must be quickly mobilized, evaluated, and replicated (Hein, 1991c). Overcoming issues of limited access, including payment and confidentiality, are basic to the provision of such preventive services. Given the latency from time of infection to disease, the vast majority of infected teenagers will not become sick until the very time when they would be joining the labor force, forming families, and entering the most economically productive years of their lives. Despite advances in early medical interventions and prophylactic medical treatments for potentially debilitating illnesses, the spectrum of HIV-related illnesses will undoubtedly become more manageable, but not necessarily curable, conditions. Even with adequate "cures" for gonorrhea and syphilis, the rates of these sexually transmitted diseases have increased in some segments of the United States population in the past few years. If HIV follows the course of other sexually transmitted diseases, the rates then would be the highest among all sexually experienced adolescents in the United States, as is already true of rates of gonorrhea and syphilis. Therefore great urgency arises about designing, implementing, and evaluating prevention strategies and services for HIV-positive youth now.

References

Arno, P. (1989, June). *The economic impact of early intervention in HIV disease* (Abstract #9573). Paper presented at the V International Conference on AIDS, Montreal, Canada.

Bell, T., & Hein, K. (1984). The adolescent and sexually transmitted disease. In K. Holmes (Ed.), *Sexually transmitted diseases* (pp. 73-84). New York: McGraw-Hill.

Brundage, J. F., Burke, D. S., Gardner, L. I. et al. (1988). HIV infection among young adults in NYC area: Prevalence and antibody screening among civilian applicants for military service. *New York State Journal of Medicine, 88,* 232-235.

Burke, D. S., Brundage, J. F., Goldenbaum, M., Gardner, L. I., Peterson, M., Visintine, R., & Redfield, R. R. (1990). Human immunodeficiency virus infections in teenagers: Seroprevalence among applicants for US military service. *Journal of the American Medical Association, 263,* 2074-2077.

Centers for Disease Control. (1991). Premarital sexual experiences among adolescent women, 1970-1988. *Morbidity and Mortality Weekly Report (MMWR), 39,* 929-932.

D'Angelo, L., Geston, P., Luban, N., & Gayle, H. (1991). HIV infection in urban adolescents. Can we predict who is at risk? *Pediatrics, 88,* 982-986.

Gayle, H., Keeling R., & Garcia-Tonon, M. (1989, June). *HIV seroprevalence on university campuses* (Abstract MAP 9 p. 79). Poster presentation at V International AIDS Conference, Montreal, Canada.

Gayle, H., Manoff, S., & Rogers, M. (1989, June). *Epidemiology of AIDS in adolescents, USA* (Abstract #MD07 p. 696). Paper presented at V International AIDS Conference, Montreal, Canada.

Hein, K. (1987). AIDS in adolescence: A rationale for concern. *New York State Journal of Medicine, 87,* 290-295.

Hein, K. (1989). AIDS in adolescence: The next wave of the HIV epidemic? *Journal of Pediatrics, 114,* 144-149.

Hein, K. (1991a). Risky business: HIV and adolescents. *Pediatrics, 88,* 1052-1054.

Hein, K. (1991b). Mandatory HIV testing of youth: A lose-lose proposition. *Journal of the American Medical Association, 266,* 2430-2431.

Hein, K. (1991c). Fighting AIDS in adolescents. *Issues in Science & Technology, 7,* 67-72.

Hevesi, D. (1989, July 18). Jobs of summer are rare rest of the year. *New York Times,* p. B1.

Hofferth, S. L., Kahn, J., & Baldwin, W. (1987). Premarital sexual activity among U.S. teenage women. *Family Planning Perspectives, 19,* 46-53.

Jaffe, L. R., Seehaus, M., Wagner, C., & Leadbeater, B. J. (1988). Anal intercourse and knowledge of acquired immunodeficiency syndrome among minority-group female adolescents. *Journal of Pediatrics, 112,* 1005-1007.

Kegeles, S., Adler, N., & Irwin, C. (1988). Sexually active adolescents and condoms. *American Journal of Pediatric Health, 78,* 460-461.

Kennedy, J. (1988, May). Testimony before the Presidential Commission on the HIV epidemic.

Mann, J. M. (1989, June). *Global AIDS into the 1990s.* Paper presented at V International Conference on AIDS, Montreal, Canada.

Moscicki, B., Millstein, S. G., Broering, J., & Irwin, C. E. (1988, January). *Psychosocial and behavioral risk factors for AIDS in adolescents.* Interim report submitted to University of California Task Force on AIDS, San Francisco, CA.

Newcomer, S. J., & Udry, J. R. (1985). Oral sex in an adolescent population. *Archives of Sexual Behavior, 14,* 41-46.

Novello, A., Wright, A., & Sondheimer, D. (1989, June). *Potential impact of HIV/AIDS on the future labor force* (Abstract). Paper presented at V International Conference on AIDS, Montreal, Canada.

Novick, L. J., Berns, D., Stricof, R. et al. (1989). HIV seroprevalence in newborns in New York State. *Journal of the American Medical Association, 261,* 1745-1750.

Novick, L., Glebatis, D., Stricof, R., & Berns, D. (1989, June). *HIV infection in adolescent child-bearing women* (Abstract WA08 p. 5). Paper presented at V International AIDS Conference, Montreal, Canada.

Quinn, T. C., Glasser, D., Cannon, R. O. et al. (1988). Human immunodeficiency virus infection among patients attending clinics for sexually transmitted diseases. *New England Journal of Medicine, 318,* 197-203.

Ramefedi, G. (1987). Adolescent homosexuality. *Pediatrics, 79,* 249-250.

Ramefedi, G. J. (Ed.). (1988). Special section on adolescent homosexuality. *Journal of Adolescent Health Care, 9.*

Sorenson, R. (1973). *Adolescents' sexuality in contemporary America.* New York: World.

Spitzer, P. G., & Weiner, N. J. (1989). Transmission of HIV infection from a woman to a man by oral sex. *New England Journal of Medicine, 320,* 251.

St. Louis, M., Hayman, C., & Miller, C. (1989, June). *HIV infection in disadvantaged adolescents in the US: Findings from the Job Corps screening program* (Abstract #MDP1 p. 711). Poster presentation at V International AIDS Conference, Montreal, Canada.

Vermund, S. V., Hein, K., Gayle, H., Cary, J., & Thomas, P. (1989). AIDS among adolescents in NYC: Case surveillance profiles compared with the rest of the U.S. *American Journal of Disease in Children, 143,* 1220-1225.

2

Monitoring Adolescents' Response to the AIDS Epidemic: Changes in Knowledge, Attitudes, Beliefs, and Behaviors

RALPH HINGSON

LEE STRUNIN

Introduction

Surveys of adolescents have varied and grown over time. During the mid-1980s, when adolescent surveys about AIDS first began, researchers were interested primarily in adolescents' knowledge of HIV transmission and in identifying the prevalence of sexual and drug use practices that might place them at risk of infection. Shortly thereafter, researchers began to compare the level of HIV knowledge and behavioral practices of different subgroups in the population, for example, males versus females, whites versus Hispanics and blacks, persons in urban versus rural areas, and persons at different age levels. They also explored whether knowledge increased over time and whether more adolescents adopted safer sexual and drug use practices. Researchers have begun also to explore the relationship among knowledge, attitudes, and beliefs about AIDS and sexual and drug use behaviors, often tapping into such social psychological models and theories as the health belief model (Janz & Becker, 1984), the theory of reasoned action (Fishbein & Azjen, 1975), problem behavior theory (Jessor, Chase, & Donovan, 1980), and social learning theory (Bandura, 1986). Researchers also have begun to explore factors other than beliefs, attitudes, and values about AIDS that may influence sexual practices and condom use, such as alcohol and drug use and beliefs about other sexually transmitted diseases and pregnancy.

Adolescents' Knowledge and Sexual Behavior Early in the AIDS Epidemic

Surveys of adolescents' knowledge about HIV transmission first began to appear in the literature in the mid-1980s. One study in 1985 of 250 students found that few high school students knew about the principle modes of HIV transmission (Price, Desmond, & Kukulka, 1985). That study, however, was conducted in a low-AIDS-incidence area. In 1986, DiClemente, Zorn, and Temoshok (1986) surveyed 1,326 students (99% of the eligible sample) in family life education classes at 19 high schools in the San Francisco school district (San Francisco was a major epicenter for the AIDS epidemic). Of those students, 92% correctly reported that HIV could be transmitted through sexual intercourse, but only 60% knew condoms could lower the risk of HIV transmission. Nearly 20% were unaware that sharing intravenous needles could allow transmission of HIV, and only 60% reported that AIDS could not be cured. Reanalysis of the 1985 survey in San Francisco by ethnicity, comparing 261 white, 226 black, and 141 Latino adolescents, revealed that white adolescents were more knowledgeable about modes of transmission than were black adolescents, who in turn were more knowledgeable than were Latino respondents, a particularly important finding because of the higher rates of infection among black and Hispanic populations (DiClemente, Boyer, & Morales, 1988).

Strunin and Hingson (1987) conducted a statewide random-digit-dial telephone survey of Massachusetts in 1986. Of the 16- to

19-year-olds surveyed ($N = 826$), only half had discussed AIDS in school, and only 45% had discussed AIDS with a parent. Even though 80% of adolescents had seen a physician in the past year, only 15% had been counseled about AIDS. Moreover, 8% of adolescents did not know about heterosexual transmission of the virus, and sizable fractions of adolescents believed that the virus could be transmitted in ways it could not, for example, from toilet seats (14%), from sharing eating and drinking utensils (37%), and by donating blood (60%). Further, 55% of the adolescents had had sexual intercourse, 13% had used drugs other than alcohol or marijuana, and 2% had injected illegal drugs. No significant differences were found in the knowledge levels of sexually active and nonsexually active adolescents or between those who used and did not use illicit drugs. School dropouts, however, were more likely to be sexually active and to use illegal drugs and were less knowledgeable about HIV transmission than were adolescents still in school. Of particular importance, only 15% of the sample reported behavioral changes in response to the AIDS epidemic, with only 3% adopting condom use or sexual abstinence.

Taken together, these studies indicated that substantial proportions of adolescents had misperceptions about how HIV is transmitted, that misperceptions were more common among minority groups and school dropouts, and that misperceptions were as high among those who were sexually active and those who used illicit drugs.

These findings all pointed to a need for education in schools about AIDS and HIV transmission. In the summer of 1986, the U.S. Surgeon General called for schools to offer educational programs in cities across the nation. Since then, 31 states have passed laws mandating the offering of HIV education in junior and senior high schools. The Centers for Disease Control were given responsibility for assisting nationwide state and local education agencies to provide effective HIV education for youth. In 1987, 15 national organizations, 15 state education agencies, and 12 local education agencies in areas with the highest cumulative AIDS cases were awarded federal funds to increase the capacities of schools and other youth-serving organizations to provide effective HIV education. School-based surveys were implemented throughout the nation in an attempt to measure HIV-related knowledge (Kann, Nelson, Jones, & Kolbe, 1989).

Increases in Knowledge
and Behavioral Changes

Subsequent statewide random-digit-dial surveys in Massachusetts were implemented in 1988 (Hingson, Strunin, & Berlin, 1990) (N = 1,762; response rate 82%) and in 1990 (Hingson et al., 1990) (N = 1,152; response rate 87%). Both surveys used sampling procedures and knowledge and behavioral questions identical to those used in 1986. The authors reported that by 1988 almost all adolescents had learned the principal modes of HIV transmission and misperceptions about HIV transmission had diminished. Nonetheless many misperceptions persisted about transmission even in 1990 (Hingson et al., 1990).

These surveys found that the proportion of adolescents who used drugs other than alcohol or marijuana declined from 13% to 7%, who used IV drugs decreased from 1% to <1%, and who adopted condom use specifically because of the AIDS epidemic increased from 2% to 14%. By 1990, however, only 37% of sexually active adolescents reported consistent condom use. Further, an 11% increase occurred in the proportion of adolescents who were sexually active: from 55% in 1986 to 66% in 1990. Consequently nearly as many adolescents had unprotected intercourse in the later surveys as in the earlier surveys. Also, while illicit drug use was declining, the reductions were confined to those adolescents who remained in school. Among those who had dropped out— 15% of those surveyed—drug use did not decline and was three times higher than among adolescents who remained in school. Of note, the proportion of adolescents who had discussed AIDS with parents increased from 44% to 63%. Also the proportion who were educated about AIDS in schools increased from 52% to 83%. Even in 1990, however, only 15% had been counseled about AIDS by a physician.

Similar findings were identified in data collected from CDC in 1989 among high school students by departments of education in 30 states, 10 cities, and 2 territories (Centers for Disease Control, 1990). Those surveys revealed higher levels of knowledge than earlier surveys: 56% of adolescents had discussed AIDS with their parents or other adults in their families; 98% knew HIV infection could be spread by sharing needles used to inject drugs, although somewhat fewer knew the virus could be spread from having sexual intercourse without using a condom (88%); 3% reported ever injecting cocaine, heroin, or other illegal drugs, and just under 1% reported sharing needles to inject illegal drugs; and 56% reported having had sexual intercourse.

A national survey of adolescent males ages 15-19 in 1988 ($N =$ 1,880) revealed that 99% and 98% of males respectively, knew AIDS could be transmitted through shared hypodermic needles and through intercourse between two men or through intercourse between men and women (Sonenstein, Pleck, & Ku, 1989). The proportion of male adolescents who reported using a condom during their most recent sexual encounter rose markedly when compared with a 1979 survey, increasing from 21% to 58%. As was noted in the Massachusetts survey, the proportion of adolescent males who had sex (data available for ages 17-19 only) increased from 66% to 76%, partially offsetting the increase in condom use. Data from the National Survey of Family Growth similarly indicated that the proportion of teenage women who reported condom use increased from 22% in 1982 to 32% in 1988 (Mosher, 1990).

Thus it appears that most adolescents have learned the major modes of HIV transmission and that as knowledge about HIV transmission has increased, so too has condom use. Just as many people continue to smoke despite knowledge of smoking's adverse health affects, many teenagers continue to engage in unprotected sex despite knowledge of the risk behaviors associated with HIV transmission. It should be noted also that while nearly all adolescents are now aware of the principal modes of HIV transmission, the few who do not may be found disproportionately among groups in which the risk of exposure to the virus may be particularly high.

DiClemente and his colleagues (1991) found lower levels of HIV-prevention knowledge in a sample of incarcerated adolescents in San Francisco, compared with a school-based population. Adolescents in the detention center were less likely to be aware that they could reduce their chances of becoming infected with HIV by not having sexual intercourse (62% vs. 80%) and by using condoms during sexual intercourse with someone who injects illegal drugs. Incarcerated youth were much more likely to engage in behaviors that place them at risk of HIV infection. Almost all were sexually active, compared with 28% of the school-based population. Most (73%) had multiple sexual partners in the past year, compared with 8% of the school sample. Only 28% of the detention group reported consistent condom use, relative to 37% of the in-school youth, while 13% of incarcerated adolescents reported intravenous drug use, compared with 4% of in-school youth. The results of this study indicate that some small adolescent subpopulations exist that still need special educational efforts to inform them of the basic modes of HIV transmission. One such subgroup may be newly arriving immigrants to the United States.

A 1990 survey of 3,049 middle and high school students selected from a random sample of Boston public middle and high school students (Hingson, Strunin et al., 1991) also revealed that one third of adolescents were born outside the United States mainland and that one fifth arrived in the United States only within the last year. HIV knowledge of students born outside the United States was much lower than those born inside the United States. For example, among immigrant students, 24%, 15%, and 13%, respectively, did not know that HIV could be transmitted during sex between two men, during sex between a man and a woman, and by the sharing of needles while injecting drugs. The corresponding percentages for United States-born students were 16%, 6%, and 3%. Further, 57% of immigrant students believed that one could not become infected by having sex with someone who appears to be healthy. In contrast, 41% of United States-born students held that belief. Immigrant students were less likely to have had sexual intercourse (31% vs. 53%), although if they were sexually active, they were just as likely to use condoms (38% vs. 38%). Moreover, they were just as likely to have injected illegal drugs in the past month (2% vs. 2%).

Adolescents from other countries were more likely than their United States-born peers to believe that persons their age are more likely to engage in HIV-related risk behaviors. Of note, 28% of immigrant students believed that all or most people their age are injecting drugs, and 16% believed that none use condoms when they have sex. In comparison, only 12% of United States-born students believed that all or most people their age are injecting illegal drugs, and only 6% believed that no one their age uses condoms. Those students who immigrated to the United States during the year prior to the survey were the most likely to believe that everyone their age is injecting illegal drugs or not using condoms during sexual intercourse.

Between 15 and 20 million people who reside in the United States were born elsewhere, and many have relocated to such high-HIV-incidence cities as New York, Los Angeles, and Miami. When immigrant teenagers first arrive in the United States, they face unique pressures to adopt the behavioral practices of their United States-born peers (Strunin, 1991). If they believe that more United States-born are engaging in riskier behaviors than actually are, non-United States born may feel disproportionate pressure to adopt risky behavior in an attempt to fit in with their new culture.

Predictors of Safer Sexual and Drug Use Practices

The CDC national survey of middle and high school students indicates that knowledge of HIV transmission is associated with lower levels of IV drug use and risky sexual practices (CDC, 1990). While increases in knowledge about HIV transmission have been accompanied by increases in condom use among sexually active adolescents, the fact is that most adolescents who are sexually active are not using condoms. This nonuse suggests that educational efforts must move beyond simply imparting knowledge in order to achieve safer sexual practices in that age group.

The 1988 Massachusetts statewide survey of 1,762 16- to 19-year-olds (Hingson, Strunin, & Berlin, 1990) tested whether the following components of the health belief model (Janz & Becker, 1984) were independently related to consistent condom use: perceived susceptibility to HIV infection, severity of HIV if infected, effectiveness of condoms in preventing infection, barriers to condom use, and behavioral cues such as exposure to media or personal communication about AIDS. According to this model, people make a rational cost-benefit analysis in trying to decide whether to adopt preventive behavior. The study also explored whether alcohol or drug use independently predicted adolescent condom use.

Among sexually active respondents (61% of those interviewed), 31% reported always using condoms. Respondents who believed that condoms are effective in preventing HIV transmission and who worried that they could get AIDS were 3.1 and 1.8 times more likely to always use condoms. Adolescents who carried condoms and who had discussed AIDS with a physician were 2.7 and 1.7

times, respectively, more likely to use them. Those who believed that condoms do not reduce sexual pleasure and would not be embarrassed to use them were 3.1 and 2.4 times more likely to use them. Adolescents who averaged five or more alcoholic drinks daily and who used marijuana were 2.8 and 1.9 times less likely to use condoms. Among respondents who drink alcohol or use drugs, 16% used condoms less often during sex after drinking, and 25% used them less often during sex after drug use.

This study found little relation between adolescents' knowledge about HIV infection and risky sexual practices primarily because most adolescents knew the principal modes of HIV infection. Several beliefs about the likelihood and consequences of HIV, as well as the effectiveness of such preventive behaviors as condom use and such barriers to use as reduction in sexual pleasure or embarrassment, were significantly related to condom use. Similar findings have been reported among runaway youth in the New York shelters (Rotheram-Borus & Koopman, 1991), incarcerated adolescents in San Francisco (DiClemente, 1991), minority adolescents in inner-city school districts (DiClemente et al., in press), and among gay and bisexual men (Becker & Joseph, 1988). The study of runaway adolescents in New York also found desires to avoid pregnancy associated with condom use. This finding suggests that on some level adolescents engage in a rational cost-benefit analysis of whether the risk of AIDS warrants condom use. Similar findings have also been observed in general population surveys of adults (Allard, 1989). Taken together, however, the beliefs outlined in the health belief model accounted for only 10-15% of the variance in condom use (Hingson, Strunin, & Berlin 1990), suggesting that many other factors may also be important influences on condom use. Further, many adolescent sexual encounters are unplanned, and alcohol or drug use may cloud judgment or undermine the rational cost-benefit analysis of adolescents.

The survey by Hingson, Strunin, and Berlin (1990) tested whether beliefs about pregnancy, about other sexually transmitted diseases, and about the social acceptability of condom use would also predict condom use. According to the theory of reasoned action, beliefs about partner and peer preferences and desire to please partners and peers may also influence behavior (Fishbein & Azjen, 1975). Many of the same beliefs about AIDS continue to predict constant condom use. In addition, beliefs about other sexually transmitted diseases, as well as beliefs about pregnancy, also predicted condom use. Respondents who believed that people can die from gonorrhea and syphilis were 2 times more likely to always use condoms, and respondents who thought it very likely that someone could get pregnant after sex without condom use were 2 times more likely to always use condoms. Beliefs about the social acceptability of condoms also predicted use. Respondents who said their partners would not be upset and would use condoms if asked were 1.5 and 3.2 times more likely to always use them. Those asked by partners to use condoms were 2.2 times more likely to use them, and those who believed that most women are asking new partners to use condoms were 2.9 times more likely to always use them.

Similarly in the 1988 National Survey of Adolescent Males, Pleck, Sonenstein, and Ku (1991) found that greater consistency of condom use was related to perceived cost-benefits concerning pregnancy prevention, AIDS, partner expectations, embarrassment, and reduction of pleasure. The belief that males have a responsibility to avoid a female partner's becoming pregnant and less actual contraceptive pill usage by the last sexual partner or recent partner were associated with more condom use. The degree of personal concern about AIDS and the perception that a partner would appreciate condom use were associated with more consistent use of condoms. Condom use was inhibited by concerns about embarrassment and reduced sexual pleasure.

The Massachusetts and national surveys both indicated that beliefs about pregnancy were strong predictors of condom use independent of beliefs about AIDS, while the Massachusetts study indicated that beliefs about other sexually transmitted diseases can also influence condom use. These findings suggest that the most effective program to increase condom use would be one that not only provides information about AIDS but that also discusses the implications of unprotected sex for pregnancy and the transmission of other sexually transmitted diseases.

Drinking, Drug Use, and Unprotected Sex

The 1988 Massachusetts survey found that alcohol and drug use may contribute independently to unprotected sex. This finding suggests that school educational efforts must not overlook substance use as a potential factor that contributes to risk taking. Similar findings have been reported in the United Kingdom (Robertson & Plant, 1988).

It is well known that heavier drinkers and drug users are more likely to engage in unprotected sex (Plant, 1990). Numerous hypotheses could be advanced to explain these relations. According to problem behavior theory (Jessor & Jessor, 1977), heavy drinkers and drug users may be more likely to be risk takers in general and hence be less likely to use condoms. Drinking and drug use may occur in settings where strangers meet in hopes of sexual encounters; consequently they may be reluctant to ask new partners to use a condom if they think the question will break the spontaneity of sex and reduce the likelihood of its occurrence (Plant, 1990). Use of alcohol in these social contexts may lead people to deny temporarily their risk of HIV infection (McKirnon & Peterson, 1989). Many people believe that alcohol promotes uncharacteristic behavior and that one cannot be accountable for behavior when drinking. Some have conjectured that blaming inappropriate behavior in advance (anticipatory attribution) may enable questionable action (Cooper, Skinner, & George, 1990; Crowe & George, 1989). Alcohol and drugs may not only reduce sexual pleasure and interfere with orgasm, they also may reduce sensitivity to the desires of others that condoms be used. If an individual has been drinking, his or her partner may feel that attempts to persuade the partner to use condoms may be less accepted and understood and consequently be less effective.

Several studies of gay men have found that even after the advent of the AIDS epidemic, gay men were less likely to use condoms or to engage in safer sex practices after drinking than when sober (Coates, Stall, Catania, & Kegeles, 1988; McKirnon & Peterson, 1989b; Ostrow, 1987; Siegal, Mesogno, Chen, & Chiel, 1989; Stall, McKusick, Wiley, Coates, & Ostrow, 1986; Valdiserri et al., 1988). Two studies of gay men found that one fifth of those who adopted safer sex practices then relapsed into unsafe practices. Drinking and drug use were among the most frequently cited reasons for relapse particularly among men with no regular partner (Kelly, St. Lawrence, & Brasfield, 1991; Stall, Ekstrand, Pollock, McKusick, & Coates, 1990). The study by Stall and his colleagues (1990) found that white men who reduced their drinking reported a reduction in unsafe sex practices; those who maintained or increased drinking were twice as likely to continue high-risk sex. Among gay men, drinking, sexual patterns, and their interrelations have been found to change over time. As substance use and risky sexual behavior become less frequent, the relationship between substance use and unprotected sex can diminish (Martin & Haiser, 1990).

The 1990 Massachusetts adolescent survey further explored whether adolescents are more likely to have sexual intercourse after drinking and drug use because (a) they were more likely to have sex or (b) they were less likely to use condoms after substance use, or (c) both (Strunin & Hingson, 1992). In this survey, 66% of the sample were sexually active, 82% reported drinking alcoholic beverages, 19% reported smoking marijuana, and 7% reported drug use other than alcohol or marijuana. Among the sexually active, 64% reported having sex after drinking, while only 15% had sex after drug use. Also, 49% of adolescents were more likely to have sex if they or their partner had been drinking, while only 17% said they used condoms less after drinking than when not drinking. Fewer, 32%, said they would be more likely to use condoms after drug use, but only 10% said they were less likely to use condoms when they had sex after drug use. Only 37% of adolescents reported consistent condom use. Because so few adolescents consistently used condoms, the greatest risk for sexually transmitted diseases, HIV transmission, and unwanted pregnancy is the increased likelihood of having sex after drinking and drug use, not the decreased likelihood of condom use after drinking and drug use. Even among older adolescents in college, similar findings have been reported. Cooper and his colleagues (1989) found that alcohol use prior to a sexual encounter significantly increased the likelihood of selecting a casual new partner, failing to discuss intercourse prior to engaging in it, and failing to use a condom during intercourse.

Conclusions

Surveys of adolescents have been critical to our understanding of their knowledge and their attitudinal and behavioral responses to the AIDS epidemic. Despite progress made during the 1980s in educating adolescents about the modes of HIV transmission, the available survey data reveal that much work remains. During the 1980s, school-based and public information efforts succeeded in informing most adolescents about the principal modes of HIV transmission. Increases in knowledge appear to have contributed to some increases in condom use. These are important achievements. Unfortunately information about the major modes of transmission has not reached all groups of adolescents.

Knowledge about how HIV is transmitted has not reached many adolescents in immigrant groups that may not have received education about AIDS prior to coming to the United States. Language barriers in the United States may limit further their understanding of and exposure to AIDS educational materials. Because many immigrants have relocated to cities with a high incidence of AIDS, it is extremely important that education be targeted to these adolescents and their parents in languages that they can understand. Adolescents who are incarcerated are also less likely to be aware of the major modes of transmission and are much more likely to be having sex than in-school youth. Because only a fraction of persons who engage in illegal behavior are apprehended, the lower knowledge levels among incarcerated youth may be present also in larger numbers of adolescents who engage in risky sexual and drug use practices but who have not been apprehended.

While most adolescents report hearing about AIDS through the media and at school, many have not received messages or counseling from important interpersonal sources of information. Approximately one third of adolescents report not having discussions with their parents about the disease, and fewer than one fifth have received any counseling about AIDS from physicians even though more than 75% have at least one physician contact annually. If adolescents do not receive counseling about AIDS from these important interpersonal sources of communication, it may undermine the perceived importance of communications they receive from other sources.

It is also clear that despite learning the principal modes of transmission, many adolescents are continuing to engage in unprotected sex. In all surveys conducted to date, a majority of sexually active adolescents continue to engage in unprotected sexual intercourse. Further, the proportion of adolescents who are sexually active was increasing before the AIDS epidemic and has continued to increase despite the epidemic.

Data from the surveys collected in Massachusetts indicate that although concern about contracting AIDS increased from 1986 to 1988, concern has remained constant since then and that the proportion who report hearing about AIDS in the media during the week prior to the survey declined from 80% to 50%. Whether this reflects an actual decline in media attention to the problem or decreased attention by adolescents to current media is not clear. Nonetheless it is troubling that from 1988-1990, when the numbers of AIDS cases among 13- to 29-year-olds in Massachusetts doubled, the proportion of adolescents who were concerned about acquiring AIDS remained constant and the proportion who are sexually active increased.

Clearly a need exists to move beyond simply educating adolescents about the modes of HIV transmission. Surveys of adolescents have indicated that their beliefs about AIDS can influence whether they have sex without using condoms (DiClemente, this volume). Educators should discuss adolescent beliefs about AIDS and should emphasize the growing susceptibility of adolescent females to infection. They should reinforce the fact that while some drugs, such as AZT, can prolong the lives of HIV-positive persons, no cure exists and that sexual abstinence and not using injection drugs are the most effective forms of avoiding infection. For those adolescents who do not refrain from sexual activity, educators should emphasize that condom use is critical. Further, educators should demonstrate how to use condoms correctly and should indicate where condoms can be obtained. Perhaps even more important, adolescents need to receive instruction on how to negotiate safety with a potential sexual partner. Role-playing exercises might be particularly helpful in teaching these communication and negotiation skills.

While most adolescents report that they would use condoms if asked, only a minority report discussing condoms prior to intercourse. It should be pointed out to adolescents that very few of their peers would object to using condoms and that increasing numbers are using them. That is not to minimize the interpersonal obstacles to condom use. Adolescents may fear that condom use will raise questions from partners about fidelity and about whether they expect and plan to have sex and do not have strict moral values; it also may raise questions about whether partners will think that they are infected with HIV or other STDs already.

Education must stress that even adolescents who are monogamous now may have been exposed to the HIV virus through earlier sexual contact and that sex can be more relaxed and result in less anxiety if condoms are used. It should be noted that condoms can be used without reducing sexual pleasure and that use of condoms should be regarded as a symbol of caring for partners. Barriers to obtaining condoms also need to be addressed. Pharmacies should be encouraged to place condoms in an easily accessible location where a salesperson is not needed to retrieve them.

Education should not only include discussion of AIDS; it should also cover beliefs and attitudes about other sexually transmitted diseases and pregnancy. Many adolescents are unaware that some sexually transmitted diseases can be asymptomatic. Further, many may not be aware that STD infection can also increase the likelihood of HIV transmission.

Pregnancy should be included in any education about HIV. Many adolescents have not considered the risk of HIV infection from a pregnant woman to her unborn fetus. Further, the rates of unplanned pregnancy among teenagers indicate that many have not carefully considered the responsibilities of pregnancy and caring for a child. In the 1990 Massachusetts survey, one fifth of the unmarried adolescents interviewed said that they would be very happy if they or their sexual partner became pregnant, a considerable disincentive to the use of condoms.

Finally, adolescents should be warned about the risks of having unprotected sex after drinking and drug use. Adolescents who were more likely to have sex after drinking and drug use tended to have had more sexual partners and reported that they were less likely to use condoms. As a result, they are obviously at greater risk for HIV infection.

Surveys have identified clearly the need for additional education of adolescents about AIDS and have offered indications of what direction that education should take. A need still exists to expand our understanding of what factors contribute to adolescents' engaging in risky behavior or relapsing from safer practices. We need to explore such factors as self-efficacy, self-esteem, gender differences, cultural and ethnic differences in response to the AIDS epidemic, and the influence of acculturation on the adoption of behaviors that may influence transmission. Further, as treatments become more effective in prolonging the lives of persons infected with HIV, more research will be needed to learn about factors that may influence whether adolescents seek and obtain HIV testing and whether the testing and the counseling that should accompany testing will influence adolescents' sexual and drug use practices, as well as their emotional adjustments to the disclosure of their HIV status.

References

Allard, B. (1989). Beliefs about AIDS as determinants of preventive practices and support for coercive measures. *American Journal of Public Health, 79*, 448-520.

Bandura, A. (1986). *Social foundations of thought and action: A social cognitive theory.* Englewood Cliffs, NJ: Prentice-Hall.

Becker, M. H., & Joseph, J. G. (1988). AIDS and behavioral change to reduce risk: A review. *American Journal of Public Health, 78*, 394-410.

Centers for Disease Control (CDC). (1990). HIV related knowledge and behaviors among high school students: Selected U.S. sites in 1989. *Journal of the American Medical Association, 264*, 318-322.

Coates, T. J., Stall, R. D., Catania, J. D., & Kegeles, S. (1988). Behavioral factors in the spread of HIV infection. *AIDS, 1*, 239-246.

Cooper, M. L., Skinner, J. B., & George, W. H. (1990). Alcohol use and sexual risk taking among adolescents: Methodologic approaches for address. *Causal Issues in Alcohol Immunomodulation and AIDS*, 11-19, New York: Alan R. Lion.

Cooper, M. L., Skinner, J. B., George, W. H., & Brunner, L. K. (1989, April). *Adolescent alcohol use and high risk sexual behavior.* Paper presented at the Alcohol and AIDS Network Conference, Tucson, AZ.

Crowe, L. C., & George, W. H. (1989). Alcohol and human sexuality. *Review and Integration Psychology Bulletin, 105*, 374-386.

DiClemente, R. J. (1991). Predictors of HIV-preventive sexual behavior in a high-risk adolescent population: The influence of perceived peer norms and sexual communication on incarcerated adolescents' consistent use of condoms. *Journal of Adolescent Health, 12*, 385-390.

DiClemente, R. J., Boyer, C. B., & Morales, E. S. (1988). Minorities and AIDS: Knowledge, attitudes and misconceptions among black and Latino adolescents. *American Journal of Public Health, 78*, 55-57.

DiClemente, R. J., Durbin, M., Siegel, D., Krasnovsky, F., Lazarus, N., & Comacho, T. (1992). Consistent condom use among middle adolescents in a predominantly minority, inner-city school district. *Pediatrics, 89*, 197-202.

DiClemente, R. J., Lanier, M. M., Horan, P. F., & Lodico, M. (1991). Comparison of AIDS knowledge, attitudes and behavior among incarcerated adolescents in a public school sample in San Francisco. *American Journal of Public Health, 81*, 628-631.

DiClemente, R. J., Zorn, J., & Temoshok, L. (1986). A survey of knowledge, attitudes and beliefs about AIDS in San Francisco. *American Journal of Public Health, 76*, 1443-1445.

Fishbein, M., & Azjen, I. (1975). *Belief altered intervention and behavior: An introduction to theory and research.* Reading, MA: Addison-Wesley.

Hingson, R., Strunin, L., & Berlin, B. (1990). AIDS transmission: Changes in knowledge and behaviors among adolescents—Massachusetts statewide surveys 1986-1988. *Pediatrics, 85,* 25-29.

Hingson, R., Strunin, L., Berlin, B., & Heeren, T. (1990). Beliefs about AIDS, use of alcohol and drugs and unprotected sex among Massachusetts adolescents. *American Journal of Public Health, 80,* 295-299.

Hingson, R., Strunin, L., Grady, M., Strunk, N., Carr, R., Berlin, B., & Craven D. (1991). Knowledge about HIV and behavioral risks of foreign born Boston public school students. *Journal of American Public Health, 1,* 1638-1641.

Janz, N. K., & Becker, M. H. (1984). The health belief model a decade later. *Health Education Quarterly, 11,* 1-47.

Jessor, R., Chase, J. A., & Donovan, J. L. (1980). Psychosocial correlates of marijuana use and problem drinking in a national sample of adolescents. *American Journal of Public Health, 70,* 604-613.

Jessor, R., & Jessor, S. L. (1977). *Problem behavior and psycho social development: A longitudinal study of youth.* New York: Academic Press.

Kann, L., Nelson, G., Jones, J., & Kolbe, L. (1989). Establishing a system of complementary school based surveys to annually assess HIV related knowledge, beliefs and behaviors among adolescents. *Journal of School Health, 59,* 55-58.

Kelly, J. A., St. Lawrence, J. S., & Brasfield, T. L. (1991). Predictors of vulnerability to AIDS risk behavior relapse. *Journal of Consulting and Clinical Psychology, 59,* 163-166.

Martin, J. L., & Haiser, D. S. (1990). Drinking alcohol and sexual behavior in a cohort of gay men, drugs and society. *Journal of Contemporary Issues, 5,* 9-67.

McKirnon, D. J., & Peterson, P. J. (1989a). AIDS risk behavior among homosexual males: The role of attitudes and substance abuse. *Psychology and Health, 3,* 161-171.

McKirnon, D. J., & Peterson, P. J. (1989b). Psychosocial and cultural factors in alcohol and drug abuse: An analysis of a homosexual community. *Addictive Behaviors, 14,* 545-553.

Mosher, W. (1990). Contraceptive practice in the U.S. 1982-1988. *Family Planning Perspectives, 22,* 198-205.

Ostrow, D. (1987). Barriers to the recognition of links between drug and alcohol abuse and AIDS. In *Acquired Immunodeficiency Syndrome and Chemical Dependency-NIAAA* (pp. 15-20). (DHHS Publication #ADM 87 1513). Washington, DC: Government Printing Office.

Plant, M. A. (1990). Alcohol, sex and AIDS. *Alcohol and Alcoholism, 25,* 293-301.

Pleck, J., Sonenstein, F., & Ku, L. (1991). Adolescent males' condom use: Relationships between perceived cost-benefits and consistency. *Journal of Marriage and the Family, 53*(4), 733-746.

Price, J., Desmond, S., & Kukulka, G. (1985). High school students' perceptions and misperceptions of AIDS. *Journal of School Health, 55,* 107-109.

Robertson, A., & Plant, M. A. (1988). Alcohol and sexual risk of HIV infection. *Drug and Alcohol Dependency, 22,* 75-78.

Rotheram-Borus, M., & Koopman, C. (1991). Sexual risk behaviors, AIDS knowledge and beliefs about AIDS among runaways. *American Journal of Public Health, 81,* 208-210.

Siegal, K., Mesogno, F., Chen, J., & Chiel, G. (1989). Factors distinguishing homo-sexual males practicing risky and safe sex. *Social Science and Medicine, 28,* 561-569.

Sonenstein, F., Pleck, J., & Ku, L. (1989). Sexual activity, condom use and AIDS awareness among adolescent males. *Family Planning Perspectives, 21,* 152-158.

Stall, R., Ekstrand, M., Pollock, L., McKusick, L., & Coates, T. J. (1990). Relapse from safer sex: The next challenge for AIDS prevention efforts. *Journal of Acquired Immune Deficiency Syndrome, 3,* 1181-1187.

Stall, R., McKusick, L., Wiley, J., Coates, T., & Ostrow, D. (1986). Alcohol use and drug use during sexual activity and compliance with safe sex. *Health Education Quarterly, 13,* 359-371.

Strunin, L. (1991). Adolescents' perceptions of risk for HIV infection: Implications for future research. *Social Science and Medicine, 32,* 221-228.

Strunin, L., & Hingson, R. (1987). Acquired immunodeficiency syndrome and adolescents: Knowledge, beliefs, attitudes and behaviors. *Pediatrics, 79,* 825-832.

Strunin, L., & Hingson, R. (1992). Alcohol, drugs and adolescent sexual behavior. *International Journal of the Addictions, 27,* 129-146.

Valdiserri, R., Lajter, D., Kevitor, L., Callahan, C., Knightly, L., & Renaldo, C. (1988). Variables influencing condom use in a cohort of gay and bi-sexual men. *American Journal of Public Health, 78,* 801-805.

3

Psychosocial Determinants
of Condom Use Among Adolescents

RALPH J. DiCLEMENTE

Introduction

Although sexual abstinence is the most effective method to prevent the transmission of HIV, as well as other sexually transmitted diseases, few adolescents adopt this HIV-preventive behavior once they have become sexually active. The primary HIV-prevention strategy for adolescents who are sexually active is to use condoms consistently during sexual intercourse. While condoms prohibit the transmission of viral pathogens, including human immunodeficiency virus (HIV), their effectiveness as a risk-reduction strategy is dependent on appropriate and consistent use. Unfortunately, increasing the consistent use of condoms among adolescents has been a formidable challenge.

A major barrier to developing more effective condom promotion programs has been our inability to understand the factors that reinforce adolescents' decisions to use condoms. Condom use is a complex social and interpersonal behavior. As such, a myriad of factors—psychological, social, interpersonal, developmental, and cultural—have been hypothesized to play prominent and interactive roles in influencing an adolescent's decision to use condoms. Consequently, understanding the influences underlying an adolescent's decision to use condoms has been difficult, in large part because many of these factors are not easily defined, isolated, or quantified. Although it is challenging, identifying and understanding the interrelationships between the determinants of condom use within the context of the HIV epidemic, are of paramount importance if we are to develop more efficacious risk-reduction programs.

This chapter will review studies that evaluated the relative influence of a number of factors to predict condom use among adolescents. Studies that examined the predictors of condom use in populations other than adolescents are not included in this review. Studies that did not measure or isolate condom use as the dependent variable are omitted as well. For example, three recent reports evaluated the role of demographic and psychosocial factors on adolescents' AIDS-related risk-taking behavior (Keller et al., 1991; Walter, Vaughn, & Cohall, 1991; Walter et al., 1992). The dependent variable in these studies was operationalized along a risk continuum. While informative, this procedure precludes isolating the effects of predictors as they relate specifically to condom use. The reader is directed to these reports, however, as they are both timely and informative.

Each study will be reviewed in turn, and an overarching synthesis of the findings will be described in a summary section. Methodological limitations inherent in the design of these studies also will be discussed. Finally, recommendations for developing more effective HIV-prevention interventions will be presented.

Review of the Literature

In one of the earliest investigations, Catania and his colleagues (Catania et al., 1989) examined a broad spectrum of psychosocial beliefs as they related to condom use among women attending a family planning clinic. The study sample consisted of 114 adolescent females ranging in age from 12-18 (mean age 17.9 years). The sample was predominantly white (92%), heterosexual (96%), and unmarried (100%).

The investigators used a self-administered questionnaire to explore the predictors of female adolescents' condom use with a primary sexual partner within the 2 months prior to completing the study questionnaire. The psychosocial variables assessed included egocentrism, susceptibility, AIDS anxiety, enjoyment of condoms, health benefits of condoms, self-efficacy, general and condom-specific communication, and condom norms. A hierarchical logistic regression analysis was computed with the dependent variable—condom use—dichotomized into condom use and nonuse. Results indicate that greater enjoyment of condoms and greater willingness to request partners to use condoms were significantly associated with condom use ($p = .008$ and $p = .0001$, respectively). All other predictors were nonsignificant.

In another study conducted at a family planning clinic, Weisman and her colleagues (Weisman et al., 1989) explored the relationship among knowledge about AIDS, perceived personal risk, and preventive behavior for 404 sexually active women who completed an interview as part of a baseline assessment. Adolescents ranged in age from 11-18, with a mean age of 16 years. Approximately 81% of the participants were black.

Results indicate that AIDS knowledge was high. On average, subjects gave correct answers to seven out of nine items (median = eight). Perceived risk of contracting AIDS was assessed using a 5-point Likert scale ranging from "very sure it will not happen" to "very sure it will happen." Forty-seven percent reported that they were "very sure" they would not get AIDS in the next 5 years. This variable was dichotomized to facilitate analyses contrasting adolescents who perceived any risk of AIDS acquisition with those who perceived none.

Other variables assessed included demographics (age, race), behaviors (past pregnancy, history of STDs, current male partner more than 5 years older, use of illicit drugs, total number of male partners), communication with sex partner about using condoms, and knowledge about condom efficacy to prevent AIDS. Multiple logistic regression analysis was used to identify the predictors of condom use at last intercourse.

Results indicate that the best predictor of condom use was communication with a sex partner requesting condom use. Adolescents who had ever asked their sex partners to use condoms were 2.66 times more likely to report condom use at last intercourse ($p<.05$). Conversely, having a sex partner more than 5 years older and a history of pregnancy significantly reduced the likelihood that condoms were used at last intercourse (odds = 0.31, $p<.05$ and 0.32, $p<.05$, respectively). Perceived risk of AIDS (odds = 0.85) was not related to condom use, while knowledge of condom efficacy was marginally associated with use (odds = 1.9, $p<.10$).

In a statewide telephone survey of Massachusetts adolescents (16 to 19-year-olds), adolescents were asked to respond to a survey that was based primarily on constructs located in the health belief model (Hingson, Strunin, Berlin, & Heeren, 1990). These constructs included demographic factors, behavioral indices, efficacy of condoms, susceptibility-severity beliefs, barriers to action (e.g., condoms are difficult and embarrassing to obtain, condoms reduce pleasure), cues to action, and alcohol and marijuana use. Of the 1,773 adolescents participating in the survey, 61% reported being sexually active in the previous year, and of these, 31% reported always using condoms during sexual intercourse.

Using stepwise logistic regression analysis to assess which beliefs were the best predictors of consistent condom use (always using condoms), alcohol/marijuana use and a number of demographic beliefs variables were identified as significantly associated with consistent condom use. Whites and younger adolescents (age 16 vs. 19) were more likely to report consistent condom use, with odds ratios (OR) of 2.1 and 2.9 for whites versus blacks, and whites versus other races, respectively, and an odds ratio of 2.48 for adolescents 16 years of age, compared with those 19 years of age. Susceptibility-severity and condom efficacy were also predictive of consistent condom use (OR = 1.8 and 3.1, respectively). The most powerful predictors, however, were perceived barriers of use. Three variables—condoms do not reduce pleasure (OR = 3.1), carrying condoms (OR = 2.7), and not being embarrassed to ask that condoms be used (OR = 2.36)—were related to consistent use. Having discussed AIDS with a physician, considered a cue to action, was also an important predictor of consistent use (OR = 1.67).

With respect to the effects of potential moderating variables, adolescents who did not drink (versus those who drank five or more drinks daily) or who did not use marijuana (in the past month) were 2.8 and 1.9 times, respectively, more likely to use condoms consistently during sexual intercourse. Further, 16% of adolescents who said that they had sex after drinking reported using condoms less often after drinking than when not drinking. Similarly, 25% of adolescents who said that they had sex after drug use reported using condoms less often after using drugs.

A recent large-scale surveillance survey monitoring adolescents' AIDS knowledge, beliefs, and behaviors has been conducted by the Centers for Disease Control (Kann, Nelson, Jones, & Kolbe, 1989). In this survey, a national probability sample of students in grades 9-12 completed self-administered questionnaires. Of the eligible students, 83% (n = 8,098) completed questionnaires. The questionnaire assessed demographic characteristics, knowledge about AIDS, exposure to HIV/AIDS instruction, attitudes and beliefs, and behaviors relevant to HIV transmission and prevention.

As one component of this project, Anderson et al. (1990), using logistic regression analyses to control for other demographic characteristics, examined the relationship between HIV/AIDS knowledge and consistent condom use. Other determinants of consistent condom use, such as beliefs, attitudes, and behavioral measures, which the research literature has shown are important predictors, were not assessed.

Results indicate that AIDS knowledge (summary score), male gender, younger age, and white race were all significantly associated with condom use ($p<.05$). Having received HIV/AIDS instruction, however, was not related to condom use.

The only national probability sample for which data are available is the National Survey of Adolescent Males (NSAM), conducted between April and November 1988 (Pleck, Sonenstein, & Ku, 1991). The sample is representative of the noninstitutionalized, never-married male population aged 15 to 19 and was stratified to overrepresent black and Hispanic adolescents. All adolescents completed in-person interviews. This analysis employed 1,263 males, 67.2% of the total sample, who reported sexual intercourse at least once.

Condom use was defined by adolescents' estimate of the percentage of time they used a condom. *Condom consistency* was collapsed into four categories: 0%, 1-50%, 51-99%, and 100%. Two measures were operationalized: condom consistency with last partner, and condom consistency with recent partners. *Consistency with last partner* was defined as "having had a sex partner in the last year and having had sexual intercourse twice or more often" ($n = 880$). Adolescents who reported having had sexual intercourse only once ever ($n = 124$) were excluded, as well as those who reported having no sexual partner in the last year.

Condom consistency with recent partners was derived for all adolescents who reported at least two episodes of sexual intercourse in the last year with the last partner, or at least one episode per partner with each of two partners. In effect, this measure reflects condom consistency in the last year if only one partner was reported during this period, or with the last two partners if the male reported more than one partner in the past year.

The interview assessed the subjective expected utility (cost-benefits) of condom use in four areas: (a) *preventing pregnancy: personal costs-benefits* (i.e., "If you use a condom, the girl will not get pregnant") and *preventing pregnancy: normative beliefs* (i.e., a 5-item scale assessed the belief that males should bear responsibility for contraception, especially in the context of pregnancy prevention); (b) *avoiding AIDS* (AIDS worry, AIDS perceived risk); (c) *partner expectation* ("If you used a condom, she would appreciate that") and AIDS discounting (i.e., "Using condoms is more trouble than it's worth" and "Even though AIDS is a fatal disease, it is uncommon and it's not really a big worry"); and (d) *embarrassment and reduction of pleasure associated with condom use.*

To assess the influence of these potential predictors on consistency of condom use with last partner and recent partners, such other factors as demographic, sociocultural, and psychological constructs were controlled in the analysis. The investigators utilized a standardized ordered logistic regression analysis employing the unweighted sample to predict level of condom use.

Results indicate that of the measures concerning cost-benefits of condom use, seven had significant independent associations with condom use. With respect to consistency of condom use with last partner, normative beliefs regarding male responsibility (beta = .19, $p<.01$), sex partner using birth control pills (beta = $-.18$, $p<.01$), frequency of worry about AIDS (beta = .22, $p<.01$), partner appreciating condom use (beta = .39, $p<.001$), embarrassment related to condom use (beta = $-.21$, $p<.01$), parents may find out (beta = .22, $p<.05$), and reduction in sexual pleasure (beta = $-.31$, $p<.001$) were associated with condom use. A nearly identical predictor profile was identified with respect to consistency of condom use with recent partners.

Biglan and his colleagues (1990) examined the interrelationship between antisocial behaviors and the association of family coercive processes and peer influences on adolescents' high-risk sexual behavior, including nonuse of condoms. Two separate samples of adolescents in grades 8-12 were recruited through newspaper advertisements, public service announcements, and leaflets distributed at local high schools and other places where adolescents congregate. Adolescents completed a self-report questionnaire that was distributed in same-sex groups. The two samples were predominantly white; 90% and 92%, respectively.

The questionnaire assessed three conceptual domains: sexual behavior, problem and prosocial behavior, and family and peer context. A *sexual behavior* index was developed, based on adolescents' responses to six items, one of which was the frequency of intercourse without the use of a condom. *Problem (antisocial) behavior* was assessed by adolescents' response to items that inquired into their aggressive behavior and delinquent actions, such as vandalism and theft, as well as school difficulties, cigarette smoking, alcohol consumption, and illicit drug use. *Prosocial behavior* assessed participation in school organizations. *Family and peer context* was assessed by developing a measure of family structure that reflected the degree to which parents were psychologically and physically available to the adolescents. Related to familial context, four aspects of parenting practices were assessed: coercive exchange occurring in the family, parental monitoring of adolescents' activities, social support, and family problem-solving skill. Data on peers' behavior, both delinquent and prosocial, and alcohol and drug use also were collected to assess their influence on adolescents' engagement in high-risk sexual behavior.

Hierarchical regression analysis was used to identify significant predictors of nonuse of condoms for sexually active adolescents.

Results for one sample ($n = 84$) who reported ever having sexual intercourse indicate that prosocial behavior is associated negatively with nonuse of condoms ($p = .001$), while smoking was associated positively with nonuse ($p = .02$). In the other sample ($n = 61$), only smoking behavior contributed significantly to the prediction of nonuse of condoms ($p = .005$).

Nonuse of condoms and its relation to social context variables were assessed for those adolescents reporting sexual intercourse in the prior year. In this analysis, sexually active adolescents in each sample ($n = 83$ and $n = 56$) who were less likely to use condoms were those with less family availability ($p<.05$; $p<.01$, respectively). This association was also a significant predictor of other high-risk sexual behavior.

A recent school-based study by Brown and his colleagues (Brown, DiClemente, & Beausoleil, under review) used the theory of reasoned action as the framework to identify predictors of consistent condom use and behavioral intentions to use condoms among high school students ($n = 1,049$) completing self-administered questionnaires. The sample was predominantly white (67%) and female (52.1%). The mean age of the sample was 16.2 years, and most were college bound (74.5%).

Of the total sample, 52% reported being sexually active, and half of these students reported sexual intercourse in the past month. Of those who reported sexual intercourse in the past month, 27% reported consistent condom use. *Consistent condom use* was operationally defined as "always used a condom when having sexual intercourse during the prior month."

The questionnaire assessed the following constructs: AIDS knowledge, fear of HIV infection, tolerance toward Persons Living with AIDS, behavioral intentions to practice low-risk sexual behaviors, a generalized scale assessing attitudes toward engaging in risky not HIV-related behaviors, past history of risk taking, and perceptions of friend's use of condoms (included as a measure of perceived peer normative behavior).

Data analysis, based on bivariate contingency table analyses, consisted of screening for potential predictors of consistent condom use in the past month. Significant predictors then were entered into a multivariate logistic regression model to adjust for the effect of each variable.

Results indicated that males, safe behavioral intentions, and a history of low-risk behavior were significantly associated with consistent condom use, the adjusted odds ratios being 3.0, 4.2, and 2.0, respectively. As behavioral intentions to practice safer sex was the best predictor of consistent condom use, a second logistic model was constructed that sought to identify the best predictor of safe behavioral intentions. With similar variables, only one factor—perceived referent-group normative behavior (perceptions of friend's use of condoms)—was significant. Adolescents who perceived their friends as using condoms were 2.6 times more likely to be consistent condom users themselves.

A series of studies exploring the determinants of adolescents' consistent use of condoms has been conducted in the San Francisco Bay Area. While the adolescent populations and measurement instruments varied among studies, a core of constructs was common to each study. This commonality allowed for assessing the relative predictive utility of these constructs in different populations. As each study used the same data analytic strategy, the statistical methodology, described below, is relevant for all studies. Deviations from the specified data analytic strategy are highlighted.

The statistical strategy used bivariate tests of proportions to evaluate whether individual factors were associated with consistent condom use. Factors identified as significantly associated with consistent condom use in the bivariate analyses were entered into a logistic regression analysis to assess the independent contribution of each factor in predicting condom use. Adjusted odds ratios (OR) and confidence limits (CL) were calculated to assess the magnitude of association between factors and condom use.

In the first study, students from three inner-city, predominantly nonwhite junior high schools completed an anonymous self-report questionnaire assessing HIV-related demographic, psychosocial, and behavioral factors (DiClemente et al., 1992). Students who reported being sexually active (n = 403) composed the sample for analysis.

All measures were derived from a self-report questionnaire. The questionnaire assessed the following: demographics, AIDS knowledge, transmission knowledge, condom efficacy, perceived costs of condom use, perceived susceptibility to HIV infection, and sexual and drug-related behaviors. Condom use, the outcome variable, was assessed by use of a 4-point Likert scale ranging from "always" to "never." Approximately 37% of the sample reported consistent condom use (always used condoms). Adolescents reporting condom use as "sometimes," "rarely," or "never" were categorized as infrequent condom users.

Adolescents' perceived costs of condom use was assessed by use of an 8-item scale. Each scale item reflected physical, emotional, or accessibility costs associated with condom use; for example, condoms are too embarrassing to use, they are too expensive to purchase, they reduce sexual pleasure, and so on. Responses were summed across the eight items and yielded a summary score. Scores were divided into three groups: low, intermediate, and high perceived costs. Adolescents categorized in the high perceived cost group were significantly less likely to be consistent condom users relative to their peers in the intermediate and low perceived costs groups ($p<.01$); however, no statistical difference was found in the proportion of consistent condom users in the intermediate and low perceived costs groups, and these groups were collapsed into a single category (i.e., low perceived costs).

Adolescents' perceptions of condoms' efficacy in preventing HIV transmission were assessed by use of a Likert scale. Adolescents' responses were recoded into two categories: high perceived condom efficacy ("condoms work very well" and "condoms work pretty well to prevent AIDS") and low perceived condom efficacy ("condoms work only slightly" and "condoms don't work at all").

Adolescents reporting low perceived costs associated with condom use were almost twice as likely to use condoms consistently during sexual intercourse as peers reporting high perceived costs (OR = 1.9; 95% CL = 1.1-3.3). Number of lifetime sexual partners was inversely related to frequency of condom use. Adolescents with a history of three or more sex partners were approximately half as likely to use condoms consistently (OR = 0.46; 95% CL = .21-.88). Perception of condoms' efficacy was the most powerful determinant of consistent condom use. Adolescents who perceived condoms as effectively preventing HIV transmission were more than twice as likely to be consistent users (OR = 2.21; 95% CL = 1.2-4.2). Interaction effects between adolescents' number of lifetime sex partners, perceived costs of condom use, and perceived condom efficacy were examined and found not to be significant.

In another cross-sectional survey (DiClemente & Fisher, 1992), all students enrolled in family life education classes, a required course, in nine primary high schools in the San Francisco Unified School District were asked to participate in the Centers for Disease Control (CDC) surveillance survey of adolescents' HIV-related knowledge, attitudes, and risk behaviors by completing an anonymous self-report survey. Developed as an epidemiologic survey instrument, the questionnaire contained 49 items with predefined response categories. The response categories for each item used binary responses (Yes-No), categorical responses (True-False-Unsure), or a Likert scale response format to increase readability and to facilitate administration. As all measures were derived from the self-report questionnaire, it is important to note that the questionnaire was designed for epidemiologic surveillance, and test-retest reliability has not been established.

Condom use was assessed on a 4-point scale, with 32.5%, 28.1%, 14.5%, and 25.0% of adolescents, respectively, reporting frequency of use as "always," "sometimes," "rarely," or "never." Condom use was categorized into two levels: consistent ("always") or infrequent (the latter including the responses "sometimes," "rarely," or "never"). Potential correlates of consistent condom use, based on constructs located in the health belief model, were identified. Constructs assessed included age, gender, general HIV knowledge, knowledge of HIV risk-reduction strategies, adolescents' perceived susceptibility to HIV infection, age at sexual debut, number of lifetime sex partners, and number of partners in the prior year.

This model was expanded to include two social influence measures: adolescents' perceptions of peer norms supporting condom use, and communication with sex partner about AIDS. Adolescents' perceptions of peer norms, based on responses to the question, "How many persons your age do you think are using condoms during sexual intercourse?" were assessed. Adolescents responded on a 5-point Likert scale of "almost all," "most," "half," "few," and "none." Based on the distribution of consistent condom use at each level, the scale was dichotomized into two levels, with the response categories "almost all" and "most" collapsed into a single category defined as "high" perceived peer support for condom use. The remaining categories were collapsed into a single category defined as "low" perceived peer support for condom use.

Adolescents' communication with sex partners about AIDS was assessed by their response to the question, "Because of AIDS, have you ever talked with your boyfriend or girlfriend about AIDS before having sexual intercourse?"

Among sexually active adolescents ($n = 270$), logistic regression analysis identified four factors associated with condom use: Adolescents discussing AIDS with sex partners and those who perceive peer norms as supporting condom use were 5.2 and 4.3 times more likely to report consistent condom use, respectively. Fewer lifetime sex partners and male gender also were associated with reported consistent condom use.

Table 3.1   Stepwise Logistic Model Predicting Consistent Condom Use

Step	Variables in Model	Step χ^2	DF	p-value
1	Gender; Lifetime number sex partners	14.6	2	.0007
2	Perceived peer norms; Talk with sex partner	27.0	2	.0000

The behavioral variable (number of sex partners) and demographic characteristic (gender) then were entered as the initial step in a stepwise logistic regression model to identify the relative influence of these variables, compared to social influence variables. The results are displayed in Table 3.1.

As can be readily observed, while behavioral and demographic variables were associated with consistent condom use, from a behavioral intervention standpoint these factors preclude modification. Social influence variables, on the other hand, even though entered following these elemental variables, make a more significant contribution to explaining condom use. As important, social influence variables are modifiable targets and thus of particular interest for future behavioral risk-reduction research.

Based on the findings demonstrating the predictive potential of social influences, another study examined whether social influence factors, in the presence of other demographic, behavioral, and psychosocial factors, would remain significant predictors of consistent condom use among a high-risk adolescent population: adolescents incarcerated in a juvenile detention facility (DiClemente, 1991).

Incarcerated adolescents completed the same survey instrument developed by the Centers for Disease Control. The variables assessed were identical to those described in the previous study, as was the mode of survey administration. Sexually active adolescents ($n = 112$) also were categorized into condom use groups by use of the previously described procedure (see DiClemente & Fisher, 1992, above).

Three factors were identified as associated with consistent condom use: nonblacks (OR = 10; $p = .005$), adolescents who communicate with their sex partners about AIDS (OR = 15.3; $p = .0006$), and those who perceive peer norms as supporting condom use

(OR = 6.7; p = .01) were significantly more likely to be consistent condom users.

The potential interaction between ethnicity (black vs. nonblack) and perceived peer norms and communication with sex partners about AIDS was examined and found not to be significant (p = .45 and p = .91, respectively). Moreover no interaction was found between sexual communication and perception of peer norms (p = .59).

In a fourth study (DiClemente & Horan, 1992), we examined the effects of alcohol disinhibition on adolescents' consistent use of condoms. While evidence was ample that alcohol use reduces the consistency with which condoms are used, less data described which psychosocial factors that alcohol exerts its influence on to effect behavior.

A sample of 455 sexually active adolescents was drawn from a pool of 1,920 students enrolled in 10th-grade family life classes and 11th-grade social studies classes in the San Francisco Unified School District (SFUSD) in February 1989. All students completed a revised CDC surveillance instrument (1989 version). Administration protocols and determination of consistent condom use were identical to previously described studies (see DiClemente & Fisher, 1992, above).

Factors assessed in this survey included age, gender, general HIV knowledge, knowledge of HIV risk-reduction strategies, adolescents' perceived susceptibility to HIV infection, resistance self-efficacy, perceived condom efficacy to prevent HIV transmission, communication with parents and with friends about AIDS, age at sexual debut, number of lifetime sex partners, and number of partners in the prior year.

A number of bivariate determinants of condom use were identified: alcohol disinhibition (p = .0001); *condom self-efficacy*, defined as "the ability to insist on condom use" (p = .0001); general HIV knowledge (p = .0001); condom efficacy to prevent HIV infection (p = .001); age of sex onset (p = .01); *resistance self-efficacy*, defined as "the ability to refuse high-risk sex" (p = .001); and number of sex partners in the year prior to completing the survey (p = .0004).

When these factors were entered into a multivariate logistic regression model, only two remained significant: (a) Adolescents who have high self-efficacy to insist on condom use were 8.8 times as likely to be consistent condom users (p = .0001). (b) Those who reported not having experienced sexual disinhibition as a result

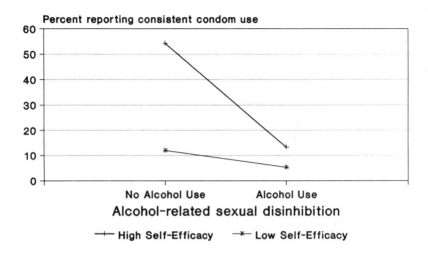

Figure 3.1. Effect of Alcohol Use on Adolescents' Ability to Insist on Condom Use During Sexual Intercourse

of being high from alcohol use were significantly more likely to use condoms consistently (OR = 6.7; p = .0001).

A significant interaction was identified, however (p = .0001). The interaction effect is displayed in Figure 3.1.

Partitioning the interaction identified a strong association between condom self-efficacy and consistent condom use for adolescents who did not report disinhibition from alcohol use (OR = 4.5; p = 0.0001). On the other hand, for adolescents who did report alcohol-induced sexual disinhibition, no relationship was found between condom self-efficacy and consistent condom use (p = .19). These findings suggest that adolescents' condom self-efficacy is affected markedly by alcohol use, increasing the likelihood that they would not be able to insist on condom use.

Summary of Findings

Though considerable variation exists in the constructs assessed, the adolescent populations studied, and research methodologies utilized, the review has identified some potentially important variables associated with condom use that warrant further investigative inquiry. With respect to demographic characteristics, males, white race, and younger adolescents were more likely to be consistent condom users. With respect to ethnic/racial differences, the findings suggest that perhaps cultural factors, not assessed, may be of critical importance in understanding condom use among multicultural adolescent populations. Moreover, the finding that male gender is associated with consistent condom use may reflect inappropriate phrasing of the questions included on interviews and self-administered measures. Younger age, on the other hand, may suggest that these adolescents may have less opportunity to demonstrate a failure to use condoms because they have fewer sex partners or a lower cumulative frequency of sexual episodes.

Behavioral variables also demonstrate predictive capability. Having a sex partner more than 5 years older, smoking, and greater number of lifetime sex partners or risk behaviors all were associated with less condom use. Interestingly, earlier onset of sexuality was not associated with less condom use.

Psychosocial constructs have a substantial impact on condom use. In particular, communication about AIDS, condom self-efficacy, and the perception of peer norms supporting condom use were strongly associated with consistent use. Another construct—negative attitudes toward condoms or the perceived costs associated with condom use (e.g., embarrassing, reduce sexual pleasure, etc.)—was strongly predictive of infrequent condom use. Conversely, enjoyment of condoms and a positive attitude (low costs of use) were highly associated with condom use. Other factors that emerged as potentially important determinants are perceived condom efficacy to prevent AIDS/HIV infection and, to a lesser extent, perceived susceptibility/worry about AIDS. A few other factors were also significant predictors of condom use; however, they were usually isolated findings not corroborated by other studies. In some cases, a particular factor was examined in only one study; thus this factor may be important but, because of the lack of confirmation from other studies reviewed, is not emphasized in this summary.

Taken as a whole, the findings strongly suggest that effective sexual communication/negotiation skills, the self-efficacy to request condom use, and the perception of HIV-preventive social norms are key factors associated with consistent use. In conjunction with more favorable attitudes toward condom use, these factors suggest that HIV-preventive efforts for promoting the adoption and maintenance of condom use should strive to incorporate program elements that directly target these critical skills, beliefs, and attitudes.

Limitations

The studies reviewed are not without limitations. First, these studies used a cross-sectional research design. Additional studies using a prospective cohort design will be necessary to evaluate the significance and the stability of identified determinants to predict consistent condom use over time. Second, while identifying potentially important determinants of condom use, these findings are based on self-report measures of behavior, particularly the frequency of condom use. Future studies also will have to include objective surrogate assessments of condom use, whenever possible, as one means of validating adolescents' self-report. One objective measure of condom use, for example, would be to assess the prevalence of sexually transmitted diseases among adolescents. Third, in many cases the sample size was small, especially in studies involving such multicultural adolescent populations as blacks and Hispanics. This small sampling may limit the utility of the findings for developing culturally appropriate HIV-prevention programs for these ethnic/racial populations. Fourth, while the research questionnaires or interviews assessed a number of relevant psychosocial constructs, operationalization and measurement of these constructs may be unreliable. Further efforts will be needed to refine our measurement instruments to ensure that they are valid and reliable measures of the constructs they purport to assess. Fifth, additional constructs, not assessed in most of the present studies, could also influence condom use. These include cultural measures, such as acculturation, developmental constructs, and psychological status. Further research should incorporate these less intensively investigated constructs.

Recommendations for HIV Prevention

The findings have implications for the development of HIV-prevention programs. Programs that emphasize the didactic transfer of information about HIV transmission or risk-reduction strategies are not likely to be effective in modifying adolescents' sexual risk behavior. Based on the present review, one recommendation would be to emphasize skills training and norm-setting activities. These activities would focus on developing and redefining communication skills around sexual negotiation and modifying adolescents' perceptions about peer norms with respect to safer sex behavior. These skill-based programs may be more effective in increasing the likelihood that adolescents will adopt or maintain HIV-preventive behaviors. In addition, increasing adolescents' belief in condom efficacy and dispelling negative attitudes about the costs associated with condom use also should be high-priority targets for behavioral intervention programs.

Conclusion

Adolescents' use of condoms is the outcome of a multifactorial decision-making process in which many influences underlie this behavior. While much more remains to be learned about factors motivating the adoption or maintenance of this HIV-preventive sexual practice, this review has highlighted several potentially important determinants of condom use. Future studies will need to define more precisely the interrelationship between determinants and their applicability for different adolescent populations.

References

Anderson, J. E., Kann, L., Holtzman, D., Arday, S., Truman, B., & Kolbe, L. (1990). HIV/AIDS knowledge and sexual behavior among high school students. *Family Planning Perspectives, 22*, 252-255.

Biglan, A., Metzler, C. W., Wirt, R., Ary, D., Noell, J., Ochs, L., French, C., & Hood, D. (1990). Social and behavioral factors associated with high-risk sexual behavior among adolescents. *Journal of Behavioral Medicine, 13*, 245-261.

Brown, L. K., DiClemente, R. J., & Beausoleil, N. (under review). Utility of a theory-driven model for understanding consistent condom use among adolescents. Manuscript submitted for publication.

Catania, J. A., Dolcini, M. M., Coates, T. J., Kegeles, S. M., Greenblatt, R. M., Puckett, S., Corman, M., & Miller, J. (1989). Predictors of condom use and multiple partnered sex among sexually-active adolescent women: Implications for AIDS-related health interventions. *Journal of Sex Research, 26*, 514-524.

DiClemente, R. J. (1991). Predictors of HIV-preventive sexual behavior in a high-risk adolescent population: The influence of perceived peer norms and sexual communication on incarcerated adolescents' consistent use of condoms. *Journal of Adolescent Health, 12*, 385-390.

DiClemente, R. J., Durbin, M., Siegel, D., Krasnovsky, F., Lazarus, N., & Comacho, T. (in press). Consistent condom use among middle adolescents in a predominantly minority, inner-city school district. *Pediatrics, 89*, 197-202.

DiClemente, R. J., & Fisher, J. D. (1992). Social influence factors associated with consistent condom use among adolescents in an HIV epicenter: Communication and perceived referent group norms. Manuscript submitted for publication.

DiClemente, R. J., & Horan, P. (1992). Effects of alcohol use on adolescents' high-risk sexual behavior in an urban AIDS center. Manuscript submitted for publication.

Hingson, R. W., Strunin, L., Berlin, B. M., & Heeren, T. (1990). Beliefs about AIDS, use of alcohol and drugs, and unprotected sex among Massachusetts adolescents. *American Journal of Public Health, 80*, 295-299.

Kann, L., Nelson, G. D., Jones, J. T., & Kolbe, L. J. (1989). Establishing a system of complementary school-based surveys to annually assess HIV-related knowledge, beliefs, and behaviors among adolescents. *Journal of School Health, 59*, 55-58.

Keller, S. E., Bartlett, J. A., Schleifer, S. J., Johnson, R. L., Pinner, E., & Delany, B. (1991). HIV-relevant sexual behavior among a healthy inner-city heterosexual adolescent population in an endemic area of HIV. *Journal of Adolescent Health, 12*, 44-48.

Pleck, J. H., Sonenstein, F. L., & Ku, L. C. (1991). Adolescent males' condom use: Relationships between perceived cost-benefits and consistency. *Journal of Marriage and the Family, 53*, 733-745.

Walter, H. J., Vaughn, R. D., & Cohall, A. T. (1991). Psychosocial influences on acquired immunodeficiency syndrome-risk behaviors among high school students. *Pediatrics, 88*, 846-852.

Walter, H. J., Vaughn, R. D., Gladis, M. M., Ragin, D. F., Kasen, S., & Cohall, A. T. (1992). Factors associated with AIDS-risk behaviors among high school students in an AIDS epicenter. *American Journal of Public Health, 82*, 528-532.

Weisman, C. S., Nathanson, C. A., Ensminger, M., Teitelbaum, M. A., Robinson, J. C., & Plichta, S. (1989). AIDS knowledge, perceived risk and prevention among adolescent clients of a family planning clinic. *Family Planning Perspectives, 21*, 213-217.

4

Incarcerated Youth at Risk
for HIV Infection

ROBERT E. MORRIS

CHARLES J. BAKER

SUSAN HUSCROFT

Introduction

Admissions to United States juvenile detention facilities nationwide continue to rise, with a 5% increase from 1987 to 1989. In 1989, a total of 1,228,000 youth were detained in 1,100 facilities. The rate of incarceration and the number of adjudicated adolescents vary widely from one region of the United States to another. The differences are accounted for by variation in age at which youngsters are considered adults, as well as by different practices regarding placement of delinquents. For example, New York defines

AUTHORS' NOTE: Supported in part by a grant from the Center for Communicable Disease Control.

a *juvenile* as a child through age 15, while in California the age is 17. Thus in 1984, New York City's three counties reported 7,417 delinquents, while Los Angeles County reported 30,870. Differences are reflected also in the 1984 custody rates for these two areas of the country. New York State had a custody rate of 171 per 100,000, while California's rate was 529 per 100,000. Vermont had the lowest rate—34 per 100,000—while the District of Columbia had the highest rate—808 per 100,000. Rates of offending also vary from location to location, which would affect the number of delinquents (Allen-Hagen, 1991).

Ethnic, Gender, and Offense Distribution Among Incarcerated Youth

Ethnic minorities are disproportionately represented in detention centers, accounting for 60% of all presently detained youth. Black adolescents account for 42% of the detainee population, while Hispanics and Native Americans or Pacific Islanders account for 15% and 2%, respectively.

The daily census of United States youth correctional facilities was 49,443 in 1989, of which only 6,680 (14%) were females. The majority of detained youth were between ages 14-17 (44,894), with only 3,276 below age 14.

Violent personal offenses increased 8% from 1987 to 1989, and a 150% increase occurred in drug and alcohol offenses from 1985 to 1989. The proportion of juveniles incarcerated for drug or alcohol offenses increased 58%, so that they comprised 12% of the custody population, compared with only 8% in 1987. A 4% decline occurred in serious property offenses from 1987 to 1989; however, this still represents the largest offense category among incarcerated youth (41%). Only 1% of the detained population were held because the youngsters were abused or neglected, and 4% were status offenders (runaway, truant, incorrigible).

The economic cost for both state and local governments is high. In 1989, it cost $1.67 billion to provide for incarcerated youth. This represents a 14% increase in expenditures from 1987. The average per year cost to house a detainee was $29,600 in 1988, with a range from $17,600 to $78,800.

Health Status of Incarcerated Youth:
Sexually Transmitted Diseases

Many adolescents enter detention with serious unmet health needs, including skin diseases, congenital deformities, orthopedic injuries, and infections, especially sexually transmitted diseases (STDs) (Council on Scientific Affairs, 1990; Farrow, 1984). In Los Angeles, 45-50% of females entering the juvenile halls have an STD, and two thirds of these have a second or even third concurrent infection. The comparable STD rate for males in Los Angeles is 15-20% (Brady, Baker, & Neinstein, 1988). Other cities on the East and West coasts report similarly high STD rates for incarcerated adolescents (Alexander-Rodriguez & Vermund, 1987; Bell et al., 1985). While geographic variation exists in the prevalence of STDs among incarcerated youth, delinquent youth usually have rates substantially higher than the general adolescent population.

Knowledge and Attitudes Regarding HIV
Among Incarcerated Youth

Despite the high prevalence of sexually transmitted diseases among this adolescent population, few cross-sectional surveys have assessed adolescents' HIV-related knowledge, attitudes, and beliefs. Longitudinal and comparative studies are even less common.

Cross-Sectional Surveys

Those surveys limited to incarcerated juveniles' responses regarding AIDS provide epidemiologic data on the prevalence of risk-taking behaviors (Baker et al., 1991; Huscroft et al., 1990; Rolf et al., 1989; Zeljkovic et al., 1991). Most studies report a high prevalence of sexual intercourse (90%), with early onset of sexual activity (13-14 years) common, and condom use during sexual intercourse as infrequent. For example, although 66% of incarcerated juveniles knew condoms helped prevent HIV infection, only 15% had used them during their last sexual encounter (Rolf et al., 1989). Drug abuse is also high. Whether injection drug use or other illicit drugs (e.g., crack cocaine) are involved, incarcerated adolescents have a high prevalence of polydrug use. Crack use by this population may result in an increased likelihood of unsafe sexual practices (Fullilove, Fullilove, Bowser, & Gross, 1990).

Comparative Studies

Nader and his colleagues (1989) compared incarcerated adolescents with urban and suburban high school students, as well as with gay youth. They report that incarcerated youth scored lower on all scales, including knowledge, agreement with health guidelines, perceived personal threat of AIDS, personal efficacy to prevent AIDS, and perceived norms of safe sex practices. Another study compared incarcerated adolescents with a control population of youth recruited from the school district in the same city (DiClemente, Lanier, Horan, & Lodico, 1991). Although school-based and incarcerated adolescents were similarly knowledgeable about modes of HIV transmission, incarcerated adolescents knew less about risk-reduction methods, with 56-75% having correct responses for risk-reduction strategies, compared with school-based adolescents, for which a larger proportion had correct responses to these questions (72-85% correct).

While HIV knowledge of the two populations was similar, substantial differences were identified with respect to the prevalence of HIV related risk behaviors. Almost all incarcerated youth reported being sexually experienced, compared with 28% of the school sample. Most incarcerated youth (73%) reported two or more sex partners during the past year, compared with 8% of the school sample. A larger proportion of incarcerated youth initiated sex at an early age, as approximately 52% and 26% of the detained and school samples, respectively, reported sexual onset by age 12. Condom use among both samples is inconsistent, although incarcerated youth reported less condom use. Injection drug abuse is more prevalent among incarcerated youth, though roughly similar proportions of intravenous drug users in each sample reported sharing needles.

Geographic differences in incarcerated adolescents' knowledge, attitudes, and risk behaviors also have been assessed (Lanier, DiClemente, & Horan, 1991). Delinquents from high-risk (San Francisco) and low-risk (Alabama) locales had similar levels of HIV knowledge, with some variation in understanding specific risk factors. For example, on the one hand, incarcerated adolescents in San Francisco were more likely to identify condoms correctly as an HIV preventive strategy, compared with delinquents from Alabama: 76%, compared with 61%, respectively. On the other hand, the Alabama youth (94%) were more accurate in identifying injection drug use as an HIV-risk practice, compared with San Francisco youth (86%). In addition to cognitive differences, variations also occurred in risk behavior between these populations. Generally Alabama teens reported fewer sex partners and more condom use. The prevalence of IV drug use and needle sharing was similar. This study provides some insight into geographic differences that may have implications for planning local HIV-prevention programs by targeting gaps in knowledge and identifying risk behaviors that are more prevalent relative to other incarcerated adolescent populations.

Repeated Cross-Sectional Surveys

To assess changes in incarcerated adolescents' HIV-related risk behaviors, the Juvenile Court Health Services of Los Angeles County has conducted an extensive interview survey, as well as clinical evaluation for presence of STDs and antibody to human immunodeficiency virus (HIV-1) among newly admitted adolescents, over the past 3 years. While data are incomplete for 1991, we present findings comparing changes in the prevalence of HIV-related risk behaviors and STDs for 1989 and 1990. Overall the findings reveal a high prevalence of many risk behaviors, although fluctuation has occurred in the rates of risk behaviors between 1989 and 1990.

Prevalence of HIV-Related
Risk Behaviors

In 1989, 1,045 minors were interviewed; 18.9% female, 81.1% male. A similar survey was conducted in 1990 in which 1,754 detainees were interviewed; 14.3% female, 85.7% male. The ethnic/racial distribution in 1989 was 39% black, 42% Hispanic, 15% white, 1% Asian, and 3% other. Some shifts occurred in this distribution in 1990, with black, Hispanic, white, Asian, and other ethnic/racial groups representing 34%, 51%, 7%, 1.5%, and 5%, respectively, of the incarcerated population.

In 1989, the prevalence of self-reported sexual activity was 97% for both boys and girls. The average number of lifetime sex partners was 16. Average age of onset of sex activity was 12.8 years. In 1990, 97% of males and 94.4% of females were sexually active, with an average of 15 lifetime sexual partners and a sexual debut of 13.1 years. Exposure to multiple sex partners appears to be common for detained juveniles.

The 1989 and 1990 surveys revealed low overall prevalence of condom use, with 65% and 67% of respondents, respectively, never using condoms, and only 7% and 4%, respectively, consistently using condoms (always used condoms during sexual intercourse). Those who reported consistent condom use were significantly less likely to have had an STD (5.4%, compared with 54% for noncondom users).

The lifetime prevalence of pregnancy was high; 43% of females had a previous pregnancy, while 5% were pregnant at the time of the intake interview. Of the males, 8% reported that a present or previous sexual partner is currently or was pregnant as a consequence of their sexual activity. These rates were stable between the 2 years.

Same-sex sexual activity differed markedly by gender. In 1989 and 1990, respectively, 8% and 6.7% of females reported same-sex partners, compared with only 2.7% and 1.2% of males in the same years. The number of males who admitted to trading sex for drugs or favors increased from 7.4% to 11.7% from 1989 to 1990. The proportion of females engaging in prostitution or trading sex for drugs decreased from 1989 (14.7%) to 1990 (6.8%).

Among heterosexual males and females, vaginal intercourse was frequent: 81% in 1989, increasing to 96% in 1990. The proportion reporting any frequency of condom use for vaginal intercourse was substantially smaller; 40% of males and 46% of females reported some condom use in 1989, while in 1990, 32% of males and 47% of females reported using condoms some of the time during vaginal intercourse. Anal intercourse was not uncommon. In 1990, 13.1% of males reported insertive anal intercourse, and 1.8% reported receptive anal sex. Only 21% of those engaging in this high-risk sexual practice, however, reported any condom use. Among females, slightly more than half who reported engaging in anal intercourse in 1990 reported that their sex partners used condoms.

Homosexual/bisexual males in 1989 reported a higher prevalence of STDs, compared with exclusively heterosexual males (36% vs. 27.5%). This rate continued to be high in 1990, with 44% of homosexual/bisexual males having had an STD, compared with 21% for the general incarcerated adolescent population.

The reported prevalence of STDs was not uniform across ethnic/racial groups. In 1989, 40% of blacks, 25% of whites, 18% of Hispanics, and 0% of Asian youth had an STD. In 1990, prevalence among black youth declined to 28%, while the prevalence among Asian youth increased to 4.2%. White and Hispanic youth had a lower prevalence in 1990—20.6% and 16%, respectively. HIV seroprevalence from Los Angeles juvenile halls also has varied between years, from 2.6 per 1,000 in 1989 to 0.8 per 1,000 in 1990.

In 1989, 20% of females and 10% of males reported sexual intercourse with an injection drug user. This decreased to 14.8% for females and 5.6% for males in 1990. In 1989, sex with an HIV-positive person was rare—1% for females and 0.7% for males. In 1990, only three persons reported having sex with a seropositive individual.

In 1989 and 1990, drug use was common, with equal percentages of males and females (74%) reporting drug use. Only 10% of females and 5% of males admitted to IV drug use in 1989, declining to 8% and 4%, respectively, in 1990. Alcohol was used by 61% of females and 76% of males in 1989, and in 1990 by 56% and 74% of females and males, respectively. In 1989, 63% of females and 58% of male drinkers got drunk, and these figures rose in 1990 to 84% for both sexes. Crack use increased from 1989 to 1990 in all racial/ethnic groups except black males and females (Morris, Baker, Huscroft, Evans, & Zeljkovic, 1991). A recent phenomenon associated with crack use consists of females "hanging out" in crack houses, trading sex for crack cocaine. This new form of prostitution may have lead to the dramatic increase in the rate of syphilis.

Despite the continuing AIDS crisis, these data suggest that incarcerated youth have not sufficiently modified high-risk behaviors associated with STD/HIV infection. This large reservoir of risk-taking youth already manifests the danger for HIV spread by the high rate of other STDs. If educational programs do not or cannot curtail these risky behaviors, the rate of HIV infection eventually will increase in this population.

HIV-Prevention Education
for Incarcerated Youth

Incarcerated adolescents present special problems that must be considered before developing and implementing an HIV-risk-reduction educational program, such as limited intellectual ability, lack of future orientation, poor self-image, limited moral reasoning, and lack of perceived value from modifying risk behaviors (Lane, 1980; McKay & Brumback, 1980; Meltzer, Roditi, & Fenton, 1986; Schuster & Guggenheim, 1982). External problems also are caused by the constraints of the facilities in which incarcerated youth are detained. Some of these problems include bans forbidding discussion of sex or drugs, reluctance of officials to allow distribution of condoms, limited financial/personnel/physical resources, and the perception that delinquents are incorrigible (Leyser & Abrams, 1982).

While these issues directly affect program development and implementation, once programs are implemented, difficulties inherent in the correctional setting may arise that severely limit evaluating their effectiveness. The transient nature of short-term incarcerated hall populations makes follow-up difficult. Many studies depend on self-report of risk behavior, such as sexual activity and illicit drug use; such reports may be unreliable. Study participants often receive multiple behavior change interventions, which make isolating the effect of a specific intervention difficult to ascertain. Constructing adequate control groups is difficult because the records of incarcerated individuals are scanty with regard to socioeconomic status, intelligence, school performance, and previous education. Last, many HIV-prevention programs are based on the premise that improved knowledge leads to behavior change. This assumption has not been validated across a range of adolescent and adult populations (Becker & Joseph, 1988).

Issues in the Design
of HIV-Prevention Programs

Programs demonstrating increased knowledge acquisition alone may not predict actual reduction of risky behavior (Brown & Fritz, 1988; Tucker & Cho, 1991). Education not coupled with increased availability of relevant medical services may not lead to increases in HIV-preventive sexual practices (Kirby, 1984), while programs that provided appropriate linkage of these components have resulted in decreased pregnancies and improved contraceptive use among students in an inner-city high school (Edwards, Steinman, & Hakanson, 1980). The objectives of any HIV-education program include (a) improving adolescents' motivation to reduce risk, (b) providing the skills to use knowledge, and (c) imprinting the perception of vulnerability (Rotheram-Borus, Koopman, Haignere, & Davis, 1991). A long-term goal should be to change social sexual norms (i.e., using condoms is "cool") and drug use norms (clean needles are "OK"). The provision of condoms at the time of release may be one strategy that would have a positive impact on decreasing risky sexual behavior.

In addition, special areas of concern exist, such as high levels of alcohol consumption; tattooing; blood-sharing rituals, such as becoming "blood brothers"; sexual intercourse with prostitutes/ strawberries (prostitution for crack cocaine) and successive (gang) rapes; higher risk of anal sex with male or female partners, often used as a contraceptive method by females; sexual activity while detained; and not uncommon ritualistic abuse and satanic rituals.

Communication Skills. Adolescents need skills in order to put knowledge to work. Practicing proper condom use and needle cleaning techniques ensures that they can successfully accomplish these tasks. Communication techniques that will allow an adolescent to negotiate safer sex and drug refusal must be learned and practiced in order that knowledge can be applied to risk situations (Schinke, Gilchrist, Snow, & Schilling, 1985).

Peer-Assisted HIV Education

Peer education leads to greater personalization of the dangers of HIV-risk behavior (Rickert, Jay, & Gottlieb, 1991). Peer groups serve a very important function for all adolescents (Conger, 1977) and especially delinquent adolescents, as evidenced by gang activity. The use of peer counselors for this population, though largely untested, is especially important and calls for further research. Education provided one-to-one during pre- and post-HIV-test counseling and during the apprehensive waiting period between blood drawing and result reporting takes advantage of a special vulnerable period of enhanced susceptibility to education.

Multisession, adult-led classroom presentation is the current standard for HIV education. Presenting educational programs during a single session is not as effective (Bell et al., 1990). Health educators also must improve adolescents' attention by utilizing participants in such activities as role playing, discussions, and personal risk assessments. Videotapes, interactive video programs, and audiotapes augment learning, compared with lecture alone (Rickert, Gottlieb, & Jay, 1990).

Actual physical interaction may lead to confrontations between minors and should be avoided or carefully planned. Many delinquents have learning problems, so materials should contain a minimum of simple reading and a maximum of pictorial content preferably in bright colors (Lane, 1980; McKay & Brumback, 1980; Meltzer et al., 1986; Schuster & Guggenheim, 1982). A catalogue and abstracts of 25 written curricula specifically developed for high-risk youth are provided by Laszlo and Johnson (1990) in *AIDS Education for High-Risk Youth: Assessing the Present, Planning for the Future.*

HIV Education in Los Angeles

In Los Angeles juvenile halls, HIV education takes several forms. The Reproductive Awareness Project consists of four 2-hour sessions, the last of which concerns STDs and HIV infection. An optional fifth session of 1 hour is devoted exclusively to HIV. Project educators feel that education provided in long-term camps allows more flexibility in teaching and follow-up when compared with short-term incarceration settings.

As part of an HIV detection and risk reduction grant, individual sessions of 45 minutes each are presented in the juvenile hall classrooms and long-term camps. After each session, adolescents are offered the opportunity to talk privately with a health educator about HIV issues. Those volunteering for this phase answer a lengthy questionnaire detailing their high-risk behaviors. After pretest counseling, the educator offers HIV testing if appropriate. Posttest counseling also provides an opportunity for education.

A third program makes short videotape programs produced by a team of five to six adolescents who write and act in the video.

Health educators assist in script production, and professional video crews record and edit the program. By advocating behaviors that they might not naturally carry out themselves, the peer educators producing these programs are more likely to change their behavior, when compared with subjects who sit passively absorbing the message (Firpo et al., 1991).

Factors Affecting the Decision to Test Minors for HIV Infection

Many legal and social interests need to be addressed before deciding to test detained juveniles for HIV infection. These must be considered in light of local customs, laws, and attitudes toward HIV infection. Despite these nonmedical concerns, the fact remains that HIV patients benefit from early intervention. A recent report from Baltimore noted that 50% of newly diagnosed HIV patients had CD4 cell counts below 500 and therefore needed treatment with zidovudine (ZVD) (Hutchinson et al., 1991). During the past 2 years in Los Angeles juvenile halls, three out of four newly diagnosed HIV patients had CD4 counts below 500. This fact makes routine testing for medical treatment purposes a very important consideration.

Special Issues for Pre- and Post-HIV-Test Counseling

All incarcerated adolescents should consent to HIV testing only after receiving appropriate pretest counseling. Only five states explicitly allow minors to consent to HIV testing: California, Colorado, Iowa, Michigan, and Washington. All states allow minors to consent to treatment of venereal disease, but most states do not list HIV as a venereal disease. Despite this, North (1990) concluded that sufficient legal authority exists for physicians to test mature, competent adolescents who give permission. In jurisdictions in which the detention health care worker may feel unsure, guidance should be sought from the juvenile court. Posttest counseling is also vital regardless of whether the test result is positive or negative.

Pretest counseling includes the following: (a) assessment of actual risk of HIV infection, based on previous behaviors, (b) discussion of the test and its limits, (c) discussion of the implications of a positive or a negative test result, (d) consideration of legal and financial repercussions, (e) planning for whom the patient would tell about a positive result, and (f) identification of support persons. In the detention setting, the pretest counselor emphasizes the implications of a positive test. The counselor must be sure to inform the adolescent who will be told the results of a positive test. If adverse consequences from a positive test are inevitable, the adolescent should be informed. The institution's policy regarding treatment of HIV disease should be explained carefully so that the adolescent has realistic expectations.

Posttest Counseling

When an adolescent's HIV test result is negative, the posttest counselor places the results in the context of beginning or continuing safe practices. In many cases, a follow-up test will be needed because of recent unsafe behavior. Giving a positive HIV result to a teenager causes psychic distress for both the counselor and the adolescent. It is helpful for the counselor to remember that early HIV identification and treatment will prolong and ultimately may save a life. The same topics are discussed with incarcerated and nonincarcerated juveniles, but special areas are stressed in detention. Dividing the facts to be discussed into specific blocks, described below, that can be discussed all at once or over several days may facilitate understanding (Green & McCreaner, 1989).

In the first block, *AIDS/HIV Block,* discussion immediately after giving a positive HIV test result unfolds as the patient asks questions about the disease. Counselors describe the biology of the disease and emphasize that HIV seropositivity does not necessarily equate to having AIDS. Counselors next provide a general description of medical treatment. Most incarcerated adolescents are medically ignorant and require simple, short explanations of complex facts. They also need repeated explanations about their disease. Sometimes repeated questions over time are hidden requests for reassurance that they will be cared for and not abandoned.

Next, in the *Transmission Block,* transmission is placed in perspective for the seropositive adolescent by discussing his or her
specific sexual and drug-use practices. A complete catalogue of
safe and unsafe behaviors is identified during this dialogue.

In the *Infection Control Block,* both the adolescent's primary
sexual relationship, as well as occasional sexual partners, must be
discussed from the viewpoint of keeping safe. Modifying adolescents' sexual practices has to be fun in order to have compliance.
Many professionals who work with delinquents worry about how
to handle an HIV-positive adolescent who will not take steps to
protect others from infection through sex or intravenous drug use.
Some advocate warning partners without the consent of the infected adolescent. Continuing incarceration of defiant adolescents
also has been suggested. A rational approach to this problem rests
with understanding that "safer sex" is the responsibility of both
partners, not just the HIV-positive person.

Implementation of forced partner notification or incarceration
of an occasional noncompliant HIV-positive adolescent conveys
the message that coercion may be used against any or all infected
youth. High-risk adolescents who perceive others undergoing
adverse consequences after testing HIV-positive are apt to refuse
voluntary testing, thus driving other potentially infected adolescents into hiding. Continued counseling of recalcitrant adolescents regarding moral and legal obligations may result in their
consent to modify risk behaviors associated with viral transmission without the physician having to resort to coercive measures
(Dickens, 1988a, 1988b; Moreno, 1989). As a last resort, exceptions
to confidentiality laws may allow a health care worker to notify
an individual who is at risk from a person known to be HIV-positive
(Dickens, 1988a, 1988b; Gostin, 1990a; Walters, 1988).

Disclosure, or *informing others about their serostatus,* is important
because it focuses on whether the HIV-positive adolescent will
decide to notify the primary sexual partner, occasional partners,
and parents about his or her health condition. After deciding
whom to tell, "how to tell" can be planned. Medical personnel can
arrange a meeting between the patient and his or her parents and,
if possible, between the minor and his or her primary sex part-
ner(s). The health care provider (posttest counselor) may be the
best person to facilitate any meetings between incarcerated adolescents and their families or sexual partners. Under these unusual

circumstances, the authorities may be willing to modify rules concerning visits to the minor.

Notification need not include distant past homosexual partners, but a heterosexual contact who may not be aware of his or her HIV risk should be contacted (Walters, 1988). In detention settings, some officials may need to be told because of policy or law. We try to involve the adolescent in the process. Officials who will be notified of possible HIV-positive adolescents should be warned also about the penalties for disclosing confidential information (Walters, 1988). Incarcerated adolescents should refrain from indiscriminately announcing their serologic status because widespread knowledge can be detrimental to the inmate. Giving the adolescent access to a trusted individual helps prevent inappropriate divulging of HIV status.

Finally the *Keeping Well Block* focuses discussion on general attitudes about health and wellness. Adolescents should avoid certain foods (raw meat, raw fish, raw eggs), smoking, and excess alcohol. They also should avoid exposure to cats, especially stray cats, and cat feces.

Special Considerations
for Pregnant HIV-Positive Adolescents

Pregnant adolescents require extensive counseling. The decision regarding disposition of the pregnancy is based on the usual concerns plus additional complications brought about by the adolescent's positive serostatus. Risk of HIV infection for the fetus is not 100%. During the mid-stages of the mother's illness, the risk is 20-40%. During the time of primary infection, advanced disease, or delivery of a previous HIV-positive baby increases the risk substantially (Van de Perre et al., 1991). The female will need also to consider if she is well enough to care for a baby and to have realistic plans available for her baby if she becomes incapacitated. Regardless of the mother's decision, she will need ongoing support and counseling to deal with worries surrounding the termination or completion of her pregnancy (Green & McCreaner, 1989).

Emotional Response of HIV-Positive Adolescents

The knowledge that they are HIV-positive causes a variety of strong, negative emotions among adolescents. Care providers, especially the primary providers, can predict the range of emotions adolescents may experience. As these feelings—shock, anger, guilt, decreased self-esteem, loss of identity, loss of security, loss of control, fear, sadness—arise, the care providers discuss these feelings by placing them into context, that is, real versus imaginary problems. Methods of coping with the feelings can be explored. Even after a satisfactory adjustment, an adolescent may relapse and require renewed help. The provision of mental health services should be available before beginning a testing program.

Ethical, Legal, and Financial Considerations When Providing Primary Care for HIV-Positive Incarcerated Adolescents

Treatment of HIV disease must meet community standards. Physicians involved in detention medicine have a duty to maintain expertise in HIV infection or to develop an appropriate referral plan for HIV-positive adolescents (Emanuel, 1988; Gostin, 1990a, 1990b). In many cases, responsibilities for care will be shared between an HIV specialist and the detention facility's primary care physician. Inclusion of a medical center-based specialist for HIV consultation allows utilization of the center's ancillary services, such as social work, psychiatry, support groups, and other medical specialists. Regardless of where medical care is rendered, it should approximate the level of care provided to the general population. In many cases, therapy for drug and alcohol abuse will be an important adjunctive therapy (Mangos et al., 1990) in order for adolescents suffering from addictions to function safely outside the detention setting. The courts have ruled that institutions should have policies in place regarding confidentiality, personnel training, infection control, and availability of appropriate equipment (Gostin, 1990b).

Treating HIV-infected adolescents is expensive. It is much less expensive to treat early HIV infection, however, than symptomatic AIDS. In financial terms, it is in the institution's interest to initiate treatment earlier to prevent disease progression, which requires a more costly level of care (Arno, Shenson, Siegel, Franks, & Lee, 1989).

The specifics of treatment change rapidly as more data accumulate. Among the many review articles, textbooks, and monographs available, *The AIDS Knowledge Base* can be recommended for its current and concise description of diagnosis and treatment of HIV disease and its complications (Cohen, Sande, & Volberding, 1990).

Housing of seropositive adolescents may be determined by institutional policy or by their medical needs. A sick or frequently medicated adolescent probably will be housed in the infirmary. Whenever possible, adolescents should continue to participate in such institutional activities as school and recreation. Limitation of activities should be based on the rational application of the Centers for Disease Control guidelines regarding risk of HIV transmission or on the patient's physical fitness.

The incarcerated HIV-positive adolescent has many nonmedical personnel involved in his or her management: defense lawyers, probation officers, prosecutors, judges, and institutional staff. The attitudes of each of these personnel toward HIV-infected individuals will affect each person's response to the adolescent and ultimately may significantly modify the judicial outcome, that is, length and type of sentence. For example, on the one hand, the probation system may prefer not to have HIV-infected adolescents in its institutions, thus leading to commutation of their sentences and early release. On the other hand, the judge or "system" may feel that HIV-infected adolescents are a risk to society and should be detained to protect society. Inadvertent disclosure of a detainee's HIV status therefore must be carefully avoided.

Summary

Delinquent youth constitute a numerically small but important segment of the adolescent population when considering the spread of HIV infection in the United States. These adolescents engage in a broad spectrum of HIV-related risk behaviors with high frequency and with numerous partners. Although they can be difficult to reach with prevention messages, the fact that they are incarcerated does provide an opportunity to access even these youth. With so much at stake, increased efforts must be made to develop effective prevention programs and to construct reliable instruments for evaluating the outcome of these programs. Moreover, detention facilities need to adopt procedures and protocols for the provision of medical care and social support services to

HIV-infected adolescents before they are needed rather than to confront a crisis situation when an HIV-infected youth is identified in the facility.

References

Alexander-Rodriguez, T., & Vermund, S. H. (1987). Gonorrhea and syphilis in incarcerated urban adolescents: Prevalence and physical signs. *Pediatrics, 80,* 561-564.

Allen-Hagen, B. (1991). Public juvenile facilities: Children in custody 1989. *Juvenile Justice Bulletin.* Washington, DC: U.S. Department of Justice, Office of Juvenile Justice and Delinquency Prevention.

Arno, P. S., Shenson, D., Siegel, N. F., Franks, P., & Lee, P. R. (1989). Economic and policy implications of early intervention in HIV disease. *Journal of the American Medical Association, 262,* 1493-1498.

Baker, C., Morris, R., Huscroft, S., Re, O., Zeljkovic, S., & Essex, A. (1991). Survey of sexual behaviors as HIV risk factors in incarcerated minors. *VII International Conference on AIDS, 1,* 414. (Abstract No. M.D. 4098)

Becker, M. H., & Joseph, J. G. (1988). AIDS and behavioral change to reduce risk: A review. *American Journal of Public Health, 78,* 394-410.

Bell, R. A., Feldmann, T. B., Grissom, S., Purifoy, F. E., Stephenson, J. J., Deines, H., Frierson, R., Gould, A., Hunt, L., & Hyde, J. (1990). Evaluating the outcomes of AIDS education. *AIDS Education and Prevention, 2,* 70-83.

Bell, T. A., Farrow, J. A., Stamm, W. E., Critchlow, C. W., & Holmes, K. K. (1985). Sexually transmitted diseases in females in a juvenile detention center. *Sexually Transmitted Diseases, 12,* 140-144.

Brady, M., Baker, C., & Neinstein, L. S. (1988). Asymptomatic *Chlamydia trachomatis* infections in teenage males. *Journal of Adolescent Health Care, 9,* 72-75.

Brown, L. K., & Fritz, G. K. (1988). AIDS education in the schools: A literature review as a guide for curriculum planning. *Clinical Pediatrics, 27,* 311-316.

Cohen, P. T., Sande, M. A., & Volberding, P. A. (Eds.). (1990). *The AIDS knowledge base.* Waltham, MA: Medical Publishing Group.

Conger, J. J. (1977). *Adolescence and youth: Psychological development in a changing world* (2nd ed.). New York: Harper & Row.

Council on Scientific Affairs. (1990). Health status of detained and incarcerated youths. *Journal of the American Medical Association, 263,* 987-991.

Dickens, B. M. (1988a). Legal rights and duties in the AIDS epidemic. *Science, 239,* 580-586.

Dickens, B. M. (1988b). Legal limits of AIDS confidentiality. *Journal of the American Medical Association, 259,* 3449-3451.

DiClemente, R. J., Lanier, M. M., Horan, P. F., & Lodico, M. (1991). Comparison of AIDS knowledge, attitudes and behaviors among adolescents in a juvenile detention facility and public schools in San Francisco. *American Journal of Public Health, 81,* 628-630.

Edwards, L., Steinman, M., & Hakanson, E. (1980). Adolescent pregnancy prevention services in high school clinics. *Family Planning Perspectives, 12,* 6-14.

Emanuel, E. J. (1988). Do physicians have an obligation to treat patients with AIDS? *New England Journal of Medicine, 318,* 1686-1690.

Farrow, J. (1984). Medical responsibility to incarcerated children. *Clinical Pediatrics, 23,* 699-700.

Firpo, R., Dugan, P., Roseman, J., Zeljkovic, S., Re, O., & Baker, C. J. (1991). AIDS education video project for incarcerated adolescents. *VII International Conference on AIDS, 2,* 451. (Abstract No. W.D. 4255)

Fullilove, R. E., Fullilove, M. T., Bowser, B., & Gross, S. (1990). Crack users: The new AIDS risk group? *Cancer Detection and Prevention, 14,* 363-368.

Gostin, L. O. (1990a). The AIDS litigation project: A national review of court and human rights commission decisions, Part I: The social impact of AIDS. *Journal of the American Medical Association, 263,* 1961-1974.

Gostin, L. O. (1990b). The AIDS litigation project: A national review of court and human rights commission decisions, Part II: Discrimination. *Journal of the American Medical Association, 263,* 2086-2093.

Green, J., & McCreaner, A. (1989). Post-test counselling. In *Counselling in HIV Infection and AIDS* (pp. 28-68). London: Blackwell.

Huscroft, S., Morris, R., Re, O., Baker, C. J., Aquino, K., & Roseman J. (1990). Survey of sexual behavior risk factors for HIV infection in incarcerated adolescents. *VII International Conference on AIDS, 2,* 436, 3016 (Abstract No. W.D. 4194).

Hutchinson, C. M., Wilson, C., Reichart, C. A., Marsiglia, V. C., Zenilman, J. M., & Hook III, E. W. (1991). CD4 lymphocyte concentrations in patients with newly identified HIV infection attending STD clinics. *Journal of the American Medical Association, 266,* 253-256.

Kirby, D. (1984). *Sexuality education; An evaluation of programs and their effects* (pp. 362-384). Santa Cruz, CA: Network Publications.

Lane, B. A. (1980). The relationship of learning disabilities to juvenile delinquency: Current status. *Journal of Learning Disabilities, 13,* 20-29.

Lanier, M. M., DiClemente, R. J., & Horan, P. F. (1991). HIV knowledge and behaviors in incarcerated youth: A comparison of high and low risk locales. *Journal of Criminal Justice, 19,* 257-262.

Laszlo, A. T., & Johnson, J. (Eds.). (1990). *AIDS education for high-risk youth: Assessing the present, planning for the future.* McLean, VA: The Circle, Inc.

Leyser, Y., & Abrams, P. D. (1982). Teacher attitudes toward normal and exceptional groups. *Journal of Psychology, 110,* 227-238.

Mangos, J. A., Doran, T., Aranda-Naranjo, B., Rodriguez-Escobar, Y., Scott, A., Setzer, J. R., Sherman, J. O., & Kossman, S. P. (1990). Pediatric AIDS: Adolescence, delinquency, drug abuse, and AIDS. *Texas Medicine, 86,* 100-103.

McKay, S., & Brumback, R. A. (1980). Relationship between learning disabilities and juvenile delinquency. *Perceptual and Motor Skills, 51,* 1223-1226.

Meltzer, L. J., Roditi, B. N., & Fenton, T. (1986). Cognitive and learning profiles of delinquent and learning-disabled adolescents. *Adolescence, 21,* 581-591.

Moreno, J. D. (1989). Treating the adolescent patient. *Journal of Adolescent Health Care, 10,* 454-459.

Morris, R., Baker, C., Huscroft, S., Evans, C. A., & Zeljkovic, S. (1991). Two year variation in HIV risk behaviors in detained minors. *VII International Conference on AIDS, 2,* 51. (Abstract No. W.D. 109)

Nader, P. R., Wexler, D. B., Patterson, T. L., McKusick, L., & Coates, T. (1989). Comparison of beliefs about AIDS among urban, suburban, incarcerated, and gay adolescents. *Journal of Adolescent Health Care, 10,* 413-418.

North, R. L. (1990). Legal authority for HIV testing of adolescents. *Journal of Adolescent Health Care, 11,* 176-187.

Rickert, V. I., Gottlieb, A., & Jay, M. S. (1990). A comparison of three clinic-based AIDS education programs on female adolescents' knowledge, attitudes, and behavior. *Journal of Adolescent Health Care, 11,* 298-303.

Rickert, V. I., Jay, M. S., & Gottlieb, A. (1991). Effects of a peer-counseled AIDS education program on knowledge, attitudes, and satisfaction of adolescents. *Journal of Adolescent Health Care, 12,* 38-43.

Rolf, J., Nanda, J., Thompson, L., Mamon, J., Chandra, A., Baldwin, J., & Delahunt, M. (1989). Issues in AIDS prevention among juvenile offenders. In J. O. Woodruff, D. Doherty, & J. G. Athey (Eds.), *Troubled adolescents and HIV infection: Issues in prevention and treatment* (pp. 56-69). Washington, DC: Georgetown University Child Development Center.

Rotheram-Borus, M. J., Koopman, C., Haignere, C., & Davies, M. (1991). Reducing HIV sexual risk behavior among runaway adolescents. *Journal of the American Medical Association, 266,* 1237-1241.

Schinke, S., Gilchrist, L., Snow, W., & Schilling, R. (1985). Skills-building methods to prevent smoking in adolescents. *Journal of Adolescent Health Care, 6,* 439-444.

Schuster, R., & Guggenheim, P. D. (1982). An investigation of the intellectual capabilities of juvenile offenders. *Journal of Forensic Sciences, 27,* 393-400.

Tucker, V. L., & Cho, C. T. (1991). AIDS and adolescents. How can you help them reduce their risk? *Postgraduate Medicine, 89,* 49-53.

Van de Perre, P., Simonon, A., & Msellati, P., et al. (1991). Postnatal transmission of human immunodeficiency virus type 1 from mother to infant. *New England Journal of Medicine, 325,* 593-598.

Walters, L. (1988). Ethical issues in the prevention and treatment of HIV infection and AIDS. *Science, 239,* 597-603.

Zeljkovic, S., Huscroft, S., Baker, C. J., Re, O., Morris, R., & Aquino, K. (1991). Survey of drug abuse behavior as HIV risk factors in incarcerated adolescents. *VII International Conference on AIDS, 2,* 436. (Abstract No. W.D. 4194)

5

HIV Infection and Disease
Among Homeless Adolescents

DIANE L. SONDHEIMER

Introduction

As the United States enters the second decade of the AIDS epidemic, concern about the spread of HIV infection to adolescents between ages 13-21 is growing. The threat of HIV infection is not uniform, however, among adolescents (Vermund, Hein, Gayle, Cary, & Thomas, 1989). One adolescent population at an increased risk of HIV infection is homeless youth. Given their residential instability, dysfunctional family history, urban geographic locality, perceived and real survival choices, and subsequent deterioration in physical and mental health, it is plausible that they may be at the greatest risk, not only for HIV infection but also for a more rapid progression from HIV to AIDS than their nonhomeless counterparts.

This chapter examines the societal, familial, and individual factors that place homeless adolescents at an unusually high degree of risk for acquiring HIV and presents the types of prevention and intervention strategies that may be the most effective in successfully meeting the unique service requirements of this population.

Operational Definition of Homelessness

A broad range of categories and terminologies is used to describe this population of homeless adolescents (e.g., runaway, throwaway, street youth, system kids) (Athey, 1991; Pennbridge, Yates, David, & MacKenzie, 1990). Because no consensus definition has been produced and because youth may move in and out of the various categories over time, the term *homeless adolescent* will be used in this chapter to include adolescents who have voluntarily or involuntarily left their living situations (e.g., traditional home, foster care, residential setting) and who spend a portion of time living either in a formal or informal shelter or on the streets either with regular, irregular, or no family contact. Adolescents are more likely to refer to themselves as *homeless*, even those who are legally defined runaways, as they believe they have no viable living situation to return to (Caton, 1986). Although problems of dimension and definition continue to plague those who study and serve homeless youth, this population is diverse, continues to increase in size, and is generally distrustful of any attempts at intervention.

Scope of Homelessness

Homelessness among youth in the United States is a problem of substantial proportion and complexity. Although the full extent of homelessness among adolescents has not been documented by use of large-scale epidemiologic studies, it is estimated that some 500,000 to 1.5 million adolescents between ages 11-18 fall into this fast-growing and understudied subpopulation of youth (Council on Scientific Affairs, 1989; Finkelhor, Hotaling, & Sedlak, 1990; Institute of Medicine, 1989; Robertson, 1990). Estimates of the number of youth permanently residing on the streets fall between 100,000-200,000, with as many as 1-2 million running away from home each year (General Accounting Office, 1990, Figures cited from the National Network of Runaway and Homeless Youth Services). Furthermore, 12 cities surveyed by the U.S. Conference of Mayors (1987) reported that approximately 4% of their homeless were composed of unaccompanied adolescents, and 9 of those cities reported increasing numbers over time. This wide variation in prevalence estimates is but one indicator of the lack of reliable information and terminology used to describe this population. In addition, most of these studies fail to include at least two groups: older homeless adolescents (ages 18-24) who are in transition from the child to the adult system, and those street youth who rarely come into contact with programs.

Demographic Characteristics

Numerous studies have been conducted over the last 5 years that attempt to document the characteristics of homeless youth (General Accounting Office, 1989; Shaffer & Caton, 1984; Shalwitz, Goulart, Dunnigan, & Flannery, 1990; Yates, MacKenzie, Pennbridge, & Cohen, 1988). Although no one study has yielded results that are generalizable to all homeless adolescents, it appears that most of these youth come from backgrounds characterized by severe emotional negligence and physical and/or sexual abuse (Adams, Gullotta, & Clancy, 1985; Chelimsky, 1982; Gullotta, 1978). Homeless youth sampled from the East and West coasts differed in ethnic makeup, socioeconomic status, and sexual preference. For example, homeless youth from New York City were primarily black and Hispanic and from lower socioeconomic backgrounds, while youth studied in San Francisco and Los Angeles were predominantly white (56-71%) and more likely to include gay male adolescents. In general, the ethnic distribution of homeless youth typically parallels the ethnic patterns of their local geographic community (Council of Community Services, 1984). Overrepresentation of whites in surveys of runaways, however, may support the idea that cultural and racial differences exist. For example, the extended black family may mediate during parent-adolescent conflicts and may at least partially explain the relatively low proportion of blacks in the runaway sample studied by Yates and colleagues (1988). Family roles also may differ among ethnic groups. Perhaps the "mundane extreme environmental stress" described by Peters and Massey (1983) may increase black family cohesiveness. Clearly, differing ethnic patterns among homeless youth require further study as multicultural and immigrant youth continue to represent a growing proportion of the overall adolescent population, particularly in large urban centers (Wetzel, 1987).

Factors Contributing to Homelessness

Just as the exact number of homeless adolescents remains undetermined, the relative contribution or interaction of various factors leading to adolescent homelessness has not been defined adequately. While family conflict and dysfunction appear to be the crux of the problem, more global conditions such as increasing levels of poverty and lack of adequate health care, education, housing, and employment may exacerbate the process (Bassuk & Rubin, 1987). Moreover, given the increasing alienation and marginality of youth in our society, one can better understand the increase in homelessness (Johnson & Carter, 1980; Nightingale & Wolverton, 1988; Schiamberg, 1986). Residential instability among adolescents in foster care, in the juvenile justice system, and in psychiatric hospitals, for example, along with concomitant serious emotional, behavioral, and mental disorders and coexisting drug and alcohol abuse, often contributes to our homeless population. To a large extent, homelessness among adolescents represents a failure of our systems of care to properly integrate and coordinate services (Stroul & Friedman, 1986). For these adolescents, the streets are often their only alternative to inadequate and often inappropriate settings. Failure of our systems of care becomes even more apparent with consistent findings of prior multiple placements in adolescents seeking emergency shelter (Mundy, Robertson, Greenblatt, & Robertson, 1989; Rotheram-Borus, 1991; Rotheram-Borus, Koopman, & Erhardt, 1991). In addition, emotional distress and psychiatric problems, for example, suicide attempts and depression, are more prevalent among homeless adolescents relative to the general adolescent population (Robertson, Koegel, Mundy, Greenblatt, & Robertson, 1988). Consequently the mental and emotional status of these youth contributes to greater participation in high-risk behaviors and may act as a barrier impeding receptivity to HIV-prevention messages and the adopting and maintaining of health-promoting behaviors (State of Washington Department of Health, 1989).

Prevalence of Risk Behaviors

Homelessness among adolescents presents multiple concerns for society. The same behaviors that increase an adolescent's likelihood of survival on the streets contribute to increased risk of HIV infection. Exposure to prostitution (Deisher, Robinson, & Boyer, 1982), pornography, and other illegal means of economic survival, along with increased abuse of alcohol and drugs, makes the risk for HIV infection pronounced in this population (Rahdert, 1988; Stein, Jones, & Fisher, 1988).

The sexual and drug and alcohol-related behavioral profiles of homeless adolescents are disturbing and demonstrate convincing evidence of risk for HIV. Contrary to popular belief, medical histories of homeless adolescents, particularly those surveyed on the East Coast, point to sexual activity with multiple partners as the predominant mode of transmission rather than injection drug use. Drug use, particularly crack, is a key cause for concern because it provides an impetus for engaging in prostitution and having multiple sex partners. Moreover, surveys of homeless adolescent males reveal that more than 50% have had greater than 10 sexual partners, compared with 7% in surveys of nonhomeless adolescents (Rotheram-Borus, Koopman, & Erhardt, 1991). Again, these data, while not representative of adolescents in general, may be applicable to the substantial number of homeless and runaway youth in this country whose environment includes frequent exposure to HIV through high-risk sexual activity and drugs (Fullilove, Fullilove, Bowser, & Gross, 1990; Stricof, Novick, Kennedy, & Weisfuse, 1988). Reporting of high prevalence of IV drug use in this population has been demonstrated primarily in cities on the West Coast (Hudson, Petty, Freeman, Holly, & Hula, 1989).

Sexual activity among homeless adolescents, especially females, is not always consensual. The rate of sexual abuse against homeless women is 20 times the rate among women in general. Moreover, about 50% of all rape victims are younger than 18 years of age (Kelly, 1985; Neinstein & Stewart, 1984). Rape among boys, although not well documented in the literature, is not uncommon among homeless adolescents (Able-Peterson, 1989).

Even when sex is consensual, the use of condoms and other forms of contraception is rare, leading to high rates of pregnancy and sexually transmitted diseases that may facilitate HIV infection in a female and her unborn child (Rotheram-Borus & Koopman, 1991b). Early initiation of sexual activity among homeless adolescents is common, with the average age at sexual debut being approximately 12.5 years. Early sexual initiation further increases the likelihood of health-threatening sequelae (Rotheram-Borus, Koopman, & Bradley, 1990).

More than half of all homeless adolescent girls become pregnant while on the streets (Deisher, Farrow, Hope, & Litchfield, 1989). Anonymous seroprevalence studies of babies born in New York City demonstrate that, of those who tested HIV-positive, a significant portion of the birth mothers were under the age of 21 (Novick et al., 1989a, 1989b). The prevalence of anal intercourse, occurring not only among gay youth but also among heterosexual adolescents with greater frequency, is yet another alarming finding among homeless adolescents (Jaffe, Seehaus, Wagner, & Leadbeater, 1988; Remafedi, 1987). It is estimated that half of the 10,000 homeless adolescents in New York City are engaged in homosexual behavior, and many of them exchange sex for money (Gross, 1987). Furthermore, gay adolescents are likely to engage in sexual activity with older gay males, a group that comprises the highest percentage of seropositivity in the United States.

Other factors, such as time living in street environment, number of runaway episodes, age, gender, and mental and emotional state, also contribute to HIV-risk status.

HIV Infection and Disease

Although the prevalence of HIV infection among homeless adolescents is unknown, it has been suggested that the rate of seropositivity in this population may be as much as 2 to 10 times higher than the rates reported for other samples of adolescents in the United States and that the risk for infection increases with age, especially for males (Stricof, Novick, & Kennedy, 1990). A recent HIV seroprevalence survey among homeless adolescents in a large city on the East Coast found that of 2,667 anonymous blood specimens collected over a 26-month period, more than 5% were antibody-positive. The prevalence rate increased to 8.6% in older adolescents. Another study of runaway and homeless adolescents frequenting shelters in several states reports that at the very least, 4% of homeless youth are infected already (Stricof, Kennedy, Natell, Weisfuse, & Novick, 1991; Stricof et al., 1990). Extrapolating these findings to the United States population of homeless youth, an estimated 60,000 may be infected with HIV.

These figures, although gathered from adolescents who presented to emergency shelters, probably grossly underestimate the actual dimensions of HIV/AIDS in this group. Because youth living on the street often receive inadequate medical care, they may be missed in case reporting. Furthermore, many may die of other causes such as accidents, homicide, or suicide, which are the leading causes of death in this age group.

Anecdotal reports from programs serving HIV-positive homeless and runaway youth document cases of rapid progression (2-3 years) from infection to death (K. Hein, personal communication, 1990). Such life stressors as social and familial alienation, especially pronounced in homeless adolescents, are often associated with the progression of HIV-related disease in adults (Holland & Tross, 1985; Martin, 1988). It is unknown, however, whether these events contribute to disease progression among adolescents. The role of other environmental or individual cofactors or the influence of endocrine or age-specific immunologic factors on the progression of disease in adolescents is unknown at this time. It is plausible that, because differences in the latency period, mean survival time, type of HIV-related illnesses, and transmission categories exist between children and adults, adolescents in general, and different subpopulations in particular, may also have a disease course that is distinct from that of other age groups.

Lack of Access to Health Care

A recurrent theme at the Surgeon General's Workshop on Children With HIV and Their Families was the inadequacy of generic programs in meeting the needs of high-risk and HIV-infected youth, specifically in services tailored to the needs of such subpopulations as minority, gay/bisexual, and homeless and runaway youth. For these individuals, health care typically is fragmented, crisis oriented, and underfinanced. For the majority of HIV-infected teenagers, few special treatment programs exist, and those that do may not be affiliated with existing research protocols that would assist in defraying the cost of treatment of the patient. Those funded programs that are geographically available to patients may be unequipped to deal with the special psychosocial needs of adolescents. Furthermore, HIV-infected youth who are also ill and in need of treatment but cannot afford it often lack the skills necessary to negotiate the health care system on their own behalf for adequate results. Therefore viable solutions to barriers to access to care, especially for disenfranchised youth, require immediate attention on local, state, and federal levels.

Strategies for Primary and Secondary Prevention

The pathology associated with the life-styles of homeless adolescents is a compelling argument for the rapid development and implementation of appropriate prevention and intervention programs to attempt to meet their special needs both before and after they become HIV-positive.

Clearly, traditional service programs are not equipped to meet the multiple and complex needs of homeless youth. In fact, most programs will not even accept them for care due to lack of resources or an accompanying adult parent or guardian. Furthermore, engaging street youth, most of whom develop a general mistrust of adults, has been extremely difficult, and those who do seek treatment in traditional institutions return rarely for follow-up.

Thus no simple strategy exists for transferring to younger adolescents the behavior change strategies that worked so well with adult gay males. This lack is largely due to the fact that, unlike their adult male counterparts who had friends and partners who were ill and dying, adolescents often remain symptom-free for long periods of time and are unlikely to be concerned about developing AIDS 5-10 years in the future. A homeless adolescent is more concerned about where he or she will sleep that night or where the next meal might come from and therefore is less likely to worry about safe sexual or drug behavior (Rotheram-Borus & Koopman, 1991a).

While short-term HIV-prevention programs increase knowledge about HIV and tend to promote positive attitudes toward responsible drug-related and sexual behavior, subsequent behavior change has not paralleled these cognitive changes among adolescents (DiClemente, 1990; Kipke, Boyer, & Hein, 1989; Miller & Lin, 1988). Homeless adolescents, while as knowledgeable about HIV prevention as their nonhomeless peers, have not demonstrated significant reductions in risk behaviors. Thus as in other adolescent subpopulations, knowledge about HIV is not sufficient to maintain safe behaviors (Des Jarlais & Friedman, 1988; Hudson et al., 1989; Rotheram-Borus & Koopman, 1991b).

While primarily knowledge-based HIV-prevention programs alone may not motivate the adoption of HIV-preventive behaviors, findings from one recent nonrandomized control study are encouraging (Rotheram-Borus, Koopman, Haignere, & Davies, 1991). In this program, homeless adolescents in New York City were exposed to an HIV-prevention program that not only provided instruction in basic knowledge about HIV/AIDS but, more importantly, emphasized coping skills, access to health care, and individual barriers to safer sex. Results at two follow-up time points—3 and 6 months after participation in the intervention—demonstrate significant differences between adolescents in the intervention as compared with their peers in the control condition. As the number of intervention sessions increased, adolescents exposed to the intervention program were more likely to increase their consistent use of condoms ($p<.05$) and to decrease high-risk sexual behaviors ($p<.05$). While the effect sizes attributable to the intervention program are not large, the findings clearly demonstrate that well-integrated and carefully implemented intervention programs can produce health-promoting behavioral changes among this population.

Based on the unique experiences of this population, effective programs seem to be more intensive and specifically targeted to the multisystem needs of homeless youth in a coordinated fashion. For example, if housing needs are not met, it is unlikely that other related efforts will be effective. Furthermore, successful interventions with high-risk, hard-to-access populations are often delivered by nontraditional street outreach workers (Froner & Rowniak, 1989; Watters et al., 1990). The needs of homeless adolescents will continue to go unmet unless traditional systems and alternative care providers join forces to create a stable, comprehensive system of care (Pires & Silber, 1991).

Adolescents who are already HIV-positive should benefit by knowledge of their HIV status. Reports show that young people frequently are requesting testing and that young mothers are having their babies tested for the HIV antibody (Athey, 1990). This is especially crucial with homeless adolescents who may have a shorter latency period in which to seek appropriate medical intervention, such as zidovudine (ZVD), dideoxyinosine (DDI), and other therapies for HIV-related illnesses. If adolescents do not have access to appropriate medical and psychological treatment, including federally funded clinical trial protocols, or are denied adequate housing due to their positive HIV status, they have no incentive to be tested.

The most successful models for treating HIV-positive adolescents are characterized by a community-based, multisystem approach and are accessible and culturally and developmentally appropriate (e.g., Montefiore Medical Center, New York; Children's Hospital, Los Angeles; University of Washington, Seattle). Other examples of community-based programs for homeless and other youth which incorporate AIDS education and counseling into the array of services they offer are Bridge Over Troubled Waters, Boston; Neon Street Center for Youth, Chicago; YouthCare, Seattle; and Youth Development, Inc., Albuquerque. These effective service delivery models are scarce, however, and must be replicated and disseminated on a national level in order to reach the growing numbers of youth who desperately need them.

Summary

Homeless adolescents represent a small but growing segment of the adolescent population. Because they lack safe and secure living environments, educational and job opportunities, appropriate adult role models, access to health care, and are exposed to a high prevalence of sexual activity and substance abuse, they are at extremely high risk for acquiring HIV and for experiencing early illness and death. Until appropriate prevention and intervention models are developed and disseminated, the problem will grow, and many otherwise promising lives will be needlessly destroyed.

Homeless youth present an array of needs that pose significant challenges to service providers and service systems. Recognizing homeless adolescents as a distinct group with special developmental needs and tailoring interventions to fit their needs are critical first steps in addressing the problem. Also knowing that homeless adolescents who are HIV-positive may not have the luxury of time that healthier groups of adolescents seem to have may help add the needed sense of urgency that currently appears to be lacking in society.

The response to the HIV epidemic in adolescents by all facets of society has not been as vigorous as it has been with children and adults with respect to the provision of adequate services and access to national clinical trial protocols, natural history studies, behavioral intervention studies, and seroprevalence surveys. In each of these areas, adults and younger children were targeted first, with adolescents only recently receiving marginal attention. This delay may be attributed to at least four important factors.

1. Adolescents frequently are grouped with younger children or adults in both statistical reporting and in clinical care settings; therefore, the distinct characteristics of this group are often obscured.

2. Adolescents are difficult research subjects for entry into virtually any type of study, and because they are hard to both access and retain, they often are excluded from research protocols altogether.

3. Given the unique legal and ethical barriers that arise in attempting to both provide care for and conduct research involving adolescents, investigators are often reluctant to study them as well.

4. Adolescents in the United States do not currently represent an age group with high morbidity and mortality attributable to HIV disease. Many young adults ages 20-29 years, however, who currently comprise 20% of all reported AIDS cases, were infected as adolescents. Consequently, without immediate and appropriate prevention and intervention strategies, prevalence of HIV among high-risk adolescent subpopulations is likely to increase rapidly (Hein, 1989).

References

Able-Peterson, T. (1989, October). *The most forgotten adolescents.* Paper presented at a conference on treatment of adolescents with alcohol, drug abuse, and mental health problems, Alexandria, VA.

Adams, G. R., Gullotta, T., & Clancy, M. A. (1985). Homeless adolescents: A descriptive study of similarities and differences between runaways and throwaways. *Adolescence, 20,* 715-724.

Athey, J. G. (1990). *Pregnancy and childbearing among homeless adolescents: A report of a workshop.* Pittsburgh: University of Pittsburgh.

Athey, J. G. (1991). HIV infection and homeless adolescents. *Child Welfare League of America, 70*(5), 517-528.

Bassuk, E., & Rubin, L. (1987). Homeless children, a neglected population. *American Journal of Orthopsychiatry, 57,* 279-286.

Caton, C. L. M. (1986). The homeless experience in adolescent years. In E. L. Bassuk (Ed.), *The mental health needs of homeless persons* (pp. 63-70). San Francisco: Jossey-Bass.

Chelimsky, E. (1982). *The problem of runaway and homeless youth.* Oversight hearing on runaway and homeless youth program, United States House of Representatives, Subcommittee on Human Resources, Committee on Education and Labor, Washington, DC.

Council of Community Services. (1984). Homeless older adolescents (16 to 21-year-olds): Needs in Albany County, Albany, New York. Albany, NY: Council of Community Services of Northeastern New York.

Council on Scientific Affairs. (1989). Health care needs of homeless and runaway youths. *Journal of the American Medical Association, 262,* 1358-1361.

Deisher, R. W., Farrow, J. A., Hope, K., & Litchfield, C. (1989). The pregnant adolescent prostitute. *American Journal of Diseases of Children, 143,* 1162-1165.

Deisher, R. W., Robinson, G., & Boyer, D. (1982). The adolescent female and male prostitute. *Pediatric Annals, 11*(4), 812-825.

Des Jarlais, D. C., & Friedman, S. R. (1988). The psychology of preventing AIDS among intravenous drug users: A social learning conceptualization. *American Psychologist, 43,* 865-870.

DiClemente, R. J. (1990). Adolescents and AIDS: Current research, prevention strategies and public policy. In L. Temoshok & A. Baum (Eds.), *Psychosocial perspectives on AIDS: Etiology, prevention, and treatment* (pp. 51-64). Hillsdale, NJ: Lawrence Erlbaum.

Finkelhor, D., Hotaling, G., & Sedlak, A. (1990). *Missing, abducted, runaway and throwaway children in America.* Washington, DC: U.S. Department of Justice.

Froner, G., & Rowniak, S. (1989). The health outreach team: Taking AIDS education on the streets. *AIDS Education and Prevention, 1,* 105-118.

Fullilove, R. E., Fullilove, M. T., Bowser, B. P., & Gross, S. A. (1990). Risk of sexually transmitted disease among black adolescent crack users in Oakland and San Francisco, CA. *Journal of the American Medical Association, 263,* 851-855.

General Accounting Office. (1989). *Homelessness: Homeless and runaway youth receiving services at federally funded shelters.* Washington, DC: Author.

General Accounting Office. (1990, May). *AIDS education: Programs for out-of-school youth slowly evolving* (HRD-90-111, p. 2). Washington, DC: Author.

Gross, J. (1987). AIDS threat brings new turmoil for gay teen-agers, *New York Times,* p. B1.

Gullotta, T. P. (1978). Runaway: Reality or myth? *Adolescence, 13,* 543-549.

Hein, K. (1989). AIDS in adolescence: Exploring the challenge. *Journal of Adolescent Health Care, 10,* 10S-35S.

Holland, J., & Tross, S. (1985). The psychosocial and neuropsychiatric sequelae of the acquired immunodeficiency syndrome and related disorders. *Annals of Internal Medicine, 103,* 760-764.

Hudson, R. A., Petty, B. A., Freeman, A. C., Holly, C. E., & Hula, M. A. (1989, June). *Adolescent runaways' behavioral risk factors, knowledge about AIDS and attitudes about condom usage.* Paper presented at V International Conference on AIDS, Montreal, Canada.

Institute of Medicine. (1989). *Research on children and adolescents with mental, behavioral and developmental disorders.* Washington, DC: National Academy Press.

Jaffe, L. R., Seehaus, M., Wagner, C., & Leadbeater, B. J. (1988). Anal intercourse and knowledge of acquired immunodeficiency syndrome among minority-group female adolescents. *Journal of Pediatrics, 112,* 1005-1007.

Johnson, R., & Carter, M. M. (1980). Flight of the young: Why children run away from their homes. *Adolescence, 15,* 483-489.

Kelly, J. T. (1985). Trauma: With the example of San Francisco's shelter programs. In P. W. Brickner, L. K. Scharer, B. Conanan et al. (Eds.), *Health care of homeless people* (pp. 77-92). New York: Springer.

Kipke, M., Boyer, C., & Hein, K. (1989, June). *An evaluation of an AIDS risk reduction education and skills training program (ARREST) for adolescents.* Paper presented at V International Conference on AIDS, Montreal, Canada.

Martin, J. (1988). Psychological consequences of AIDS-related bereavement among gay men. *Journal of Consulting Clinical Psychology, 56,* 856-862.

Miller, D., & Lin E. (1988). Children in sheltered homeless families: Reported health status and use of health services. *Pediatrics, 81,* 668-673.

Mundy, P., Robertson, J., Greenblatt, M., & Robertson, M. (1989). Residential instability in adolescent inpatients. *Journal of the American Academy of Child and Adolescent Psychiatry, 28,* 176-181.

Neinstein, L. S., & Stewart, D. C. (1984). *Adolescent health care: A practical guide.* Baltimore: Urban and Schwartzenberg.

Nightingale, E. O., & Wolverton. L. (1988). *Adolescent rolessness in modern society.* New York: Carnegie Corporation of New York.

Novick, L. F., Glebatis, D., Stricof, R., & Berns, D. (1989, June). *HIV infection in adolescent childbearing women* (meeting abstract). V International Conference on AIDS, Montreal, Canada.

Novick, L. F., Berns, D., Stricof, R., Stevens, R. et al. (1989). HIV seroprevalence in newborns in New York State. *Journal of the American Medical Association, 261,* 1745-1750.

Pennbridge, J. N., Yates, G. L., David, T. G., & MacKenzie, R. G. (1990). Runaway and homeless youth in Los Angeles County, California. *Journal of Adolescent Health, 11,* 159-165.

Peters, M. F., & Massey, G. (1983). Mundane extreme environmental stress: The case of black families in white America. *Marriage and Family Review, 6,* 193-218.

Pires, S. A., & Silber, J. T. (1991). *On their own: Runaway and homeless youth and programs that serve them.* Washington, DC: Georgetown University Child Development Center.

Rahdert, E. R. (1988). Treatment services for adolescent drug abuse: Analysis of treatment research. In E. R. Rahdert & J. Grabowski (Eds.), *National Institute on Drug Abuse Monograph #77* (pp. 1-3). Rockville, MD: National Institute on Drug Abuse.

Remafedi, G. (1987). Adolescent homosexuality: Psychosocial and medical implications. *Pediatrics, 79*, 331-337.

Robertson, M. J. (1990). Homeless youth: An overview of the recent literature.
Homeless children and youth. New Brunswick, NJ: Transaction Books.

Robertson, M. J., Koegel, P., Mundy, P., Greenblatt, M., & Robertson, J. (1988,
November). *Mental health status of homeless adolescents in Hollywood.* Paper presented at the American Public Health Association meeting, Boston, MA.

Rotheram-Borus, M. J. (1991). Mental health issues with homeless and runaway
youth. *Family and Community Health, Vol. 1, 14*(3), 67-76.

Rotheram-Borus, M. J., & Koopman, C. (1991a). HIV/AIDS prevention among
adolescents. *Journal of Primary Prevention, 12*(1), 65-82.

Rotheram-Borus, M. J., & Koopman, C. (1991b). Sexual risk behaviors, AIDS knowledge, and beliefs about AIDS among runaways. *American Journal of Public Health,
81*, 208-210.

Rotheram-Borus, M. J., Koopman, C., & Bradley, J. S. (1990). Barriers to successful
AIDS prevention programs with runaway youth. In J. O. Woodruff, D. Dougherty,
& J. G. Athey (Eds.), *Troubled adolescents and HIV infection: Issues in prevention
and treatment* (pp. 37-55). Washington, DC: CASSP Technical Assistance Center.

Rotheram-Borus, M. J., Koopman, C., & Ehrhardt, A. A. (1991). Homeless youths
and HIV infection. *American Psychologist, 46*, 1188-1197.

Rotheram-Borus, M. J., Koopman, C., Haignere, C., & Davies, M. (1991). Reducing
HIV sexual risk behaviors among runaway adolescents. *Journal of the American
Medical Association, 266*, 1237-1241.

Schiamberg, L. B. (1986). A family systems approach to adolescent alienation. In G.
K. Leigh & G. W. Peterson (Eds.), *Adolescents in families* (pp. 277-307). Cincinnati:
South-Western.

Shaffer, D., & Caton, D. (1984). *Runaway and homeless youth in New York City: A report
to the Ittleson Foundation.* New York: Ittleson Foundation.

Shalwitz, J. C., Goulart, M., Dunnigan, K., & Flannery, D. (1990, June). *Prevalence of
sexually transmitted diseases (STD) and HIV in a homeless youth medical clinic in San
Francisco.* Paper presented at the VI International Conference on AIDS, San
Francisco, CA.

State of Washington Department of Health. (1989). *Out of home adolescents: HIV
infection and disease* (DOH-PUB #410-002). Olympia, WA: Author.

Stein, J. B., Jones, S. J., & Fisher, G. (1988). AIDS and IV drug use: Prevention
strategies for youth. In M. Quackenbush, M. Nelson, & K. Clark (Eds.), *The AIDS
challenge* (pp. 273-295). Santa Cruz, CA: Network.

Stricof, R. L., Kennedy, J. T., Natell, T. C., Weisfuse, I. B., & Novick, L. F. (1991). HIV
seroprevalence in a facility for runaway and homeless adolescents. *American
Journal of Public Health, 81*(Supplement), 50-53.

Stricof, R., Novick, L. F., & Kennedy, J. (1990, June). *HIV-1 seroprevalence in facilities
for runaway and homeless adolescents in four states: Florida, Texas, Louisiana and New
York.* Paper presented at VI International Conference on AIDS, San Francisco,
CA.

Stricof, R., Novick, L., Kennedy, J., & Weisfuse, I. B. (1988, November). *HIV seroprevalence of adolescents at Covenant House/under 21 in New York City* (meeting
abstract). American Public Health Association Conference, Boston, MA.

Stroul, B. A., & Friedman, R. M. (1986). *A system of care for severely emotionally disturbed children and youth*. Washington, DC: Georgetown University Child Development Center.

U.S. Conference of Mayors. (1987). *The continuing growth of hunger, homelessness and poverty in America's cities: 1987*. Washington, DC: Author.

Vermund, S. V., Hein, K., Gayle, H., Cary, J., & Thomas, P. (1989). AIDS among adolescents in NYC: Case surveillance profiles compared with the rest of the US. *American Journal of Disease in Children, 143*, 1220-1225.

Watters, J. K., Cheng, Y., Segal, M., Lorvick, J., Case, P. K., & Carlson, J. (1990, June). *Epidemiology and prevention of HIV in intravenous drug users in San Francisco, CA, 1986-1989*. In abstracts of VI International Conference on AIDS, San Francisco, CA.

Wetzel, J. (1987). *American youth: A statistical snapshot*. New York: William T. Grant Foundation.

Yates, G., MacKenzie, R., Pennbridge, J., & Cohen, E. (1988). A risk profile comparison of runaway and non-runaway youth. *American Journal of Public Health, 78*, 820-821.

PART II

Prevention: Theory, Design, and Evaluation

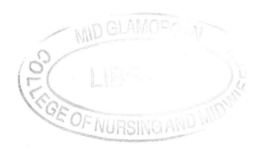

6

A Social Cognitive Approach
to the Exercise of Control
Over AIDS Infection

ALBERT BANDURA

Introduction

Prevention of infection with the AIDS virus requires people to exercise influence over their own motivation and behavior. Social efforts designed to control the spread of AIDS have centered mainly on informing the public about how the human immunodeficiency virus (HIV) is transmitted and how to safeguard against such infection. Unfortunately information alone does not necessarily exert much influence on refractory health-impairing habits. It has not slimmed the obese, eradicated cigarette smoking despite its acknowledged health hazard, or made a substantial dent on nutritional patterns that create high risk of cardiovascular disease in those who need to change most. It certainly will not make the sexually active celibate and impel intravenous drug users to renounce drugs, which are the two major modes of HIV transmission.

To achieve self-directed change, people need to be given not only reasons to alter risky habits but also the means, resources, and social supports to do so. Effective self-regulation of behavior is not achieved by an act of will. It requires certain skills in self-motivation and self-guidance (Bandura, 1986). Moreover, a difference exists between possessing self-regulative skills and being able to use them effectively and consistently under difficult circumstances. Success requires not only skills but also strong self-belief in one's efficacy to exercise personal control.

Perceived Self-Efficacy

Perceived self-efficacy is concerned with people's beliefs that they can exert control over their motivation, behavior, and social environment. People's beliefs about their capabilities affect what they choose to do, how much effort they mobilize, how long they will persevere in the face of difficulties, and whether they engage in self-debilitating or self-encouraging thought patterns. When lacking a sense of self-efficacy, individuals do not manage situations effectively even though they know what to do and possess the requisite skills. Self-inefficacious thinking creates discrepancies between knowledge and self-protective action. Numerous studies have been conducted linking perceived self-efficacy to health-promoting and health-impairing behavior (Bandura, 1986, 1991; O'Leary, 1985). The results show that perceived efficacy can affect every phase of personal change—whether people even consider changing their health habits, how hard they try should they choose to do so, how much they change, and how well they maintain the changes they have achieved.

Translating health knowledge into effective self-protection action against HIV infection requires social and self-regulative skills and a sense of personal power to exercise control over sexual situations. As Gagnon and Simon (1973) have correctly observed, managing sexuality involves managing interpersonal relationships. Thus risk reduction calls for enhancement of interpersonal efficacy rather than simply targeting a specific infective behavior for change. The major problem is not teaching people safer sex guidelines, which is easily achievable, but equipping them with skills that enable them to put the guidelines consistently into practice in the face of counteracting influences. Difficulties arise in following safer sex practices because self-protection often conflicts with interpersonal pressures and sentiments. In these interpersonal situations, the sway of coercive threat, allurements, desire for social acceptance, social pressures, situational constraints, and fear of rejection and personal embarrassment can override the influence of the best of informed judgment. The weaker the perceived self-efficacy, the more such social and affective factors can increase the likelihood of risky sexual behavior.

Exercise of personal control over sexual situations calls on skills and self-efficacy in communicating frankly about sexual matters and protective sexual methods and ensuring their use. Some of the people who perceive a personal risk of sexually transmitted disease are reducing the number of sexual partners and are more wary of engaging in sex with casual partners. Ignorance of a partner's sexual and drug activities has become a new risk factor. To rest self-protection on partners' reports of their sexual and drug history, however, is a hazardous safeguard. Sexual ardor and impression management can readily expurgate risky histories in personal disclosures. Survey studies reveal that even a majority of "monogamous" relationships are so in name rather than in actual practice. Because the AIDS virus is transmittable heterosexually, occasional sex with partners outside a monogamous relationship, especially those who have had bisexual or drug involvements, expands the range of potential risk.

Subjective risk appraisal for AIDS infection is highly unreliable because infected individuals remain asymptomatic for a long time and their sexual and drug histories often remain a private matter. Lacking knowledge of the behavioral history and serostatus of sexual partners, people tend to make their risk appraisals on the basis of social and physical appearances, which can be highly misleading. In light of evidence that most males would lie about their sexual history to gain sex (Keeling, 1989), seeking protection through probing inquiry provides illusory safety. Indeed, the stronger that people believe in their personal efficacy to assess by inquiry the risk status of a new partner, the more likely they are to engage in unprotected intercourse (O'Leary, Goodhart, Jemmott, & Boccher-Lattimore, 1992).

Even people who are well informed on safer-sex guidelines often err in their subjective appraisal of the extent to which they are putting themselves at risk of HIV infection. Bauman and Siegel

(1987) found that gay men who practice hazardous sex underestimate the riskiness of their behavior as judged against epidemiologically established linkage to seropositivity. Misappraisals of riskiness of one's sexual practices tend to be associated with underestimation of personal susceptibility to infection and with misbeliefs that risky sex with a few regular partners is safe and that behavioral precautions actually having no protective value (showering before and after sexual contact, healthful regimens, inspecting partners for lesions) will render risky sex safe. Such findings underscore the need for risk-reduction messages to describe not only risky sexual practices but also the common misbeliefs about factors that invest risky practices with false safety.

In managing sexuality, people have to exercise influence over themselves, as well as over others. This requires self-regulative skills in guiding and motivating one's actions. Self-regulation operates through internal standards, affective reactions to one's conduct, use of motivating self-incentives, and other forms of cognitive self-guidance. Self-regulative skills thus form an integral part of risk-reduction capabilities. They partly determine the social situations into which people get themselves, how well they navigate through them, and how effectively they can resist social inducements to potentially risky behavior. It is easier to wield control over preliminary choice behavior that may lead to troublesome social situations than to try to extricate oneself from such situations while enmeshed in them. This is because the *antecedent phase* involves mainly anticipatory motivators, which are amenable to cognitive control; the *entanglement phase* includes stronger social inducements to engage in high-risk behavior, which are less easily manageable.

In some countries in Africa, Latin America, and the Caribbean, AIDS is almost exclusively a heterosexually transmitted disease, with untreated venereal diseases increasing susceptibility to HIV infection. In Europe and the United States, the route of heterosexual transmission is mainly via bisexuals and intravenous drug users infected by sharing contaminated needles. Southern Asian countries are witnessing a rapid spread of infection among intravenous drug users, which then spreads to heterosexual partners and their newborns (Des Jarlais & Friedman, 1988b). Control of the spread of the AIDS virus by intravenous drug users requires risk-reduction strategies aimed at both drug and sexual practices.

Relatively little effort has been devoted to developing interventions to prevent infection among intravenous drug users. This is a serious neglect because infected male drug users are transmitting the virus heterosexually to their female sexual partners, who in turn run a high chance of infecting their infants through perinatal transmission. As a result, AIDS is taking an increasingly heavy toll on women and children, especially among ethnic minorities in impoverished environs where drug use is prevalent. Those who continue to inject drugs intravenously despite cognizance of the threat of AIDS infection need access to sterile needles and knowledge on how to disinfect needles to safeguard against transmission of the virus. They need to be taught protective sexual practices to avoid infecting their sexual partners and persuaded to use them consistently.

Perceived Self-Efficacy and Adoption of Health Practices

People's beliefs that they can motivate themselves and regulate their own behavior play a crucial role in whether they even consider altering habits detrimental to health. They see little point to even trying if they believe they cannot exercise control over their own behavior and that of others. Even people who believe their detrimental habits may be harming their health achieve little success in curtailing their behavior unless they judge themselves as having some efficacy to resist the instigators to it. This observation is corroborated in a longitudinal study conducted by McKusick, Wiley, Coates, and Morin (1986) of gay men's sexual behavior. Several psychological factors that could influence sexual risk-taking behavior were assessed. These included perceived threat that one is potentially at risk of exposure to the AIDS virus, degree of peer support for adopting safer sexual behavior, social skills necessary to negotiate protective sexual behavior, level of self-esteem, and perceived self-efficacy that one can take protective actions that lessen the risk of AIDS infection. Belief in one's personal efficacy to exercise control over one's sexual behavior emerged as the best predictor of sexual risk-taking behavior. The lower the perceived self-efficacy, the higher the likelihood of engagement in sexual practices that carry a high risk of AIDS infection. Men who frequented bars and bathhouses had a lower sense of efficacy than those who were committed to a monogamous relationship. Social skill in negotiating self-protective sexual activity also was associated with low-risk sexual practices.

The role of perceived self-efficacy in the adoption and maintenance of self-protective behavior is corroborated in other lines of research. Even though individuals acknowledge that safer sex practices reduce risk of infection, they do not adopt them if they believe they cannot exercise control in sexual relations (Siegel, Mesagno, Chen, & Christ, 1989). Perceived self-efficacy to negotiate condom use predicts safer sex practices in adolescents (Rosenthal, Moore, & Flynn, 1991) and adults (Brafford & Beck, 1991; O'Leary et al., 1992). Alcohol and drug use in the context of sexual activity fosters risky sex. Drugs and alcohol lower perceived self-efficacy to adhere to safer sex practices (Rosenthal et al., 1991).

The spreading threat of AIDS has produced substantial changes in sexual practices in the gay community, as shown in reduction of high-risk sexual acts and number of sexual partners. In the study of longitudinal predictors, McKusick and his colleagues (McKusick, Coates, Morin, Pollack, & Hoff, 1990) found that a strong sense of efficacy to exercise self-protective control, association with groups that made safer sex the norm, and knowledge of serostatus were the significant predictors of enduring reductions in high-risk sexual practices. The reductions in high-risk practices accompanying each of these three sources of influence are summarized in Figure 6.1. These longitudinal predictors underscore the importance of self-efficacy enhancement through skill development and alterations of subcommunity norms in programs designed to produce long-term behavior change.

Components of Effective Self-Directed Change

Social cognitive theory explains human functioning in terms of triadic reciprocal causation (Bandura, 1986). In this causal model, which is summarized schematically in Figure 6.2, Behavior; Personal determinants in the form of cognitive, affective, and biological factors; and Environmental influences all operate as interacting determinants of each other. An effective program of widespread change in detrimental life-style practices includes four major components devised to alter each of the three classes of interacting

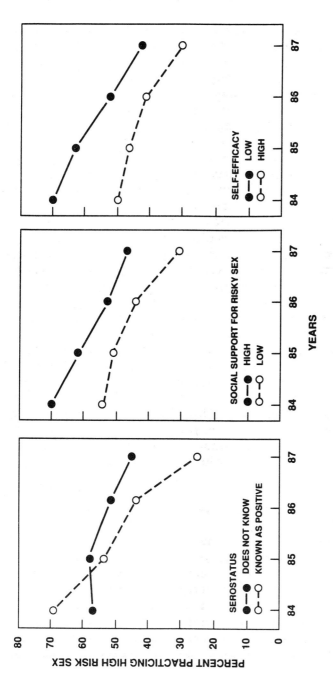

Figure 6.1. Changes in Percentage of Homosexual Respondents Practicing High-Risk Sexual Behavior Over Time as a Function of Knowledge of Seropositive Status, Perceived Self-Efficacy to Adhere to Self-Protective Behavior, and Perceived Number of Friends and Acquaintances Following a Norm of Risky Sexual Activities

SOURCE: Plotted from data of McKusick, Coates, & Morin, 1989.

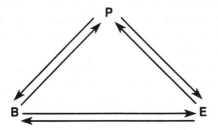

Figure 6.2. Schematization of Triadic Reciprocal Causation
NOTE: B signifies behavior; P the cognitive, biological, and other internal events that affect perceptions and action; and E the external environment.

determinants. The first component is informational, designed to increase people's awareness and knowledge of health risks. The second component is concerned with development of the social and self-regulative skills needed to translate informed concerns into effective preventive action. The third component is aimed at skill enhancement and building resilient self-efficacy by providing opportunities for guided practice and corrective feedback in applying the skills in high-risk situations. The fourth component involves enlisting and creating social supports for desired personal changes. Let us consider how each of these four components would apply to self-directed change of behaviors that pose high risk of AIDS infection.

Informational Component

Efforts to encourage people to adopt health practices rely heavily on persuasive communications in health education campaigns. In such health messages, appeals to fear by depicting the ravages of disease are used often as motivators, and recommended preventive practices are provided as guides for action. People need enough knowledge of potential dangers to warrant action, but they do not have to be scared out of their wits to act, any more than homeowners have to be terrified to insure their households. Rather, what people need is sound information on how AIDS is transmitted, guidance on how to regulate their behavior, and firm belief in their personal efficacy to turn concerns into effective preventive actions. Responding to these needs requires a shift in emphasis from trying to scare people into healthy behavior to empowering them with the tools for exercising personal control over their health habits.

The influential role of people's beliefs in their personal efficacy in adopting preventive health practices is shown by Beck and Lund (1981). They studied the persuasiveness of health communications in which the seriousness of a disease and susceptibility to it were varied. Patients' perceived self-efficacy that they could stick to the required preventive behavior was a good predictor of whether they adopted the preventive practices. Fear arousal had little effect on whether they did so. Analyses of the mechanisms through which mass media health campaigns exert their effects similarly reveal that perceived self-efficacy plays an influential role in the adoption of health practices (Maibach, Flora, & Nass, 1991; Slater, 1989). The stronger the preexisting perceived self-efficacy and the more the media campaigns enhance people's self-regulative efficacy, the more likely people are to adopt the recommended practices. The relationship remains even when multiple controls are applied for a host of other possible influences.

To be most effective, health communications should instill in people the belief that they have the capability to alter their health habits and should instruct them on how to do it. Communications that explicitly do so increase people's determination to modify habits detrimental to their health (Maddux & Rogers, 1983). Entrenched habits rarely yield to a single attempt at self-regulation. Success usually is achieved through renewed effort following failed attempts. To strengthen the staying power of self-beliefs, health communications should emphasize that success requires perseverant effort, so that people's sense of efficacy is not undermined by a few setbacks. Faultless self-regulation is not easy to come by even for pliant habits, let alone for addictive and sexual behaviors. A strong sense of controlling efficacy is built by overcoming setbacks through perseverant effort. Unfortunately the possibility that the AIDS virus is transmittable to the immunologically vulnerable through a few sexual contacts with infected partners or sharing a few contaminated needles does not leave much room for carelessness or occasional reversions to risky habits.

An increased research effort is needed to determine how preventive health communications should be framed to maximize their impact on perceived self-regulative efficacy. Self-efficacy theory provides one set of guidelines (Bandura, 1986). I shall consider later how symbolic modeling influences should be structured to maximize their psychosocial impact. Decision theory regarding risk perception and risky decisions provides other suggestions (Tversky & Kahneman, 1981). For example, people interpret information regarding risky activities in terms of potential gains and potential losses. Persuasive communications have differential impact on perceived self-efficacy, depending on whether they are framed in terms of gains or losses. Communications phrased in terms of benefits are less effective in altering detrimental habits than are communications phrased in terms of personal losses. Examination of possible mediating mechanisms shows that the more persuasive messages achieve their effects by raising perceived self-efficacy rather than by heightening fear or perceived threat (Meyerowitz & Chaiken, 1987). In designing national education campaigns, we need to exploit our knowledge of social-influence processes and the cognitive and affective mechanisms governing human motivation and behavior.

The preconditions for change are created by increasing people's awareness and knowledge of the profound threat of AIDS. They need to be provided with a great deal of factual information about the nature of AIDS, its modes of transmission, what constitutes high-risk sexual and drug practices, and how to achieve protection from infection. This is easier said than done. Our society does not provide much in the way of treatment of drug addiction, nor is it about to provide refractory drug users with easy access to sterile needles and other drug paraphernalia. It has little experience in how to reach and educate drug users on how to disinfect needles to reduce the risk of AIDS infection.

In the sexual domain, our society has always had difficulty talking frankly about sex and imparting sexual information to the public at large. Because parents generally do a poor job of it as well, most youngsters pick up their sex education from other, often less trustworthy and reputable, sources outside the home or from the consequences of uninformed sexual experimentation. To complicate matters further, some sectors of the society lobby actively for maintaining a veil of silence regarding protective sexual practices on the belief that such information will promote indiscriminate sexuality. In their view, the remedy for the spreading

AIDS epidemic is a national celibacy campaign for unweds and gays and faithful monogamy among the wedded. They oppose educational programs in the schools that talk about sex methods that provide protection against AIDS infection.

The net result is that many of our public education campaigns regarding AIDS are couched in desexualized generalities that leave some ignorance in their wake. To those most at risk, such sanitized expressions as "exchange of bodily fluids" is not only uninformative but may invest safe bodily substances with perceived infective properties. Even those more skilled in deciphering medical locutions do not always know what the preventive messages are talking about. For example, an intensive campaign spanning a full week, conducted at a university campus, included public lectures, numerous panel discussions, presentations in dormitories, and condom distribution, all of which were widely reported in the campus newspaper. A systematic assessment of students' beliefs and sexual practices conducted several weeks later revealed that more than a quarter of the students did not know what constitutes "safer sex," and some of them had misconceptions of safer sex practices that in fact would present high risk of infection (Chervin & Martinez, 1987). Other findings of this study, which will be reviewed later, document the severe limitations of efforts to change sexual practices by information alone.

The informational component of the model of self-directed change includes two main factors: the informational content of the health communications, and the mechanisms of social diffusion. Detailed factual information about AIDS must be socially imparted in an understandable, credible, and persuasive manner. Social cognitive theories provide a number of guidelines on how this might be best accomplished (Bandura, 1986; McGuire, 1984; Zimbardo, Ebbesen, & Maslach, 1977). Developing effective AIDS-prevention programs, however, is only the first step; they must also be disseminated. Unlike other health-risk-reduction campaigns that involve relatively prosaic habits, the risky habits for AIDS infection are laden with matters of illegalities and judged immoralities.

Informative health messages, however well designed, cannot have much social impact without effective means of dissemination. Because of their wide reach and influence, the mass media, especially television, can serve as major vehicles of social diffusion of information regarding health guidelines. A variety of diffusion vehicles, however, must be enlisted in a public health campaign for several reasons. High costs and restricted access to television limit its availability. Moreover, television networks typically adopt a conservative stance on controversial matters. They have resisted getting into the act for fear that talk of protective sex practices will jeopardize advertising revenue by arousing the wrath of some sectors of their viewing audience. This resistance would have weakened if the AIDS virus had spread rapidly heterosexually across all sectors of society, thus making it a general societal problem rather than one confined to gays and drug users. It is unlikely, however, that the television industry will offer much help as long as AIDS remains mainly a disease of poor minorities. Existing social, religious, recreational, occupational, and educational organizations can serve as highly effective disseminators of preventive health guidelines. Wide cultural diversity requires that the messages of risk-reduction campaigns for AIDS be tailored to socioeconomic, racial, and ethnic differences in value orientations and be disseminated through multiple sources to ensure adequate exposure (Mantell, Schinke, & Akabas, 1988).

Nontraditional social networks must be enlisted for high-risk groups who are beyond the reach of the usual community organizations. For example, in outreach programs, streetwise counselors have been highly successful in reaching drug populations (Watters et al., 1990). After the counselors become known in the social circles of drug users, they help the users with referrals to drug treatment programs. They offer them explicit instruction in safer sex practices. They teach intravenous drug users how to reduce the risk of AIDS by disinfecting needles with ordinary household bleach, which kills the HIV virus. The disinfection procedure, which drug users rarely used before, was widely adopted and consistently applied. Although this outreach program also increased the use of condoms, the drug users were much more conscientious in disinfecting needles than in protecting their sexual partners against sexually transmitted infection. Such findings underscore the need for sexual partners to exercise personal control in protecting their own health.

A comprehensive national program regarding the growing AIDS threat must address broader social issues, as well as risky health practices. This is because the AIDS epidemic has far-reaching social repercussions. One of these issues concerns the widespread public fear of AIDS infection. Many people continue to believe that the AIDS virus can be transmitted by casual contact or by insect transmission and food handling despite evidence to the contrary. Efforts by health professionals to dispel misapprehensions are discounted by many of those who are alarmed on the grounds that what is proclaimed safe currently may be discovered to be risky later. Recurrent disputes among researchers in the public media regarding risk factors for other diseases have eroded some of the credibility of medical expertise. Widespread public fear gets translated into advocacy of laws requiring sweeping mandatory blood testing and identification and social restriction of those with antibodies to the HIV virus.

In public perceptions of the AIDS threat, risky behavior gets transformed to risky groups. As AIDS imposes mounting financial burdens on society and strains medical and social service systems, members of high-risk groups may become targets of growing public hostility. Once entire groups get stigmatized because some of their members behave in high-risk ways, those who do not also become the objects of fear and hostility. The way in which they are treated socially may be dictated more by group identity than by their personal characteristics. Public alarm, fueled by many misbeliefs, enhances such stigmatization. Policy debates on how to control the spread of AIDS have become highly politicized. Prohibitionists argue that public health campaigns promote indiscriminate sex. Their critics argue that knowledge does not foster sexuality and that prohibitionists are intent at curtailing sex practices they find morally objectionable rather than at increasing the safety of sex. Uninformed public reactions to the AIDS threat require serious attention, as do the risky health practices themselves, because they help shape public policies and impose constraints on health education programs. Even societies that possess the necessary scientific knowledge, resources, and expertise can be immobilized by conflicts of values and morals from establishing psychosocial programs that can help stem the tide of infection.

Development of Self-Protective Skills and Controlling Self-Efficacy

It is not enough to convince people that they should alter risky habits. Most of them also need guidance on how to translate their concerns into efficacious actions. In the campus survey mentioned earlier (Chervin & Martinez, 1987), after exposure to the intensive educational campaign, fewer than half of the students who were sexually active used safer sex methods designed to prevent infection with sexually transmitted diseases. Most of them even avoided talking about the matter with their sexual partners. Studies conducted on other campuses similarly reveal that most sexually active students who are knowledgeable about AIDS do not adopt safer sex practices (Edgar, Freimuth, & Hammond, 1988). McKusick, Horstman, and Coates (1985) found that gay men were uniformly well informed about safer sex methods for protecting against AIDS infection, but those who had a low sense of efficacy that they could manage their behavior and sexual relationships were unable to act on their knowledge.

The ability to learn by social modeling provides a highly effective method for increasing human knowledge and skills. A special power of modeling is that it can simultaneously transmit knowledge and valuable skills to large numbers of people through the medium of videotape modeling. Knowledge of modeling processes identifies a number of factors that can be used to enhance the instructive power of modeling (Bandura, 1986). Applications of modeling principles to AIDS prevention would focus on how to manage interpersonal situations and one's own behavior in ways that afford protection against infection with the AIDS virus. Both self-regulative and risk-reduction strategies for dealing with a variety of situations that promote risky behavior would be modeled to convey general guides that can be applied and adjusted to fit changing circumstances.

We saw earlier that human competency requires not only skills but also self-belief in one's capability to use those skills well. Indeed results of numerous studies of diverse health habits and physical dysfunctions reveal that the impact of different methods of influence on health behavior is partly mediated through their effects on perceived self-efficacy (Bandura, 1991). The stronger the self-efficacy beliefs they instill, the more likely are people to enlist and sustain the effort needed to change habits detrimental to health. Modeling influences therefore should be designed to build self-assurance, as well as to convey strategies for how to deal effectively with coercions for risky practices. The influence of modeling on beliefs about one's capabilities relies on comparison with others. People judge their own capabilities in part from how well those whom they regard as similar to themselves exercise control over situations. People develop stronger belief in their capabilities and more readily adopt modeled ways if they see models similar to themselves solve problems successfully with the modeled strategies than if they see the models as very different from themselves (Bandura, 1986). To increase the impact of modeling, the characteristics of models, such as their age, sex, and status, the type of problems with which they cope, and the situation in which they apply their skills, should be made to appear similar to the people's own circumstances.

Enhancement of Social Proficiency and Resiliency of Self-Efficacy

Proficiency requires extensive practice, and this is no less true of managing the interpersonal aspects of sexuality. After people gain knowledge of new skills and social strategies, they need guidance and opportunities to perfect these skills. Initially people practice in simulated situations in which they need not fear making mistakes or appearing inadequate. This is best achieved by role playing in which they practice handling the types of situations they have to manage in their social environment. They receive informative feedback on how they are doing and the corrective changes that need to be made. The simulated practice is continued until the skills are performed proficiently and spontaneously.

Not all the benefits of guided practice are due to skill improvement. Some of the gains result from raising people's beliefs in their capabilities (Bandura, 1988). Experiences in exercising control over social situations serve as self-efficacy builders. This is an important aspect of self-directed change because if people are not fully convinced of their personal efficacy, they undermine their efforts in situations that tax capabilities and readily abandon the skills they have been taught when they fail to get quick results or suffer reverses. The important matter is not that difficulties rouse self-doubts, which is a natural immediate reaction, but rather the degree and speed of recovery from setbacks. It is resiliency in perceived self-efficacy that counts in maintenance of changes in health habits. The higher the perceived self-efficacy, the greater the success in maintenance of health-promoting behavior (Bandura, 1991).

The influential role played by perceived self-efficacy in the management of sexual activities is documented in studies of contraceptive use by teenage women at high risk because they often engage in unprotected intercourse (Levinson, 1986). Such research shows that perceived self-efficacy in managing sexual relationships is associated with more effective use of contraceptives. The predictive relation remains when controls are applied for demographic factors, knowledge, and sexual experience.

Gilchrist and Schinke (1983) applied the main features of the multicomponent model of personal change to teach teenagers how to exercise self-protective control over sexual situations. The teens received essential factual information about high-risk sexual behavior and self-protective measures. Through modeling, they were taught how to communicate frankly about sexual matters and contraceptives, how to deal with conflicts regarding sexual activities, and how to resist unwanted sexual advances. They practiced applying these social skills by role playing in simulated situations and received instructive feedback. The self-regulative program significantly enhanced perceived self-efficacy and skill in managing sexuality. A program incorporating many elements of a self-regulative model produced significant AIDS risk reduction in black male adolescents (Jemmott, Jemmott, & Fong, 1992). Those who had the benefit of the program were more knowledgeable about infective risks, less accepting of risky practices, and reported engaging in lower risky sexual behavior with fewer sexual partners in follow-up assessments than did those in a control condition.

Research by Kelly and his colleagues attests to the substantial value of self-regulative programs for AIDS risk reduction (Kelly, St. Lawrence, Hood, & Brasfield, 1989). Gay men were taught through modeling, role playing, and corrective feedback how to exercise self-protective control in sexual relationships and to resist coercions for high-risk sex. Multifaceted assessments showed that they became more skillful in handling sexual relationships and coercions, markedly reduced risky sexual practices, and used condoms on a regular basis. As shown in Figure 6.3, these self-protective practices were fully maintained in follow-up assessments. In contrast, a matched control group of gay men continued to engage in unprotected high-risk sexual practices.

Combining factual information about health risks with development of risk-reduction efficacy produces good results. Because

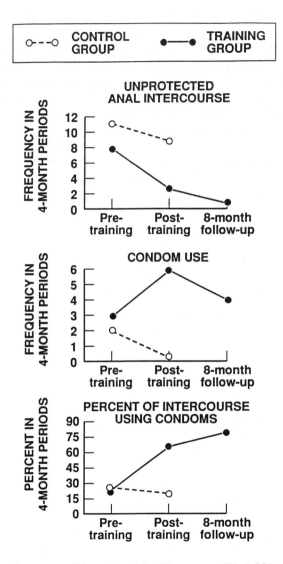

Figure 6.3. Frequency of Unprotected Anal Intercourse, Digital/Anal Activities, and Proportion of Condom Use During Intercourse by Gay Men Who Received the Self-Regulative Program and Those in a Control Group Who Did Not

SOURCE: From "Behavioral Intervention to Reduce AIDS Risk Activities" by J. A. Kelly, J. S. St. Lawrence, H. V. Hood, and T. L. Brasfield, 1989, *Journal of Consulting and Clinical Psychology,* 57, 60-67. Copyright 1989 by the American Psychological Association. Reprinted by permission. NOTE: Each data point represents the average rate for each 2-week period.

people learn and perfect effective ways of behaving under lifelike conditions, problems of transferring the new skills to everyday life are reduced. The mastery-modeling approach is readily adaptable in audiotape or videocassette format to self-protective behavior with regard to AIDS. Large-scale applications of self-regulative programs sacrifice the guided role-playing component. Instruction in imaginal rehearsal, however, in which people mentally practice dealing with prototypic, troublesome situations, boosts perceived self-efficacy and improves actual performance (Bandura, 1986; Kazdin, 1978). Maibach (1990) tested the incremental benefits of cued cognitive rehearsal of self-protective strategies imbedded in videotaped modeling of how to manage potentially risky sexual activities. Cognitive rehearsal enhanced the power of symbolic modeling to strengthen a sense of personal efficacy to exercise self-protective control. The self-regulative approach, designed in a format suitable for mass distribution, has been shown to achieve some success in changing other refractory health-impairing behavior (Sallis et al., 1986).

Because of the high level of unprotected sexual activity and experimentation with drugs by adolescents, they are vulnerable to becoming a high-risk group as transmitters of the AIDS virus (Mantell & Schinke, in press). Training materials need to be developed to assist parents and teachers on how to educate youngsters about AIDS. Winett and his colleagues, using modeling and cued rehearsal of self-protective skills, devised a video prototype for use in the home by parents and their teenagers (Winett et al., in press). This home-based program increased knowledge about HIV transmission and prevention, fostered more open communication between parents and their teenagers regarding sexuality, increased family problem-solving skills, and taught teenagers strategies on how to manage common risk situations. Further efforts to increase the power of this familial approach are centered on augmenting the skill development component. The mastery-modeling program developed by Gilchrist and Schinke (1983) provides a good prototype for application in schools. Other channels of dissemination, however, must be created to reach teenagers who live in dysfunctional families and receive little guidance from school because of factional opposition to educational efforts that address self-protective behavior in an explicitly informative manner. A major segment of the teenage population can be reached by making informative audiotapes and videocassettes readily available in the settings they frequent, such as music and video stores.

AIDS infection is spreading rapidly among intravenous drug users and to their sexual partners and offspring. Efforts to control this source of infection are directed mainly at curtailing the supply of drugs, instituting risk-reduction programs focused on disinfection and exchange of drug injection equipment, developing non-reusable syringes, and treating addictive conditions. These efforts must be supplemented by AIDS-prevention programs designed to reduce the demand for drugs. As in other areas of habit change, informational campaigns alone will not do it. A comprehensive preventive effort must provide knowledge about the determinants, precipitants, and immediate and long-term consequences of drug use, must alter the valuation of drugs, must develop self-regulative and social skills to resist social pressures to use drugs, and must cultivate social norms that discourage experimentation with and use of drugs. These features are best achieved by school-based primary prevention programs that have proven effective in other areas of health promotion and risk reduction (Flora & Thoresen, 1988; Killen et al., 1989).

The prototypic skills enhancement program developed by Gilchrist and Schinke (1985) has been successfully extended to the prevention and reduction of drug abuse by adolescents. This type of program informs adolescents about drug effects, provides them with interpersonal skills for managing personal and social pressures to use drugs, lowers drug use, and fosters self-conceptions as a nonuser (Gilchrist, Schinke, Trimble, & Cvetkovich, 1987). These findings are all the more interesting because they were achieved with ethnic and minority youth among whom substance abuse is prevalent. Adoption of a self-conception as a nonuser can produce profound life-style changes. This is most likely to occur when the emergent new self-conception leads to severance of social ties with substance abusers and sufficient social support is provided for immersion in nonuser social networks (Stall & Biernacki, 1986).

Social Supports for Personal Change

People achieve self-directed change when they understand how personal habits threaten their well-being, are taught how to modify them, and believe in their capabilities to marshall the effort and resources needed to exercise control. Personal change, however, occurs within a network of social influences. Depending on their nature, social influences can aid, retard, or undermine efforts at personal change. This is especially true in the case of sexual and drug practices, which are subjected to strong social normative influences.

In social cognitive theory, normative influences regulate behavior through two regulatory processes: social sanctions, and instated self-sanctions (Bandura, 1986). Norms influence behavior anticipatorily by the social consequences they provide. Behavior that violates prevailing social norms brings social censure or other punishing consequences, whereas behavior that fulfills socially valued norms is approved and rewarded. People do not act like weather vanes, constantly shifting their behavior to conform to whatever others might want. Rather they adopt certain standards of behavior for themselves and regulate their behavior anticipatorily through self-evaluative consequences. Social norms convey standards of conduct. Adoption of personal standards creates a self-regulative system that operates partly through internalized self-sanctions. People behave in ways that give them self-satisfaction, and they refrain from behaving in ways that violate their standards because it will bring self-censure. Anticipatory self-sanctions thus keep conduct in line with internal standards.

Normative consensus strengthens both its modeling and sanctioning functions. The normative influences that foster preventive measures center on the behavioral practices by which the virus is transmitted and on the cultural patterning of social relationships. Because of their proximity, immediacy, and prevalency, the interpersonal influences operating within one's immediate social network claim a stronger regulatory function than do general normative sanctions, which are more distal and applied only infrequently to the behavior of any given individual because unfamiliar others are not around to react to it. Even when unfamiliar others are around, if the norms of one's immediate network are at odds with those of the larger group, the reactions of outsiders carry lesser weight, if not disregarded altogether.

People who are fully informed on the modes of HIV transmission and effective self-protective methods acquire the virus only if they allow it to happen. They often allow it to happen because interpersonal, sociocultural, religious, and economic factors operate as constraints on self-protective behavior. Some of those most at risk must contend with sociocultural obstacles to the use of prophylactic methods that afford protection against HIV infection. The major burden for self-protection against heterosexually transmitted diseases usually falls on women. Unlike protection against pregnancy, for which women can exercise independent control, use of condoms requires them to exercise control over the behavior of men. Those men who possess coercive power over their partners resist the use of condoms if in their view it reduces their sexual pleasure, threatens their sense of manliness and authority, casts aspersions on their faithfulness, and carries the frightening implication that they may be carriers of disease. It is difficult for women, especially those of poor and minority status who are most at risk, to press the issue in the face of emotional and economic dependence, coercive threat, and subcultural prescription of compliant roles for them (Mays & Cochran, 1988). Women who are enmeshed in relationships of imbalanced power need to be taught how to negotiate protected sex nonconfrontationally. Women who are well equipped with condoms run the risk of being viewed as promiscuous.

At the broader societal level, attitudes and social norms must be altered to increase men's sense of responsibility for the social consequences of their sexuality. In societies in which the virus is spread heterosexually through prostitution, economic conditions that thrust women into prostitution and drug dependencies that drive them to sell sex for drugs create major impediments to preventive efforts. In short, if AIDS prevention programs are to achieve much success, they must address the sociocultural realities that impose constraints on the exercise of self-protective measures.

In the case of high-risk sexual behavior, strong involvement in a social network supportive of self-protective practices increases knowledge of risky behaviors, beliefs of efficacy, and adoption of safer sex practices (Fisher, 1988; McKusick et al., 1990). Risk reduction through alteration of subcommunity norms is an especially important vehicle for curbing the spread of AIDS among intravenous drug users because drug use is often a socially shared activity. Restricted access to drug injection equipment and the legal problems of being caught with it promote risky shared use of drug paraphernalia. Shooting galleries involving widespread sharing of contaminated needles provide the most fertile ground for spreading the virus. Preventive efforts aimed at drug subcultures show that drug users are reachable and instructable in safer practices. Thus provision of protective information by outreach workers about AIDS transmission, needle-exchange programs, and instruction on how to sterilize syringes can substantially reduce risky injection practices, which lowers infection rates among those who continue the drug habit (Des Jarlais & Friedman, 1988a; Watters et al., 1990). Needle-exchange programs do not propagate drug use, as some people have feared it might (Buning, van Brussel, & van Santen, 1988). As Des Jarlais notes, most drug users now know about the modes of AIDS transmission, but many are inadequately informed or misinformed about risk reduction techniques. For example, some dutifully wash needles in water or in other ways that do not kill the virus. Emerging subcommunity norms against needle-sharing behavior are a good predictor of reduction in risky injection practices among intravenous drug users (Des Jarlais & Friedman, 1988a). Although the subcommunity approach also serves as an excellent vehicle for enlisting drug users in treatment programs, outreach workers can offer them little because of the scarcity of treatment services.

Social influences rooted in indigenous sources generally have greater impact and sustaining power than those applied by outsiders for a limited time. A major benefit of community-mediated programs is that they can mobilize the power of formal and informal networks of influence for transmitting knowledge and cultivating beneficial patterns of behavior. A community-mediated approach is a potentially powerful vehicle for promoting both personal and social change in several ways. It provides an effective means for creating the motivational preconditions of change, for modeling requisite skills, for enlisting natural social incentives for adopting and maintaining beneficial habits, and for establishing protective practices as the normative standards of conduct. Generic principles of effective programs are readily adaptable at the subcommunity level to sociocultural differences in the populations being served. In the social diffusion of new behavior patterns, indigenous adopters usually serve as more influential exemplars and persuaders than do outsiders. Moreover, behavioral practices that create widespread health problems require group solutions that are best achieved through community-mediated efforts.

In their pioneering health-promoting programs, Farquhar and Maccoby have drawn heavily on existing community networks for transmitting knowledge and cultivating beneficial patterns of health behavior (Farquhar, Maccoby, & Solomon, 1984). This work provides a model of how to mobilize community resources to disseminate health information and to convey explicit guides on how to change refractory health habits. A program of self-directed change should be applied in ways designed to create self-sustaining structures within the community for promoting behavioral practices conducive to health. Persons in the community who serve as local organizers are taught how to design, coordinate, and implement the programs. By teaching persons in communities how to take charge of their own change, self-directedness is fostered at the community level, as well as at the personal level.

The substantial reductions in high-risk sexual practices by gay subgroups were achieved largely through effective self-empowering organization (McKusick et al., 1990; Stall & Paul, 1989). For example, in the unprecedented social and behavioral changes brought about by the gay community in San Francisco, the members educated themselves, made safer sex practices the social norm, devised and implemented their own instructional programs to prevent HIV transmission, established mechanisms for diffusing this knowledge, issued regular updates on new research findings and available treatments, created social support systems to counteract despair and to encourage meaningful life pursuits, and actively fostered life-style changes that might enhance immune function in those infected with the virus but not yet experiencing any symptoms. Some attempts have been made at self-mobilization by drug-user subgroups for self-protective change, but these have been less successful (Friedman, de Jong, & Des Jarlais, 1988). Lack of educational and financial resources, illegalities surrounding drug activities, societal restrictions of the means for safer injection practices, mistrusts, and the large amount of time devoted to supporting the drug habit impede efforts at self-organization. These conditions create a greater need for external aid in subgroup organization for risk reduction.

Attitudinal Impediments to Development
of Psychosocial Models

Despite the superiority of preventive measures, psychosocial research receives only a paltry 2% of the AIDS research budget (Siegel, Graham, & Stoto, 1990). Several attitudes downgrade the priority for research into psychosocial determinants and mechanisms governing AIDS-related behavior and for effective application of existing knowledge to this deadly epidemic. One view trivializes psychosocial approaches by regarding them as merely stopgap measures until a vaccine is discovered. Such an attitude reflects how little has been learned from past experiences with behaviorally transmitted diseases.

The AIDS virus appears in many forms and mutates rapidly, thus requiring vaccines for different viral strains. It invades immune cells and not only evades destruction by the body's defense system but turns infected T-helper cells into producers of more viruses and eventually destroys the very cells that provide protective immunity. It remains latent for long periods, and it may become more virulent over time. Considering these baffling biological properties, the quest for a vaccine that will provide protective immunity against the changing forms of this virus is likely to be a lengthy and frustrating one. Because viruses merge into the host cells, the task of developing antiviral treatments that can kill the AIDS virus without destroying the host immune cells is a formidable one.

Even the more limited goal of slowing the progress of the disease or keeping it in check with antiviral drugs that do not produce toxicities creating severe and even lethal side effects presents an immense challenge. Drugs that retard reproduction of the virus but do not eradicate it must be taken continually. Thus in animals engrafted with human immune organs and infected with the HIV virus, the antiviral drug AZT reduces the virus to a very low level but when the drug is withdrawn, the infection flares (McCune, Namikawa, Shih, Rabin, & Kaneshima, 1990). Prolonged use of drugs that are beneficial in the short term by attacking nonresistant viral strains can give rise to new resistant strains and to serious physical damage that requires discontinuation of the drug. Because the HIV virus mutates rapidly, mutant strains of the virus are likely to emerge that outwit the drugs.

Sexually transmitted diseases, such as gonorrhea and syphilis, that have been with us for ages have thwarted vaccine development. Discovery of effective treatments lowers the prevalence rates of a disease but does not eradicate it. With the development of a simple treatment for venereal disease, support for psychosocial control programs was curtailed, with a resultant rise in infection rates (Cutler & Arnold, 1988). The history of efforts to control diseases transmitted by behavior underscores the need for a multifaceted approach combining medical treatments with psychosocial preventive programs. Contrary to the commonly voiced view, it is not that psychosocial preventive programs are of value because they provide the only means available to stem the spread of AIDS in the absence of vaccines or effective treatments. Rather, psychosocial programs constitute an integral part of a multifaceted public health strategy not only before but even after effective treatments are found. The lessons from the past concerning behaviorally transmitted diseases should not be lost on the AIDS problem. Whether our advanced biotechnology will triumph over the AIDS virus or the mutable virus will foil our biotechnology remains to be seen. In any event, AIDS will remain with us as a continuing problem requiring psychosocial preventive measures.

Another downgrading view rests on the misbelief that psychosocial influences cannot effect much change in the transmissive risky behaviors because they serve potent drives. Amenability of behavior to change differs considerably, depending on whether one seeks to eliminate certain kinds of gratifications or to alter the means of gaining those gratifications. It is much more difficult to get people to relinquish behavior that is powerfully reinforced than to adopt safer forms of the behavior that serve the same function. In the case of AIDS prevention, people who are not about to give up drugs or their preferred forms of sexuality can achieve substantial protection against HIV infection by substituting safer behaviors for risky ones. Multifaceted psychosocial programs that equip people with protective knowledge, with the means and self-beliefs to exercise effective personal control, and provide social supports for their efforts at personal change can achieve highly beneficial results. Indeed, prevention programs that incorporate many of these elements have produced substantial reductions in risky sexual and drug-injection behaviors.

References

Bandura, A. (1986). *Social foundations of thought and action: A social cognitive theory.* Englewood Cliffs, NJ: Prentice-Hall.

Bandura, A. (1988). Perceived self-efficacy: Exercise of control through self-belief. In J. P. Dauwalder, M. Perrez, & V. Hobi (Eds.), *Annual series of European research in behavior therapy* (Vol. 2). (pp. 27-59). Lisse (NL): Swets & Zeitlinger.

Bandura, A. (1991). Self-efficacy mechanism in psysiological activation and health-promoting behavior. In J. Madden, IV (Ed.), *Neurobiology of learning, emotion, and affect* (pp. 229-270). New York: Raven.

Bauman, L. J., & Siegel, K. (1987). Misperception among gay men of the risk for AIDS associated with their sexual behavior. *Journal of Applied Social Psychology, 17,* 329-350.

Beck, K. H., & Lund, A. K. (1981). The effects of health threat seriousness and personal efficacy upon intentions and behavior. *Journal of Applied Social Psychology, 11,* 401-415.

Brafford, L. J., & Beck, K. H. (1991). Development and validation of a condom self-efficacy scale for college students. *Journal of American College Health, 39,* 219-225.

Buning, E. C., van Brussel, G. H. A., & van Santen, G. (1988). Amsterdam's drug policy and its implications for controlling needle sharing. In R. Battjes & R. Pickens (Eds.), *Needle sharing among intravenous drug abusers: National and international perspectives* (Research Monograph Series No. 80) (pp. 59-74). Bethesda, MD: National Institute on Drug Abuse.

Chervin, D. D., & Martinez, A. (1987, February 19). *Survey on the health of Stanford students.* Report to the Board of Trustees, Stanford University, Stanford, CA.

Cutler, J. C., & Arnold, R. C. (1988). Venereal disease control by health departments in the past: Lessons for the present. *American Journal of Public Health, 78,* 372-376.

Des Jarlais, D. C., & Friedman, S. R. (1988a). The psychology of preventing AIDS among intravenous drug users: A social learning conceptualization. *American Psychologist, 43,* 865-870.

Des Jarlais, D. C., & Friedman, S. R. (1988b). HIV infection among persons who inject illicit drugs: Problems and prospects. *Journal of Acquired Immune Deficiency Syndromes, 1,* 267-273.

Edgar, T., Freimuth, V. S., & Hammond, S. L. (1988). Communicating the AIDS risk to college students: The problem of motivating change. *Health Education Research, 3,* 59-65.

Farquhar, J. W., Maccoby, N., & Solomon, D. S. (1984). Community applications of behavioral medicine. In W. D. Gentry (Ed.), *Handbook of behavioral medicine* (pp. 437-478). New York: Guilford.

Fisher, J. D. (1988). Possible effects of reference group-based social influence on AIDS-risk behavior and AIDS prevention. *American Psychologist, 43,* 914-920.

Flora, J. A., & Thoresen, C. E. (1988). Reducing the risk of AIDS in adolescents. *American Psychologist, 43,* 965-970.

Friedman, S. R., de Jong, W. M., & Des Jarlais, D. C. (1988). Problems and dynamics of organizing intravenous drug users for AIDS prevention. *Health Education Research, 3,* 49-57.

Gagnon, J., & Simon, W. (1973). *Sexual conduct, the social sources of human sexuality.* Chicago: Aldine.

Gilchrist, L. D., & Schinke, S. P. (1983). Coping with contraception: Cognitive and behavioral methods with adolescents. *Cognitive Therapy and Research, 7,* 379-388.

Gilchrist, L. D., & Schinke, S. P. (Eds.). (1985). *Preventing social and health problems through life skills training.* Seattle: University of Washington.

Gilchrist, L. D., Schinke, S. P., Trimble, J., & Cvetkovich, G. T. (1987). Skills enhancement to prevent substance abuse among American Indian adolescents. *International Journal of the Addictions, 22,* 869-879.

Jemmott, J. B., Jemmott, L. S., & Fong, G. T. (1992). Reducing the risk of sexually transmitted HIV infection: Attitudes, knowledge, intentions, and behavior. *American Journal of Public Health, 82,* 372-377.

Kazdin, A. E. (1978). Covert modeling: The therapeutic application of imagined rehearsal. In J. L. Singer & K. S. Pope (Eds.), *The power of human imagination: New methods in psychotherapy. Emotions, personality, and psychotherapy* (pp. 255-278). New York: Plenum.

Keeling, R. P. (Ed.). (1989). *AIDS on the college campus* (2nd ed.). Rockville, MD: American College Health Association.

Kelly, J. A., St. Lawrence, J. S., Hood, H. V., & Brasfield, T. L. (1989). Behavioral intervention to reduce AIDS risk activities. *Journal of Consulting and Clinical Psychology, 57,* 60-67.

Killen, J. D., Robinson, T. N., Telch, M. J., Saylor, K. E., Maron, D. J., Rich, T., & Bryson, S. (1989). The Stanford adolescent heart health program. *Health Education Quarterly, 16,* 263-283.

Levinson, R. A. (1986). Contraceptive self-efficacy: A perspective on teenage girls' contraceptive behavior. *Journal of Sex Research, 22,* 347-369.

Maddux, J. E., & Rogers, R. W. (1983). Protection motivation and self-efficacy: A revised theory of fear appeals and attitude change. *Journal of Experimental Social Psychology, 19,* 469-479.

Maibach, E. W. (1990). *Symbolic modeling and cognitive rehearsal: Using video to promote AIDS prevention self-efficacy.* Unpublished doctoral dissertation, Stanford University, Stanford, CA.

Maibach, E., Flora, J., & Nass, C. (1991). Changes in self-efficacy and health behavior in response to a minimal contact community health campaign. *Health Communication, 3,* 1-15.

Mantell, J. E., & Schinke, S. P. (in press). The crisis of AIDS for adolescents: The need for preventive risk-reduction interventions. In A. R. Roberts (Ed.), *Contemporary perspectives on crisis intervention and prevention.* Englewood Cliffs, NJ: Prentice-Hall.

Mantell, J. E., Schinke, S. P., & Akabas, S. H. (1988). Women and AIDS prevention. *Journal of Primary Prevention, 9,* 18-40.

Mays, V. M., & Cochran, S. D. (1988). Issues in the perception of AIDS risk and risk reduction activities by black and Hispanic/Latina women. *American Psychologist, 43,* 949-957.

McCune, J. M., Namikawa, R., Shih, C., Rabin, L., & Kaneshima, H. (1990). Suppression of HIV infection in AZT-treated SCID-hu mice. *Science, 247,* 564-566.

McGuire, W. J. (1984). Public communication as a strategy for inducing health-promoting behavioral change. *Preventive Medicine, 13,* 299-319.

McKusick, L., Coates, T. J., & Morin, S. F. (1989). *Longitudinal predictors of reductions in high risk sexual behaviors among gay men in San Francisco: The AIDS behavioral research project*. Paper presented at the 5th International Conference on AIDS, Montreal, Canada.

McKusick, L., Coates, T. J., Morin, S. F., Pollack, L., & Hoff, C. (1990). Longitudinal predictors of unprotected anal intercourse among gay men in San Fancisco. *Journal of Public Health, 80*, 978-983.

McKusick, L., Horstman, W., & Coates, T. J. (1985). AIDS and sexual behavior reported by gay men in San Francisco. *American Journal of Public Health, 75*, 493-496.

McKusick, L., Wiley, J., Coates, T. J., & Morin, S. F. (1986, November). *Predictors of AIDS behavioral risk reduction: The AIDS Behavioral Research Project*. Paper presented at the New Zealand AIDS Foundation Prevention Education Workshop, Auckland, New Zealand.

Meyerowitz, B. E., & Chaiken, S. (1987). The effect of message framing on breast self-examination attitudes, intentions, and behavior. *Journal of Personality and Social Psychology, 52*, 500-510.

O'Leary, A. (1985). Self-efficacy and health. *Behavior Research Therapy, 23*, 437-451.

O'Leary, A., Goodhart, F., Jemmott, L. S., & Boccher-Lattimore, D. (1992). Predictors of safer sexual behavior on the college campus: A social cognitive analysis. *Journal of American College Health, 39*.

Rosenthal, D., Moore, S., & Flynn, I. (1991). Adolescent self-efficacy, self-esteem, and sexual risk-taking. *Journal of Community & Applied Social Psychology, 1*, 77-88.

Sallis, J. F., Hill, R. D., Killen, J. D., Telch, M. J., Flora, J. A., Girard, J., & Taylor, C. B. (1986). Efficacy of self-help behavior modification materials in smoking cessation. *American Journal of Preventive Medicine, 2*, 342-344.

Siegel, J. E., Graham, J. D., & Stoto, M. A. (1990). Allocating resources among AIDS research strategies. *Policy Sciences, 23*, 1-23.

Siegel, K., Mesagno, F. P., Chen, J., & Christ, G. (1989). Factors distinguishing homosexual males practicing risky and safer sex. *Social Science Medicine, 28*, 561-569.

Slater, M. D. (1989). Social influences and cognitive control as predictors of self-efficacy and eating behavior. *Cognitive Therapy and Research, 13*, 231-245.

Stall, R., & Biernacki, P. (1986). Spontaneous remission from the problematic use of substances: An inductive model derived from a comparative analysis of the alcohol, opiate, tobacco, and food/obesity literatures. *International Journal of the Addictions, 21*, 1-23.

Stall, R., & Paul, J. (1989). *Changes in sexual risk for infection with the human immunodeficiency virus among gay and bisexual men in San Francisco*. (Document prepared for the World Health Organization Global Programme on AIDS). San Francisco: University of California.

Tversky, A., & Kahneman, D. (1981). The framing of decisions and the psychology of choice. *Science, 211*, 453-458.

Watters, J. K., Downing, M., Case, P., Lorvick, J., Cheng, Y., & Fergusson, B. (1990). AIDS prevention for intravenous drug users in the community: Street-based education and risk behavior. *American Journal of Community Psychology, 18*, 587-596.

Winett, R. A., Anderson, E. S., Moore, J. F., Sikkema, K. J., Hook, R., Webster, D. A., Taylor, C. D., Dalton, J. E., Ollendick, T. H., & Eisler, R. M. (in press). Family/media approach to HIV prevention: Results with a home-based, parent-teen video program. *Health Psychology*.

Zimbardo, P. G., Ebbesen, E. B., & Maslach, C. (1977). *Influencing attitudes and changing behavior*. Reading, MA: Addison-Wesley.

7

Impact of Perceived Social Norms on Adolescents' AIDS-Risk Behavior and Prevention

JEFFREY D. FISHER

STEPHEN J. MISOVICH

WILLIAM A. FISHER

Introduction

In response to the emergence of adolescence as a time of increased HIV risk, researchers have investigated various avenues for AIDS-risk reduction in this population. One of the most frequently utilized strategies involves increasing adolescents' knowledge about HIV/AIDS. Most interventions provide individuals with information about the specific means of viral transmission and about behaviors (e.g., condom use or abstinence) that can reduce AIDS

AUTHORS' NOTE: Work on this chapter was supported by NIMH grant number 1RO1MH46224-01 to the first and third authors.

risk, under the assumption that such information will increase HIV prevention. While early research indicated low levels of HIV knowl-edge among adolescents (Price, Desmond, & Kukulka, 1985), recent research has shown that adolescents have become more informed (Fisher & Misovich, 1991a), perhaps in part due to the profusion of knowledge-based HIV-risk-reduction interventions in the past de-cade, and some studies now demonstrate relatively high levels of knowledge regarding specific modes of HIV transmission (Brown, Fritz, & Barone, 1989; Fisher & Misovich, 1991a; Malavaud, Dumay, & Malavaud, 1990; Roscoe & Kruger, 1990). Nevertheless, significant deficits remain in adolescents' knowledge in some domains impor-tant for prevention (Fisher & Fisher, 1991; Hingson et al., 1989; Williams et al., in press), and knowledge levels appear to remain low in some minority groups (Bell, Feraios, & Bryan, 1990; DiClemente, Boyer, & Morales, 1988; DiClemente, Zorn, & Temoshok, 1987).

Even when adolescents' HIV knowledge is high, it has not generally translated into safer sexual practices (DiClemente, 1990; Fisher & Misovich, 1991a; Roscoe & Kruger, 1990; Ross & Rosser, 1989). In fact, it has been demonstrated consistently that adoles-cent HIV knowledge is a necessary but not a sufficient condition for adolescents adopting preventive practices (Fisher & Fisher, 1992). In spite of this, the vast majority of HIV-risk-reduction interventions for adolescents have focused and continue to focus solely on providing adolescents with HIV information.

Given the apparent limitations of knowledge-based interventions, other means of eliciting behavior change in adolescents must be inves-tigated. We have argued elsewhere (Fisher, 1988; Fisher & Misovich, 1990) that extant, anti-prevention reference group social norms consti-tute a significant cause of adolescents' (and others') HIV-risk behavior and that changing such norms in a pro-prevention direction could constitute an essential element in successful HIV-risk-reduction inter-ventions. In this chapter, we review past and more recent work by ourselves and others that focuses on the effects of reference group social norms on HIV-risk behavior and prevention and that suggests ways to change such norms in order to increase prevention.

Social Norms, Risk Behavior, and Prevention

Social science researchers have long accepted the notion that *social norms*—"expected modes of behavior and belief that are established formally or informally by a group" (Jones & Gerard, 1967)—are important determinants of group members' behavior. The mechanism by which social norms affect group members' behavior has generally been termed *normative social influence,* which occurs when members behave in a particular way in order to gain approval from their reference group or to avoid group sanctions (Deutsch & Gerard, 1955).

We would argue that, at present, normative social influence is responsible for much of adolescent HIV-risk behavior. Presently, anti-prevention reference group norms among adolescents discourage HIV prevention due to fear of social sanctions, which occur when group norms are violated. Because the normative adolescent script for sexual relations is to have them without a presex discussion regarding HIV prevention (Fisher & Misovich, 1991b; Williams et al., in press), adolescents expect sanctions for failing to conform to this script. In our work, interviews with primarily heterosexual college students suggested that they found it "easier to have [unprotected] sex than to discuss STD prevention" (Fisher & Misovich, 1990). Both males and females feared rejection by their sex partner (i.e., sanctions) if they failed to conform to group norms and discussed the topic of prevention (Fisher & Misovich, 1990; Williams et al., in press). If adolescent norms could be changed in a pro-prevention direction, adolescent HIV prevention would increase dramatically because conforming to pro-prevention norms would then be reinforced by the peer group.

In addition to research that suggests that violating social norms results in sanctions in and of itself (Schachter, 1951), attributions are more apt to be made for behaviors that violate norms than for behaviors that conform to norms (Jones & Davis, 1965). In the case of adolescents (and others) who initiate HIV prevention in the context of group norms that are inconsistent with this activity, the resulting attributions may be very damaging and may result in additional sanctions. These attributions may suggest that an individual initiating condom use is at risk for or has an STD or HIV (perhaps due to promiscuity, practicing gay or bisexual sex, or IV drug use) or that the individual initiating condom use believes the partner is at risk for or has an STD or HIV (perhaps for the same reasons) (Williams et al., in press). Other likely (and also damaging) attributions that may be associated with violating anti-prevention norms and initiating safer sex are that the initiator is "uncool," neurotic, or untrusting (Williams et al., in press).

Due to the negative social consequences for adolescents of violating HIV-prevention-relevant norms and the fact that, in contrast, conforming to such norms is rewarded, HIV-prevention-relevant social norms have been viewed as important elements in adolescents' motivation to practice prevention (DiClemente & Fisher, 1991; Fisher & Fisher, 1991). While norms regarding prevention are thought to affect HIV prevention across populations at risk for HIV, adolescents have been described as uniquely susceptible to normative pressures (White, 1987), including pressures to perform risky and safer sexual activities (Brooks-Gunn & Furstenberg, 1989; Petosa & Wessinger, 1990).

The notion that adolescent norms can strongly influence levels of risky or safer behavior has been supported in domains outside of AIDS prevention. Adolescent norms regarding contraception have been found to affect adolescent contraceptive behavior (Lowe & Radius, 1987; Stanton, Black, Keane, & Feigelman, 1990), and adolescent norms regarding drinking and driving have been found to affect the incidence of this risky behavior (e.g., McKnight, 1986). Similarly, peer norms regarding smoking have been found to be an important cause of adolescent smoking (cf. Fishbein, 1982; Grube, Morgan, & McGree, 1986; Krosnick & Judd, 1982), and the belief that drug and/or alcohol use are normative in an adolescent's peer group is a strong predictor of group members' use of these substances (Kandel, Kessler, & Margulies, 1978).

In addition to *behavior-specific* norms that may affect relatively circumscribed behaviors (e.g., norms regarding safer sex or condom use, which affect the likelihood of these behaviors; norms regarding drinking and driving, which affect the likelihood of driving while intoxicated), *general* group norms and values may affect risk-taking behavior more broadly. For instance, it is normative for people in their late teens and 20s to feel invulnerable, to believe they are impervious to negative events (Gochman & Saucier, 1982; Kreipe, 1985), and to take risks (Kitzner, 1989). Furthermore, research findings indicate that adolescents often view risk as a value and do not want to appear less risky than their peers (e.g., exhibit neurotic overconcern) (Levinger & Schneider, 1969; Wallach & Wing, 1968). It is also normative for adolescents to show little concern regarding their health (Radius, Dielman, Becker, Rosenstock, & Horvath, 1980). Taken together, these more general normative values imply that lack of HIV prevention would be widespread among adolescents and that appearing concerned about HIV would be inconsistent with norms that promote personal invincibility and risk taking and would regard neurotic overconcern as a negative trait. Among adolescents in certain social and ethnic groups, exhibiting concern about HIV would also be inconsistent with "machismo" values (Vazquez-Nuttall, Avila-Vivas, & Morales-Barreto, 1984).

Perceived Norms and HIV Prevention

A model describing the effects of social influence on HIV risk and prevention may serve as a useful framework for understanding the effects of perceived norms on these behaviors (Fisher, 1988). According to this model, to the extent that both general and behavior-specific group norms are consistent with HIV prevention, *normative social influence* processes within the group work to increase preventive behavior. Under these circumstances, members of an individual's social network provide support for engaging in HIV prevention and may even engage in sanctions against members who are risky in their sexual practices. Further, when group norms are pro-prevention, members are apt to be exposed to *informational social influence* supporting HIV-preventive behavior (e.g., information from peers about the efficacy and utility of specific prevention practices, practical how-to information from peers imparting the behavioral skills necessary for practicing risk-reduction activities, and perhaps even eroticizing HIV prevention). In effect, when group norms are pro-prevention, normative social influence is likely to work in tandem with informational social influence to foster HIV prevention. (See Figure 7.1.)

If group norms are anti-prevention, different effects may be observed. In this case, the reference group will not support HIV-preventive behavior in group members and even may engage in sanctions against individuals perceived as pro-prevention or who are engaging in preventive behaviors. To the extent that group norms are inconsistent with prevention, group-level normative social influence will be directed toward thwarting prevention and promoting whatever alternative norms exist (e.g., "casual sex"). Further, when group norms are inconsistent with prevention, the group is likely to provide informational social influence that is

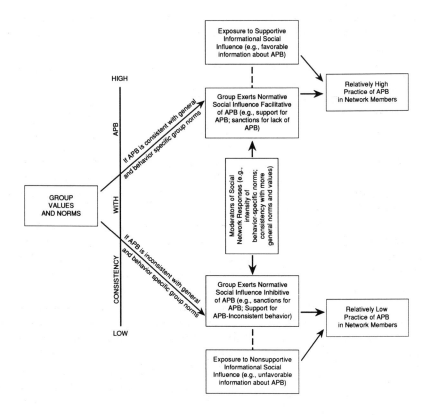

Figure 7.1. Effects of Group Norms on AIDS-Preventive Behavior (APB)

nonsupportive of risk reduction. Individuals in such groups are more apt to receive information from peers that HIV-preventive behaviors (e.g., using condoms) are either unnecessary or ineffective or that they will lead to negative physical or social consequences (e.g., the loss of sensation, rejection by partners). These elements of normative and informational social influence are likely to lead to lower levels of HIV prevention in members of such groups. The rationale for our prediction that peers will discourage prevention via normative and informational social influence when prevention is nonnormative but will encourage prevention through these means when it is normative is theoretical work (Fisher & Goff, 1986; Nadler & Fisher, in press) suggesting that social networks and reference groups are generally conservative and are motivated to protect the status quo in terms of norms and values.

The strength of the network's response in supporting or failing to support HIV prevention will depend in part on the intensity of *behavior-specific* HIV-prevention group norms. If behavior-specific norms (e.g., regarding the use of condoms) are more strongly pro-prevention, HIV prevention will be more strongly encouraged via normative and informational social influence. Conversely, if behavior-specific norms are more strongly anti-prevention, HIV prevention will be discouraged more strongly via normative and informational social influence.

In addition to the intensity of *behavior-specific* norms, the extent to which HIV prevention is consistent or inconsistent with more *general* norms and underlying values (Nadler & Fisher, in press) will affect the strength of the network's pro- or anti-prevention response (see Figure 7.1). If using condoms conflicts with behavior-specific norms and also with general underlying norms and values central to the group's belief system (e.g., the notion that risk is a value), it will be challenged more strongly via normative and informational social influence, and risky behavior will be more strongly reinforced. Unfortunately this is presently the case with adolescents, making HIV prevention in this group relatively uncommon and making normative change especially important— both with respect to behavior-specific norms regarding prevention, and also with regard to more general underlying values. On the other hand, if HIV-preventive behavior is consistent with behavior-specific norms and with general core values in a group's assumptive system (as is becoming more the case for gay men, especially those residing in major cities) (Kelly et al., 1990), it will be supported vigorously by the social network.

The Effects of Perceived Norms on HIV Prevention

Other conceptual work has suggested the powerful effect that reference group social norms may have on HIV-risk behavior in adolescents and others who are at risk for HIV. The Committee on HIV Research in the Behavioral, Social, and Statistical Sciences has stated that in addition to information and other factors, widespread behavior change may require modification of perceived norms for behavior (Miller, Turner, & Moses, 1990). Coates and his colleagues (e.g., Coates & Greenblatt, 1989; McKusick, Conant, & Coates, 1985) emphasize that for interventions to produce and sustain HIV-risk reduction, it is necessary to intervene at the community level, as well as at the individual level, to make risk behavior less socially acceptable and to increase individuals' perceptions that risk behavior will result in social sanctions. Finally, researchers have suggested the importance of changing norms to elicit behavior change in gay men (Kelly et al., 1990) and in injection drug users (DesJarlais, 1989). Changing norms also have been identified as an important prerequisite to widespread behavior change within minority populations (Mays & Cochran, 1988).

In accord with these assertions, empirical research on HIV prevention among gay men has found that changing perceived group norms regarding prevention does affect individuals' level of risk reduction. DesJarlais (1989) found that HIV-prevention programs for IV drug users frequently are able to change participants' perceptions of needle-sharing norms and reported that these changes resulted in HIV-risk-reduction behavior. In addition, Friedman et al. (1987) reported that for IV drug users in New York City, the strongest predictor of behavior change was the belief that one's friends were changing their IV drug use behavior in response to HIV.

Finally, individual differences in perceived group norms appear to predict levels of preventive behavior. McKusick, Coates, and Morin (1990) report that HIV-preventive behavior was greater among gay and bisexual men who perceived their group's social norms to support HIV-risk reduction than among those who did not; parallel findings were reported by Joseph et al. (1987). Fisher and Misovich (1990) found that men who were more involved with homophile organizations (in which norms are typically more pro-prevention) were more apt to engage in HIV prevention then men who were less involved with such organizations. Research on men who patronize gay bars (Kelly et al., 1990) also demonstrated the predicted relationship between perceived social norms for HIV-risk reduction and actual risk-reduction behavior.

College Students' Perceived Norms
for Safer Sex Practices

To determine the degree to which college age adolescents view their peers as pro- or anti-HIV-prevention and to explore the relationship between this and their actual levels of prevention, in the spring of 1990 our research team distributed a questionnaire to 284 undergraduate students. The questionnaire tapped participants' perceived peer group norms for safer sexual practices (i.e., condom use, refusing to have unsafe sex, and trying to persuade sexual partners to engage in safer sex), measured subjects' actual safer sex practices, and contained other items concerning the topic of HIV. Data on perceived peer norms were collected on a 5-point scale, with 1 indicating that it was perceived as "very true" that the peer group supported that behavior, and 5 indicating that it was perceived as "very untrue." Two months later, the same subjects completed a follow-up questionnaire that asked them, among other things, to report the extent to which they had engaged in safer sexual practices over the previous 2 months. The perceived social norm data from two different sets of peers (i.e., friends, and present or potential sexual partners) are presented in Table 7.1. Differences in students' perceptions of norms for HIV prevention among friends and sexual partners, and the differential impact of these two groups on individuals' own levels of preventive behavior (see Table 7.2) can provide us with information regarding which group of peers has the greater impact on adolescents' HIV-relevant behavior.

Table 7.1 illustrates students' perceived norms for the three preventive behaviors. For each, the percentage of subjects who believed that their friends and their sexual partners supported or did not support their performing the behavior are presented. The data indicate that for all of the preventive behaviors measured, the degree of perceived support both from friends and sexual partners was far from uniform or consistently enthusiastic. In effect, the majority of the subjects believed that friends and sexual partners did not support their performance of many HIV-preventive behaviors. Summing into a single category, the percentages of students who responded "neither true nor untrue," "somewhat untrue," or

Table 7.1   Perceived Norms for HIV-Preventive Behaviors

	Very true	Somewhat true	Neither true nor untrue	Somewhat untrue	Very untrue
My partners believe I should always use condoms					
Female	20.4%	20.4%	30.7%	12.4%	16.1%
Male	20.2%	28.7%	36.4%	7.8%	7.0%
My friends believe I should always use condoms					
Females	29.2%	21.9%	41.6%	3.6%	3.6%
Males	12.2%	29.0%	52.7%	3.1%	3.1%
My partners believe I should refuse to have unsafe sex					
Females	28.3%	15.9%	35.5%	13.0%	7.2%
Males	24.8%	25.6%	42.6%	4.7%	2.3%
My friends believe I should refuse to have unsafe sex					
Females	48.6%	13.6%	30.7%	1.4%	5.7%
Males	14.6%	23.8%	47.7%	10.0%	3.8%
My partners believe I should try to persuade my partners to practice only safer sex					
Females	23.9%	14.9%	52.2%	4.5%	4.5%
Males	14.7%	22.5%	57.4%	3.1%	2.3%
My friends believe I should try to persuade my partners to practice only safer sex					
Females	36.9%	22.0%	36.9%	1.4%	2.8%
Males	10.7%	25.2%	51.1%	9.9%	3.1%

"very untrue" with respect to a particular peer group supporting a given preventive behavior illustrates this finding. For example, 59% of the adolescent females and 51% of the adolescent males did not think it was true that their *current or potential sexual partners* felt that they should always use condoms. Forty-nine percent of the females and 59% of the males did not think it was true that their *friends* felt that they should always use condoms. Nearly half (49%) of the male subjects and more than half (56%) of the females thought that their sexual partners would not support their refusal to have unsafe sex. More than half (62%) of the males and 37% of the females perceived their friends as nonsupportive of their refusing to have unsafe sex.

A similar pattern of results emerged with the question concerning discussion of safer sexual practices. A majority of females (61%) and males (63%) thought that their present and potential sexual partners would not support their persuading them to practice only safer sex. Forty-one percent of the females and 65% of the

Table 7.2   Correlations Between Perceived Norms for Condom Use
                  and Actual Condom Use

| | Condom Use at Time 1 | | Condom Use at Time 2 | |
	Male	Female	Male	Female
Partner norm at Time 1	.48**	.42**	.57**	.52**
Friend norm at Time 1	.15	.29**	.15	.44**

**p<.01

males thought that their friends also would not support their persuading their current and potential sexual partners to practice only safer sex. These data indicate that many college students do not perceive their friends and sexual partners as being strongly supportive of their practicing safer sexual behaviors. In many instances, the students believed that their friends and partners were *unsupportive* of their performing these behaviors.

**Correlations Between Perceived Norms
and Actual Preventive Behavior**

To determine the relationship between their perceived norms for preventive behavior and students' actual sexual practices, we correlated the perceived friend and partner norms for the most essential preventive behavior—consistent condom use—with the reported level of performing this behavior (see Table 7.2). The information on students' actual condom use behavior was collected both at the time of the original administration of the norm questions and from the same subjects 2 months later so that we could investigate the relationship between perceived norms and behavior at a later date. Collecting the preventive behavior data 2 months later also helped us deal with potential response bias that could emerge when asking subjects questions about norms for behavior and about their actual behavior at the same time.

For both males and females, perceived norms of *present and potential future sexual partners* regarding condom use were associated strongly with actual frequency of condom use both at the time of the initial questionnaire (Time 1), and at the time of the follow-up (Time 2). The correlation between this norm and condom use at Time 1 was .48 for males ($p<.01$) and .42 for females ($p<.01$), indicating that perceived partner norms were related strongly to current condom use. Further, perceived partner norms measured at Time 1 were a very strong predictor of actual condom use 2 months later at Time 2: The correlations between perceived partner norms at Time 1 and condom use at Time 2 were .57 ($p<.01$) for males and .52 ($p<.01$) for females. Perceived *friend* norms for condom use had a weaker effect on actual condom use, especially among male subjects. Friends' norms for condom use at Time 1 and actual condom use at Time 1 correlated .29 ($p<.01$) for females and .15 (n.s.) for males. Friend norms for condom use at Time 1 correlated .44 ($p<.01$) with actual condom use at Time 2 among females, and .15 (n.s.) for males.

In summary, perceived norms toward condom use among one's present and potential future sexual partners strongly predicted actual condom use. Adolescents who believed their current and potential future partners supported their using condoms were more likely to use condoms consistently; adolescents who believed that their current and potential future partners did not support their condom use were less likely to engage in this essential form of prevention. For both genders, the perceived norms of one's friends were less strongly associated with condom use than were the perceived norms of sex partners; for males, perceived friend norms did not have a significant effect. In terms of interventions, this suggests that to increase condom use in both genders, it may be most useful to attempt to change perceived (or actual) prevention-related norms of present and potential future sex partners. This could be accomplished through mixed-sex interventions suggesting that potential adolescent sexual partners *expect* individuals to use condoms (Fisher & Fisher, 1991). In light of the very high extant rates of perceived *nonsupport* for HIV prevention among present and potential sex partners, a great deal of potential for change appears to exist. Because these norms appear to be predictive of preventive behavior, such a change may well translate into increased prevention among adolescents.

The study described above measured college students' perceived norms regarding prevention by assessing individuals' beliefs about how certain peers (i.e., friends and present and future sexual partners) think they should behave regarding HIV prevention. Earlier in this chapter, it was noted that beliefs about how reference group members think one should behave reflect reference group norms. Conforming or failing to conform to such beliefs (i.e., conforming to or violating group norms) elicits rewards or sanctions. In a second study (Fisher & Misovich, 1991b), we measured perceived reference group norms by simply assessing the extent to which college students believed that HIV prevention was normative within their peer group. To do this, we embedded two items in a larger questionnaire. One item measured perceived norms for HIV-preventive-behavior change at a global level by tapping the extent of subjects' endorsement of the item, "Many people I know have made changes in their lives to protect themselves against HIV." The second item measured perceived norms for college students' use of condoms in particular by indexing subjects' endorsement of the statement, "Many students are trying to protect themselves by using condoms." Both of these items then were correlated individually with a measure of actual condom use (i.e., "What percentage of your sexual relations involve the use of condoms?").

For both males and females, perceived norms for HIV-risk-behavior change at a global level were associated with condom use. For males, the global perception that HIV-risk-behavior change was normative correlated with actual condom use ($r = .33$; $p<.006$), indicating that males who believed that many people they knew had changed their behaviors in response to HIV were themselves more likely to use condoms. The same relationship, though slightly weaker, was identified for females ($r = .22$, $p<.03$). Similarly males' and females' perceptions of peer norms regarding condom use in particular were correlated significantly with reports of actual condom use. Males who felt that many students were trying to protect themselves by using condoms used condoms more frequently in their own sexual activity ($r = .25$, $p<.04$). Females showed the same pattern, with stronger perceived norms for condom use being associated with a higher percentage of condom use ($r = .26$, $p<.01$).

Both studies indicate that perceived norms regarding prevention are consistently predictive of HIV-preventive behavior. These findings are corroborated by other studies on the relation between perceived adolescent norms for prevention and actual levels of prevention. For instance, Catania et al. (1989) reported that perceived norms regarding HIV prevention predicted adolescents' number of sexual partners. Similarly, DiClemente (1990) reported that although knowledge about HIV and HIV prevention were unrelated to risk reduction among adolescents, those who believed that condom use was supported by their peers were nearly twice as likely to use condoms during intercourse. The effect of perceived normative behavior is also influential among high-risk, incarcerated adolescents (DiClemente, 1991). In this study, youth in juvenile detention facilities were almost five times as likely to report consistent condom use if they perceived peer norms as supporting condom use. Finally, in research among ethnically diverse, sexually active inner-city adolescents, those who believed their peers frequently used condoms were over four times as likely to report consistent condom use themselves (DiClemente & Fisher, 1991).

Changing HIV-Prevention Norms to Increase Prevention

The findings suggest that it may be extremely useful to institute group-level interventions to change reference group norms in a pro-prevention direction and that this ultimately may increase adolescents' HIV prevention. Unfortunately, few if any adolescent HIV-risk-reduction programs have explicitly attempted to change group norms to promote HIV-prevention activities. Nevertheless, the model that has been presented in this chapter and related conceptual work (Fisher & Fisher, 1992) generate suggestions for HIV-prevention interventions to influence adolescents through group-level techniques.

In order to change adolescents' (or any other group's) HIV-risk behaviors through group-level interventions designed to change social norms, a series of steps must be undertaken. First, it is necessary to ascertain through elicitation research (Fisher & Fisher, 1992) the HIV-prevention-relevant norms of the target group in question. This would include determining the *specific* norms for such HIV-risk-reduction behaviors as condom use and abstinence, and the relevant, underlying, *general* norms and core values (e.g., the group's beliefs regarding the valence of risky behavior in general). Once the group's HIV-relevant norms have been measured, intervention planners may use this information to determine the extent to which extant norms and/or values must be changed.

Adolescent social norms may be manipulated in interventions through a variety of techniques (Fisher & Fisher, 1991). One method of changing prevention-related norms involves the continual presence in the intervention of attractive, popular peers who continually endorse HIV prevention and attempt to make it seem like "the in thing to do." In light of the minority influence literature (Moscovici & Faucheux, 1972), it would appear that individuals who espouse preventive behaviors in a group that is generally anti-prevention will be most likely to influence majority behavior when they are (a) similar to the majority except in the particular position they are advocating, (b) consistent in their views over time, and (c) not rigid or dogmatic in upholding their views (Baron & Byrne, 1987). Workshops in which attractive undergraduate fraternity and sorority members were trained to promote prevention in fraternity and sorority members by behaving in the above-described manner were generally viewed as successful (Fisher & Misovich, 1990).

A second intervention approach to changing reference group norms involves the presentation of videotaped pro-prevention testimonials by individuals who are viewed by adolescents as especially influential referent others. The particular others who constitute the most effective referent others for changing norms in adolescents (e.g., national or local adolescent "natural opinion leaders") may be identified in elicitation research or by examining relevant literature. For example, Brown, Fritz, and Barone (1989) found that an HIV-education videotape starring a popular female teenage actress had a stronger effect on adolescent females than on adolescent males or pre-adolescents. Once optimal referent others have been identified, these individuals could convey pro-AIDS-prevention messages either live or on videotape. Similarly, research in the gay community has reported that live testimonials by attractive natural opinion leaders can change HIV-prevention norms (Kelly et al., 1991) and ultimately levels of preventive behavior.

A final normative change component may involve the changed behavior of adolescent intervention participants themselves. Once social norms in a group begin to change, other group members will observe these changes, which ultimately will reverberate throughout the group. We suspect that this process may be hastened if the intervention involves giving participants very attractive, adolescent-oriented, and professionally designed T-shirts, pens, and other artifacts with pro-prevention slogans on them. If these are sufficiently attractive and valuable that teens use them, such use may effect a change both in their own perceived norms (through a counterattitudinal advocacy, public commitment procedure) and in the perceived norms of others who observe them (to the extent that observing others wearing HIV-prevention artifacts leads HIV prevention to appear normative).

Most of the techniques presented above (e.g., including pro-HIV-prevention peers in the intervention, having influential others make pro-HIV-prevention testimonials) attempt to change *behavior-specific* norms as opposed to more *general* group norms and values. To the extent that the group that is the target of a behavior-specific norm change attempt views HIV-prevention-related issues as conflicting with general core norms and values (e.g., to the extent the target group views risk as a value or perceives itself to be invulnerable to negative events), behavior-specific normative change attempts may be resisted. In addition, attempts to change the group's behavior-specific norms may have less of an enduring effect unless general norms and core values inconsistent with HIV prevention are weakened. For adolescents, who view risk as a value, who have little concern for their health (Radius et al., 1980), and who feel relatively invulnerable to negative events, including HIV (Gochman & Saucier, 1982), such values may need to be modified before behavior-specific pro-HIV-prevention norms and behaviors can be maintained.

While it clearly will be more difficult to change behavior-specific norms or to maintain changes in such norms when underlying general core values are not consistent, it is possible to change these norms without modifying underlying values. For example, it is conceivable that through the techniques described above, through aggressive advertising, or by pairing condom use with rewards highly valued by adolescents, condom use could become the "in" thing to do, without changing adolescents' belief in risk as a value or in their perceived invulnerability. At the limit, condom use could become the norm in the same way that athletic shoes that "pump up" are currently the norm, and condoms would then be used simply because they are associated with social rewards, regardless of whether adolescents retain more general beliefs in risk as a value. For instance, if condom use were paired for adolescents with the same rewards that are associated in advertising with drinking beer, a large-scale increase in HIV-prevention behavior would occur in adolescent males regardless of whether condom use conformed to more general prevention-related values of adolescents.

Before concluding, a few caveats are in order. While we believe that interventions that change adolescents' social norms would impact strongly on HIV prevention, intervention elements that affect such other factors as adolescents' attitudes toward prevention, their perceived vulnerability to HIV, and the perceived efficacy of HIV prevention should be incorporated into attempts to reduce HIV risk among adolescents. Like perceived norms, many of these factors affect individuals' motivation to practice prevention (Fisher & Fisher, 1992). Another important element for behavior change in adolescents is training in the behavioral skills necessary for prevention. Unfortunately, components affecting motivation and behavioral skills have generally been excluded from HIV-education programs targeted at adolescents, which tend to focus merely on imparting HIV-relevant information (Fisher & Fisher, 1992). Because recent research has demonstrated that actual levels of HIV prevention among adolescents are a function of their levels of information, motivation, and behavioral skills (Fisher & Fisher, 1992), it is important for interventions encompassing all three of these elements to become the norm in the future.

References

Baron, R. A., & Byrne, D. (1987). *Social psychology: Understanding human interaction.* Boston: Allyn & Bacon.

Bell, D., Feraios, A., & Bryan, T. (1990). Adolescent males' knowledge and attitudes about HIV in the context of their social world. *Journal of Applied Social Psychology, 20,* 424-448.

Brooks-Gunn, J., & Furstenburg, F. F. (1989). Adolescent sexual behavior. *American Psychologist, 44,* 249-257.

Brown, L. K., Fritz, G. K., & Barone, V. J. (1989). The impact of HIV education on junior and senior high school students. *Journal of Adolescent Health Care, 10,* 386-392.

Catania, J. A., Dolcini, M. M., Coates, T. J., Kegeles, S. M., Greenblatt, R., Puckett, S., Corman, M., & Miller, J. (1989). Predictors of condom use and multiple partnered sex among sexually active adolescent women: Implications for HIV-related health interventions. *Journal of Sex Research, 26,* 514-524.

Coates, T. J., & Greenblatt, R. M. (1989). Behavioral change using community level interventions. In K. Holmes (Ed.), *Sexually transmitted diseases* (pp. 1075-1080). New York: McGraw-Hill.

DesJarlais, D. C. (1989). HIV prevention programs for intravenous drug users: Diversity and evolution. *International Review of Psychiatry, 1,* 101-108.

Deutsch, M., & Gerard, H. B. (1955). A study of normative and informational social influences on individual judgment. *Journal of Abnormal and Social Psychology, 51,* 629-636.

DiClemente, R. J. (1990). Adolescents and AIDS: Current research, prevention strategies and public policy. In L. Temoshok & A. Baum (Eds.), *Psychological aspects of AIDS and HIV disease* (pp. 52-64). Hillsdale, NJ: Lawrence Erlbaum.

DiClemente, R. J. (1991). Predictors of HIV-preventive sexual behavior in a high-risk adolescent population: The influence of perceived peer norms and sexual communication on incarcerated adolescents' consistent use of condoms. *Journal of Adolescent Health, 12,* 385-390.

DiClemente, R. J., Boyer, C. B., & Morales, E. (1988). Minorities and AIDS: Knowledge, attitudes and misconceptions among black and Latino adolescents. *American Journal of Public Health, 1,* 55-57.

DiClemente, R. J., & Fisher, J. D. (1991). *Predictors of HIV-preventive sexual behavior among adolescents in an HIV epicenter: The influence of communication and perceived referent group norms on frequency of condom use.* Unpublished manuscript, University of California, San Francisco.

DiClemente, R. J., Zorn, J., & Temoshok, L. (1987). The association of gender, ethnicity, and length of residence in the Bay area to adolescents' knowledge and attitudes about acquired immune deficiency syndrome. *Journal of Applied Social Psychology, 17,* 216-230.

Fishbein, M. (1982). Social psychological analysis of smoking behavior. In J. R. Eiser (Ed.), *Social psychology and behavioral medicine* (pp. 179-197). Chichester, UK: Wiley.

Fisher, J. D. (1988). Possible effects of reference group-based social influence on HIV-risk behavior and HIV prevention. *American Psychologist, 43,* 914-920.

Fisher, J. D., & Fisher, W. A. (1991). *A general social psychological technology for changing HIV risk behavior.* Unpublished manuscript, University of Connecticut, Storrs, CT.

Fisher, J. D., & Fisher, W. A. (1992). A general social psychological model for changing HIV risk behavior. *Psychological Bulletin, 111,* 455-474.

Fisher, J. D., & Goff, B. A. (1986, July). *Social support, life events, and change: Blood may be thicker than water, but is it always better?* Paper presented at the International Conference on Personal Relationships, Herzalia, Israel.

Fisher, J. D., & Misovich, S. J. (1990). Social influence and HIV-preventive behavior. In J. Edwards, R. S. Tindale, L. Heath, & E. J. Posevac (Eds.), *Social influence processes and prevention* (pp. 39-70). New York: Plenum.

Fisher, J. D., & Misovich, S. J. (1991a). Evolution of college students' HIV-related behavioral responses, attitudes, knowledge, and fear. *HIV Education and Prevention, 2,* 322-337.

Fisher, J. D., & Misovich, S. J. (1991b). *Perceived peer support for HIV prevention and condom use among college students.* Unpublished manuscript, University of Connecticut, Storrs, CT.

Friedman, S. R., DesJarlais, D. C., Sotheran, J. L., Garber, J. Cohen, H., & Smith, D. (1987). HIV and self-organization among intravenous drug users. *International Journal of the Addictions, 22,* 201-220.

Gochman, D. S., & Saucier, J. (1982). Perceived vulnerability in children and adolescents. *Health Education Quarterly, 9,* 142-155.

Grube, J. W., Morgan, M., & McGree, S. T. (1986). Attitudes and normative beliefs as predictors of smoking intentions and behaviors: A test of three models. *British Journal of Social Psychology, 25,* 81-93.

Hingson, R., Strunin, L., Craven, D. E., Mofenson, L., Mangione, T., Berlin, B., Amaro, H., & Lamb, G. A. (1989). Survey of HIV knowledge and behavior changes among Massachusetts adults. *Preventive Medicine, 18,* 808-818.

Jones, E. E., & Davis, K. E. (1965). From acts to dispositions: The attribution process in person perception. In L. Berkowitz (Ed.), *Advances in experimental social psychology* (Vol. 2). (pp. 219-266). New York: Academic Press.

Jones, E. E., & Gerard, H. B. (1967). *Foundations of social psychology.* New York: John Wiley.

Joseph, J. G., Montgomery, S. B., Emmons, C., Kessler, R. C., Ostrow, D. G., Wortman, C. B., O'Brien, K., Eller, M., & Eshleman, S. (1987). Magnitude and determinants of behavioral risk reduction: Longitudinal analysis of a cohort at risk for HIV. *Psychology and Health, 1,* 73-96.

Kandel, D. B., Kessler, R. C., & Margulies, R. Z. (1978). Antecedents of adolescent initiation into stages of drug use: A developmental analysis. *Journal of Youth and Adolescence, 7,* 13-40.

Kelly, J. A., St. Lawrence, J. S., Brasfield, T. L., Stevenson, L. Y., Diaz, Y. Y., & Hauth, A. C. (1990). HIV risk behavior patterns among gay men in small southern cities. *American Journal of Public Health, 80,* 416-418.

Kelly, J. A., St. Lawrence, J. S., Diaz, Y. E., Stevenson, Y., Hauth, A. C., Brasfield, T., Kalichman, S. C., Smith, J. E., & Andrew, M. E. (1991). HIV risk behavior reduction following intervention with key opinion leaders of population: An experimental analysis. *American Journal of Public Health, 81,* 168-171.

Kitzner, M. D. (1989). HIV prevention and education: Recommendations of the work group. *Journal of Adolescent Health Care, 10,* 45s-47s.

Kriepe, R. E. (1985). Normal adolescent development: Helping teenagers cope with change. *New York State Journal of Medicine, 5,* 214-217.

Krosnick, J. A., & Judd, C. M. (1982). Transitions in social influence at adolescence: Who induces cigarette smoking? *Developmental Psychology, 18,* 359-368.

Levinger, G., & Schneider, D. (1969). A test of the risk-as-a-value hypothesis. *Journal of Personality and Social Psychology, 11,* 165-169.

Lowe, C. S., & Radius, S. M. (1987). Young adults' contraceptive practices: An investigation of influences. *Adolescence, 22,* 291-304.

Malavaud, S., Dumay, F., & Malavaud, B. (1990). HIV infection: Assessment of sexual risk, knowledge, and attitudes towards prevention in 1,586 high school students in the Toulouse Education Authority Area. *American Journal of Health Promotion, 4,* 260-265.

Mays, V. M., & Cochran, S. D. (1988). Issues in the perception of HIV risk and risk reduction activities by black and Hispanic/Latina women. *American Psychologist, 43,* 949-957.

McKnight, J. A. (1986). Intervention in teenage drunk driving. *Alcohol, Drugs, and Driving Abstracts and Reviews, 2,* 17-28.

McKusick, L., Coates, T. J., & Morin, S. (1990). Longitudinal predictors of unprotected anal intercourse among gay and bisexual men in San Francisco: The HIV Behavioral Research Project. *American Journal of Public Health, 80,* 978-983.

McKusick, L., Conant, M. A., & Coates, T. J. (1985). The HIV epidemic: A model for developing intervention strategies for reducing high risk behavior in gay men. *Sexually Transmitted Diseases, 12,* 229-234.

Miller, H. G., Turner, C. F., & Moses, L. E. (Eds.). (1990). *HIV: The second decade.* Washington, DC: National Academy.

Moscovici, S., & Faucheux, C. (1972). The effects of consensus-breaking and consensus-preempting partners on reduction of conformity. *Journal of Personality and Social Psychology, 11,* 215-223.

Nadler, A., & Fisher, J. D. (in press). Volitional personal change in an interpersonal perspective. In Y. Klar, J. D. Fisher, J. M. Chinsky, & A. Nadler (Eds.), *Initiating self-changes: Social, psychological, and clinical perspectives.* New York: Springer-Verlag.

Petosa, R., & Wessinger, J. (1990). The HIV education needs of adolescents: A theory-based approach. *HIV Education and Prevention, 2,* 127-136.

Price, J. H., Desmond, S., & Kukulka, G. (1985). High school students' perceptions and misperceptions of HIV. *Journal of School Health, 55,* 107-109.

Radius, S. M., Dielman, T. E., Becker, M. H., Rosenstock, J. M., & Horvath, W. J. (1980). Adolescent perspectives on health and illness. *Adolescence, 15,* 375-384.

Roscoe, B., & Kruger, T. L. (1990). HIV: Late adolescents' knowledge and its influence on sexual behavior. *Adolescence, 25,* 39-48.

Ross, M. W., & Rosser, B. R. S. (1989). Education and HIV risks: A review. *Health Education Research: Theory and Practice, 4,* 273-284.

Schachter, S. (1951). Deviation, rejection and communication. *Journal of Abnormal and Social Psychology, 46,* 190-207.

Stanton, B., Black, M., Keane, V., & Feigelman, S. (1990). HIV risk behaviors in young people: Can we benefit from 30 years of research experience? *HIV and Public Policy Journal, 5,* 17-23.

Vazquez-Nuttall, E., Avila-Vivas, Z., & Morales-Barreto, G. (1984). Working with Latin American families. *Family Therapy Collections, 9,* 74-90.

Wallach, M., & Wing, C. (1968). Is risk a value? *Journal of Personality and Social Psychology, 9,* 101-106.

White, J. L. (1987). *The troubled adolescent.* Elmsford, NY: Pergamon.

Williams, S. S., Kimble, D. L., Hertzog, N. B., Newton, K. J., Fisher, J. D., & Fisher, W. A. (in press). College students use implicit personality theory instead of safer sex. *Journal of Applied Social Psychology.*

8

Using Mass Media for Prevention
of HIV Infection Among Adolescents

DANIEL ROMER

ROBERT C. HORNIK

Introduction

Mass media often are recommended as channels for dissemination of health information, especially regarding HIV (e.g., Freudenberg, 1989; Office of Technology Assessment, 1988). Nevertheless deliberate use of mass media for HIV education in the United States has been limited and as a result has yet to reach its potential. Although mass media have played a key role in informing Americans about HIV disease, much of this influence probably has been delivered through news reports and other informal educational channels. The national campaign for HIV education ("America Responds to AIDS") did not appear on television until late 1987, and the national mailing of HIV information to all households in the country ("Understanding AIDS") did not occur until mid-1988 (Shikles, 1988). Despite the slowness of these educational efforts, condom sales appeared to increase rapidly in 1987 (Moran, Janes, Peterman, & Stone, 1990). This surge in sales appeared to be attributable to the Surgeon General's 1986 endorsement of condoms for preventing HIV transmission and to the news and feature articles stimulated by the endorsement (Moran et al., 1990) rather than to the content of formal educational messages (Freimuth, Hammond, Edgar, & Monahan, 1989; Singer, Rogers, & Glassman, 1991).

It is in the context of underuse of the mass media for HIV education that we discuss the role of mass media as channels for HIV prevention in young people. We begin by contrasting the use of mass media for health promotion with the variety of channels that are available for health education.

Mass Media
as Health Communication Channels

Communication channels are systems for delivering messages to audiences. Channels include the materials on which the messages are recorded (e.g., books, audiotape, pamphlets), the distribution mechanisms for delivering the messages (e.g., schools, radio, clinics), and the people who deliver the messages (e.g., teachers, disc jockeys, nurses). Two types of channels can be distinguished— personal and mass communication—depending on whether messages are delivered between individuals who know each other or between a communicator and large audiences unknown to the communicator (Kotler & Roberto, 1989). *Mass communication* includes broadcasting (television and radio programming), print (magazines, newspapers, direct mail, etc.), displays (billboards, posters, etc.), mass-marketed recordings (audio and video tapes, films, records, etc.), and staged events (street theater, music festivals, etc.). *Personal communication* includes face-to-face interaction (health counseling, school teaching, community outreach, etc.), as well as mediated interaction (telephone conversation, mail correspondence, etc.).

One can also distinguish between a channel and the particular program that it carries. The same message may be delivered in many ways on any channel, depending on the format and length of the particular program. For example, one may dramatize the effects of HIV infection on a single episode of a regularly scheduled program. Alternatively one may reach the same audience with a 30-second message that can be shown on many episodes of the show. Although these are both uses of the same channel, they are different education programs that can have a differential impact on the audience.

In an ideal world, health educators would select the best channels to accomplish their goals in the same way they select messages, themes, and other education materials. Channels, however, often are selected because program planners have access to one or another intervention site and feel comfortable using that channel. As a result, research is seldom used to select channels, and education tends to be directed through channels that may not be optimal for program goals.

The most comprehensive criterion for evaluating health education is cost effectiveness. Mass media are among the most cost-effective channels for health education (DeJong & Winsten, 1989; Warner, 1987), and they should be used more frequently to encourage the prevention of HIV infection, to correct misinformation about the infection, and to create more sympathetic attitudes toward HIV-infected persons. The schools are probably the only other channel that can reach large numbers of young people. If we rely on the schools alone, however, we may not reach all young people effectively, and we may still not reach parents and other adults. The mass media not only have wide reach, they also have the power to promote the social changes that can help control the epidemic. To support this argument, we first will review how the cost-effectiveness of a channel is determined and why mass media are often superior to other channels. We then will review some recent uses of mass media for health promotion, including HIV education. Finally some barriers to using mass media for HIV education will be considered.

Evaluating Channels for Health Education

Any message potentially can be delivered across a variety of channels. In designing education programs, planners should consider the overall cost-effectiveness of alternative channels. *Cost-effectiveness* is composed of three components: (a) the ability to expose the audience to the message, (b) the ability to influence the audience that is exposed to the message, and (c) the ability to accomplish (a) and (b) in the most feasible and low-cost manner. Effective channels not only expose audiences to messages but also enhance the ability of those messages to influence audiences and to maintain this influence over time. Furthermore, the lower the cost and the more feasible it is to operate channels, the more education can be delivered with limited resources.

The cost-effectiveness of alternative channels can be compared by calculating a cost-effectiveness ratio (CER). The CER indexes the cost of achieving education goals for the average audience member. In the case of HIV education, these goals might be adoption of safer sex or safe needle practice for a specified period of time. A more stringent goal might be prevention of HIV transmission or of acquisition of some other sexually transmitted disease. The CER is a function of the total cost of an education program divided by the number of people for whom the education goal is met. The number of people for whom the goal is met is in turn a function of the exposure and influence of the program:

$$CER = (Cost\ of\ Program)/(Exposure \times Influence)$$

The CER can be compared across channels if the messages transmitted, the audiences targeted, and the education goals are the same. The lower the CER, the more effective a channel is per unit of cost (cf. Altman, Flora, Fortmann, & Farquhar, 1987; Weinstein, Graham, Siegel, & Fineberg, 1989).

The use of the CER for evaluating program alternatives can be illustrated by use of research on the effectiveness of smoking prevention and cessation programs. Research on smoking prevention has progressed to the point where cost-effectiveness calculations have been performed for a number of programs. For example, Altman et al. (1987) compared CERs for three smoking cessation programs: (a) class instruction over a period of eight sessions, (b) contests publicized over several channels with prizes for successful quitters, and (c) self-help kits that could be distributed at clinics or mailed to requestors. Self-help kits tended to produce the least audience influence; that is, kits tended to influence the smallest percentage of persons exposed to the program, while classes tended to influence the largest percentage of persons exposed to the program. Nevertheless classes were quite expensive, time consuming, and required a great deal of effort from both audience members and trainers. As a result, kits were the most cost-effective, producing the most change per unit of cost.

Although this analysis was not strictly a channel comparison, the three programs were probably most appropriate for different channels. Classroom instruction involves a personal channel, whereas the other two could be delivered along mass-communication channels. Furthermore, the example illustrates a common outcome of cost-effectiveness analyses: The program or channel that is least effective at the level of audience influence (i.e., percentage of audience influenced) may nevertheless be the most cost-effective (Hornik, 1989; Warner, 1987). This can occur for two reasons. First, audience exposure may be sufficiently greater for the less influential channel and may produce an overall greater impact per unit of cost. Second, if exposure across channels is held constant, the cost of reaching each audience member may be sufficiently low that the CER is still lower for the less influential channel.

Cost-effectiveness may not be the only criterion for choosing channels. Channels may differ in absolute reach, or budget considerations may rule out certain channels even if they are more cost-effective. Unless program designers evaluate all three components of the CER, however, they will be unlikely to select the best channel option. The most compelling argument for the use of personal channels is their greater influence among those persons exposed to the program. Because of their wider exposure and lower cost per person reached, however, mass media are often more effective in changing social standards and norms regarding novel behavior. To the degree that "safer sex" and compassion for HIV-positive persons are still novel behaviors, mass media would seem to be well suited for increasing our acceptance of these behaviors.

In the next section, we identify some of the major factors that determine cost-effectiveness, and we review some of the issues to consider as program planners consider choices among channels for delivering health messages.

Audience Exposure

Three factors make mass media channels effective at exposing audiences to messages: the ability to reach wide audiences, the ability to reach them frequently, and the ability to stimulate additional message exposure through informal social networks. Each factor is discussed in turn.

Reach. Reach can be quantified as the percentage of the target audience that can be exposed to the message at least once during a fixed period (e.g., the first year of the program). Mass media are among the most powerful sources of rapid social change in our culture. Because large audiences can be exposed to messages, the collective awareness and meaning of such novel concepts as safe sex can be transmitted quickly. Mass media not only have the ability to educate but also to change social norms (Fisher, 1988). Personal channels are limited in their ability to diffuse messages and require more time to do so.

Reach can be assessed readily for many mass communication channels by conducting surveys of media use (or by consulting available listener or readership data) that determine the times of day and programs that are watched or listened to, the newspapers and magazines that are read, and the ages and sex of the audience for these channels (e.g., Alcalay & Taplin, 1989). Appropriately selected mass media will have greater reach than personal channels within reasonable time periods.

Frequency. In addition to reaching the audience at least once, channels differ in their ability to send messages repeatedly over time. Repeated message exposure is critical for the adoption of novel behavior. Repetition makes messages more familiar and acceptable. It also increases the salience and importance of messages, making it more likely to set the audience's agenda and to increase the interest value of health recommendations.

Mass media tend to have regular audiences that can be reached repeatedly over time. As a result, they are ideally suited for delivering messages repeatedly. Of course, particular uses of mass media may not permit more than one or two exposures to a message. For example, if a television drama is to educate young people about the dangers of HIV infection, then the show may have wide reach but it will not be able to support repeated viewing without costly efforts to develop new plots and extended story lines. On the other hand, some personal channels that appear to afford ample frequency, such as school health education, may be less effective than supposed because important groups of children leave school during the year or attend irregularly.

Ability to Activate Informal Social Networks. Although formal channels for distributing messages are critical for message exposure, continued discussion through informal social networks can increase the chances of messages reaching the entire audience. Because mass media can increase the salience and importance of health topics, audience members are more likely to discuss messages with each other and, in the case of young people, with their parents. This increased discussion permits the initial messages to diffuse through the audience and to magnify their influence (Nowak, Szamrej, & Latane, 1990; Rogers, 1983). This process also can make it more likely that the audience will see the recommended practices as normative and socially acceptable (Katz, 1980). Because of their greater reach and agenda-setting abilities, mass media are often more effective than personal communication in activating informal networks.

Message Influence

Channels also differ in their ability to influence the persons exposed to messages. Although personal channels tend to reach smaller audiences, they also tend to influence a larger proportion of the audiences reached. Several factors probably underlie this ability, including the credibility of personal channels, and their ability to involve the audience, to transmit complex information, and to tailor messages to the individual. Nevertheless mass media can be influential under the appropriate circumstances. Furthermore, another factor that affects the influence of a channel—its fidelity in transmitting messages—often favors mass media over personal channels.

Credibility. Channels differ in the credibility they lend to health messages. Personal channels may be more credible than mass media in many cases simply because they permit educators to develop rapport and trust with the audience or because educators already possess these characteristics (e.g., friends or neighbors). Schools are usually perceived by most children as credible channels; however, in the case of health education, some high-risk adolescent populations may not see schools as very credible sources of information (Nutbeam, Aar, & Catford, 1989). Homeless and runaway adolescents, for instance, are a particularly difficult audience to educate through most channels because of their distrust of authority (Dalglish, in press). Celebrity spokespersons with wide mass media appeal may, however, overcome some of these barriers.

Involvement. A channel is more effective if it has the ability to capture the audience's attention and to create involvement toward the message. Personal channels are often stronger on this dimension if only because educators have more control over the audience's attention in personal settings. Nevertheless mass media also can be involving. Scheduling health messages during the time a popular disc jockey is on the air may create more interest in HIV prevention than similar announcements in schools even though both may have the same reach and frequency.

Ability to Transmit Complex or Novel Information. Personal channels are often more effective for transmitting complex information. If messages are to educate adolescents on the use of condoms or on the benefits of safer sex, they may require channels that can carry this information with sufficient detail and interest value. Printed materials also can serve this purpose, but they may require messages on other channels to motivate attention to the more complex printed materials.

Ability to Tailor Messages to Individual Needs. Personal channels are usually superior in tailoring messages for the individual. Personal channels tend to involve more interaction with audience members and to permit message modification according to the needs of the person. Nevertheless mass communication can be targeted to distinctive segments of the audience (e.g., younger, sexually inexperienced persons versus older, more experienced persons) by using formative research in personal settings to learn about the needs of the audience.

Fidelity. Channels can differ widely in the degree to which they faithfully transmit messages as they were intended to be disseminated. If message dissemination depends on successful passage through intermediate trainers or educators, then distortion is a possible consequence. For example, teachers who are trained to administer HIV education in classroom settings may introduce their own viewpoints and biases regarding risky behaviors or preventive practices. This distortion can serve to undermine the effectiveness of the education program as it was designed. Mass media messages are subject also to distortion if the messages are delivered in a confusing or poorly executed manner. If, however, the messages are recorded or read from scripts, pretesting can help eliminate unnecessary sources of misunderstanding.

In sum, although personal channels are often stronger on message influence, mass communication channels can be credible, involving, informative, sensitive to the audience, and potentially more faithful to the communication goal.

Feasibility and Cost

The final component of cost-effectiveness is the operational feasibility and cost of the channel. Mass media are often superior on this dimension when the goal is to reach large audiences. The efficiency of mass media derives from the independence of mass media from other supports, the lower cost of setting up and maintaining mass media channels, and the fewer organizational requirements needed to implement and maintain the channel.

Independence From Other Channels. Mass media tend to be relatively independent of other supporting channels. Because these channels already have an audience, they do not require other channels to reach the audience. For example, telephone helplines are a useful channel for obtaining information, but they require other channels to publicize their presence, hours of operation, and so on. Similarly health clinics are an important place where adolescents can receive counseling or condoms, but they need publicity from other channels to maximize their use. Furthermore if the channel for distributing messages is not under the control of the program planner, then obstacles will arise to maintaining the channel. For example, if health clinic workers are to distribute educational materials to the audience, then planners may need to depend on the motivation of these workers to deliver the program. To the degree a program is dependent on other channels for success, it may require more resources to achieve the same educational impact that a more independent channel can achieve.

Cost of Materials and Personnel. Even if a channel can be sustained on its own, it is critical to evaluate the cost and feasibility of setting up and maintaining a channel. Materials must be designed, settings for disseminating messages put in place, and people supported to deliver the messages. For example, some personal channels require heavy investments in outreach workers or teacher time, resources that are difficult to sustain over time. The costs of mass media channels are often smaller because once the materials are designed, personnel needs are less intense. Mass media are also often easier to sustain simply because fewer persons are needed to deliver messages relative to the number of persons reached.

Organizational Requirements. Mass media not only require fewer personnel, but they also involve fewer management and training resources than personal channels. For example, to implement a new HIV-prevention curriculum in the schools requires teacher training and a system for coordinating the process. Unless a school system has the resources to coordinate a large-scale curriculum change, there is no guarantee it will be implemented effectively in the way it was intended. Mass media often require fewer of these resources and are easier to sustain.

Examples of Successful Mass Media Education Programs

We have argued that mass media are often more cost-effective than personal channels for delivering health education. In the next section, we review some mass media programs that have succeeded in changing behavior on a large scale, especially the behavior of young people. Although the average changes observed in these programs may often seem small, the exposure achieved by them is considerable, and the resulting effectiveness relative to cost is great. Furthermore, many health-related outcomes, such as greater use of condoms, require broad changes in the meaning of and normative support for previously unpopular behaviors. By reaching large populations, even small immediate changes can accumulate over time to produce larger shifts in social norms and behavior.

Smoking Prevention and Cessation

As noted earlier, considerable progress has been made in assessing the cost-effectiveness of smoking education. Many programs have been developed and tested over the years. Flay's (1987a, 1987b) reviews of these programs indicate that mass media advertising and self-help clinics delivered through the media can be successful in reducing the prevalence of smoking in adults. Self-help clinics delivered through the media are modeled after clinic programs that require face-to-face attendance. Because media programs can be received in the home, the potential reach of these programs is far greater than clinic-based approaches, and the resultant costs are much lower.

The favorable influence of mass media campaigns depends on the amount of exposure, frequency of exposure, and the length of the campaign (Flay, 1987a, 1987b). If sufficient exposure is achieved for a long enough period of time, media can have a powerful effect on behavior. In some research programs, personal communication programs supplemented the mass media campaigns. For persons exposed to both communication sources, the impact was approximately double the level of media alone. The mass media programs, however, were still probably more cost-effective because of the greater reach afforded by those programs.

Mass media are primary channels for the current California tobacco control campaign (Kizer & Honig, 1990). This campaign began in 1990, with the aim of reaching young children (under age 10), older children (ages 11-18), and adults across various ethnic groups. The major messages have attempted to cast smoking as a nonglamorous and dangerous habit (especially for pregnant women) and to encourage smokers to enter cessation programs. These messages have been disseminated primarily on television, with additional use of radio, billboards, posters, and newspaper ads. Television was chosen because of its ability to reach all audiences. Radio was also an important choice for reaching young people. In various ethnic communities with large numbers of non-English speaking persons, however, newspapers have been the best channels to reach the audience.

Although evaluations of the campaign are still being conducted, initial results indicate that the campaign is achieving its goals. Two waves of data collection with in-school youth (grades 4-12) after only 2 months of the campaign indicated substantial awareness of the campaign (about 75%). A slight but significant reduction occurred in smoking prevalence (from 12.8% to 10.3%) and in intentions to begin smoking (24.6% to 21.8%). As the campaign proceeds, the opportunity will be greater for it to influence young people and for local programs sponsored by county health departments to reinforce the mass media program.

An interesting test of mass-media smoking prevention programming was conducted recently in the southeastern United States by Bauman et al. (1991). This project compared three media programs, each of which was delivered to two cities. Four additional cities served as control sites and did not receive any programming. A core campaign used radio to inform young people about seven unfavorable consequences of smoking. The messages were selected in careful formative research (Bauman et al., 1988) and were delivered over a period of 6 months. The two other campaigns also involved a sweepstakes offer designed to increase peer interaction. One of these campaigns was delivered by radio and the other by television. More than 80% of the intended audiences were exposed to the messages from 10-14 times.

A panel of more than 1,600 children aged 12-14 was surveyed before the campaigns and then again 2 years later, about 11 months after the campaigns ended. Bauman et al. (1991) were able to identify significant effects on subjective expected utilities for the seven consequences featured in the campaigns and on perceptions of peer approval for smoking. The core radio campaign devoted exclusively to the consequences messages seemed to have the greatest impact on these outcomes. Nevertheless the research design did not seem to have enough precision to isolate a significant effect of media on actual smoking rates, at least not 11 months after the campaigns ended.

Illicit Drug Use

We are currently in the middle of one of the largest mass media campaigns ever launched to promote health. Since 1987, the Partnership for a Drug-Free America has coordinated a massive media campaign to prevent the use of illicit drugs, especially among young people. The campaign receives more than $300 million annually in donated media time and space to expose a variety of ads aimed at young people and adults (American Association of Advertising Agencies, 1990).

Annual surveys conducted by the Partnership, the University of Michigan, and National Institute on Drug Abuse confirm the effects of this campaign (Black, DiPasquale, Bayer, Cirillo, & Palmerini, 1990). In areas where the ads have achieved more exposure, impact appears to be greater. For example, in areas with high exposure to the campaign, reported use of marijuana by adults has declined about 30% annually, whereas in areas with less exposure, virtually no change has occurred in marijuana use. Use of marijuana and cocaine by people ages 18-25 also has declined during the period of the campaign, and attitudes toward drug use among adolescents have become less favorable.

The first years of the campaign seemed to have greater impact on adults and younger children (ages 9-12). As a result, the campaign shifted its emphasis in 1989 toward adolescents (Black et al., 1990). This shift in strategy resulted in dramatic changes in the reported attitudes and behavior of teenagers. More adolescents recognized the risks of using such drugs as marijuana (from 64% to 72%) and cocaine (62% to 71%), and teenagers reported less use of these drugs during the previous year.

HIV-Related Behavior

Deliberate use of mass media for the prevention of HIV infection has been less frequent in the United States. The CDC campaign ("America Responds to AIDS") has focused primarily on promotion of the National AIDS Hotline (NAH). The NAH provides confidential information to the general public about HIV prevention and acts as a referral source for other services (e.g., testing and counseling). When the campaign began in October 1987, calls to the NAH more than doubled from previous levels of activity (Centers for Disease Control, 1990). Prior to the campaign, the NAH received between 50,000 and 70,000 calls a month. Following the beginning of the campaign, between 150,000 and 210,000 calls were received per month for about 9 months. The campaign used a variety of media to publicize the NAH, including television, radio, magazine ads, and mass transit posters. The level of caller volume appeared to drop following the national mailing of the Surgeon General's information brochure "Understanding AIDS" in June 1988 (CDC, 1990).

The CDC has encouraged the states to engage in their own HIV-education programs. Efforts by the states to educate young people, however, have focused on the schools. Many states now recommend sex education with a component devoted to HIV. Very few states have devised mass media campaigns to educate the public about HIV disease. One notable exception is the state of Michigan, which since 1988 has supported a large-scale mass media campaign to educate the general population, as well as young people (Moore & Associates, 1990). This campaign has had several goals: (a) to increase knowledge of HIV disease and to eliminate misconceptions about HIV transmission in the general population; (b) to increase the use of the Michigan AIDS Hotline, especially for high-risk persons; (c) to increase awareness and appropriate use of the state's free and confidential HIV-testing and counseling services; and (d) to encourage behavior change among high-risk persons.

The campaign has relied primarily on television advertising designed to reach all segments of the population. More than $2 million in media time and space has been donated or purchased for the campaign in 1988 and 1989. Adolescents also have been targeted as an important audience, and specific radio and print ads have been created for this audience. One 30-second radio spot involved an announcer saying:

> Remember how when you were a little kid your mom used to tell you, "Now, don't go out without your rubbers!" That's even better advice today. If you're going to have sex, play it safe. Use a latex condom with a spermicide containing Nonoxynol-9. For confidential help and information call 1-800-872-AIDS. This message comes to you from the Michigan Department of Public Health AIDS Prevention Program. And your mom.

The campaign has appeared to reach both adolescents and adults (Moore & Associates, 1990). Large surveys of high school students indicated increases in awareness of the AIDS Hotline from 37% before the campaign to 52% after it had been operating for a year.

In addition, a survey of out-of-school youth showed high aware-ness (65%) among this important group. Among persons over age 18, almost two thirds claimed awareness of the hotline. Calls to the hotline following the initiation of the campaign increased dramatically, and about 12% of the calls were received from ado-lescents. The general information messages in the campaign ap-peared to reduce concern about "unfounded" transmission routes. As the campaign proceeded, calls to the hotline regarding incor-rect transmission routes declined from about 16% at the beginning of the campaign to about 8% at the end of the second year of the campaign.

Adolescents also appeared to respond to the campaign by in-creasing their use of testing and counseling services. Prior to the campaign, only about 4% of the users of these services were under age 20. By the second year of the campaign, adolescents accounted for about 12% of those seeking HIV-testing and counseling ser-vices. Although requests for testing increased dramatically over the course of the campaign, no increase seemed to have occurred in inappropriate use of this service. One of the potential unwanted consequences of media attention to HIV prevention is increased use of testing by persons unlikely to be at risk of HIV infection, as occurred in the British AIDS campaign (Anderson et al., 1987).

One of the potential aims of mass media health education is the creation of norms favorable to the practice of low-risk behaviors. Surveys among high school students and out-of-school youth from ages 16-19 revealed greater perceptions of peer support for safer behavior. For example, students who were aware of the campaign agreed somewhat more than unaware students that their sexually active friends would "ask their partner about previ-ous activities before having sex" (33% vs. 26%) and would "always insist that a condom be used" (52% vs. 45%). Even stronger results were obtained for out-of-school youth.

The results of this campaign are still preliminary. More research is being conducted to evaluate the campaign, and further changes are expected as the campaign continues. Although the prevalence of safer behavior has not yet been determined, the cost-effectiveness of the campaign probably justifies its continuance. Large propor-tions of the state's adult and adolescent population have been exposed to the campaign at a cost of less than $1 per person reached. This blanket exposure to HIV education probably has helped create a more favorable climate for young people to try to maintain safer sex practices. Future research should tell us more about the effect of this education on sexual practices.

Other Successful Uses of Mass Media for HIV Education. Mass media HIV education in the United States has focused on promotion of personal communication channels, such as telephone helplines and testing/counseling services. Less emphasis has been placed on promotion of safer behavior itself. Despite this underuse of mass media, some notable campaigns have occurred in Europe that appear to increase dramatically the prevalence of safer behavior, especially among more at-risk audiences.

A series of campaigns to promote safe sex has been ongoing in the Netherlands since 1987 (deVroome et al., 1990). These campaigns have been designed for the general population of both heterosexual and homosexual persons. Although the principal aim has been to encourage use of condoms in nonsteady, new, or otherwise risky relationships, the campaigns adopted the more general theme of safe sex and attempted to educate the general population about this concept in a nonjudgmental and objective manner. The emphasis on safe sex rather than condoms was chosen in part to avoid offending those segments of the population that might view condom promotion as immoral. This focus also allowed other options, such as monogamy and nonpenetrative sex, to be discussed, and it acknowledged that condoms are not perfectly reliable for disease prevention.

At least two of the campaigns were directed toward young people. One campaign focused on the need to take precautions on holidays away from home. The other sought to debunk the rationalizations that many young people give for avoiding safe-sex practices. A number of channels were used to reach young people, including posters displayed at discos and train stations, brochures dispensed at colleges and health centers, magazine ads, radio and television announcements, and cinema ads. Random samples of persons aged 15-45 were interviewed by telephone at 6-month intervals to determine the effects of the campaigns with a total of more than 6,000 persons participating. In addition, condom sales and STD rates were followed over the course of the campaigns.

The campaigns succeeded in changing the cultural meaning of safe sex. Prior to the campaigns (in early 1987), condom use was associated spontaneously with safe sex by only 43% of the audience. This increased to as high as 82% during one campaign and leveled off at about 70% after almost 3 years. People also increasingly associated safe sex with partner reduction, beginning around 14% and ending up at around 30%, even though this was not an explicit message in any of the campaigns. In addition, associations between safe sex and contraception declined from 22% to 12%.

The meaning of the condom also changed over the course of the campaigns. Initially condoms were seen primarily as protecting against pregnancy (74%) rather than HIV infection (57%) or STDs (59%). As the campaigns progressed, however, protection from HIV infection became seen as the primary purpose of condoms (73%) rather than avoidance of pregnancy (49%) or other STDs (54%). Although condoms were seen initially as inhibiting "sensitivity" (60%), this reaction dropped to only 39% after exposure to the campaigns. Apparently this barrier to use was at least partially overcome as the social acceptance of condoms increased and their favorable association with disease prevention became more prevalent.

The most dramatic effects of the campaigns were observed among those persons most likely to be at risk of HIV infection. Of all the persons interviewed, 82% had been sexually active in the past 6 months, and 92% of this group claimed to have had intercourse with a steady partner. The other 8% who claimed to have had sex with one or more nonsteady partners were a primary target for the campaign. In this group, claimed use of condoms in the past 6 months increased dramatically (see Figure 8.1). Young people from ages 15-25 also claimed greater use of condoms during the campaign, although the absolute increase was smaller than in the group with nonsteady partners (18% vs. 31%).

Not surprisingly the absolute increase in condom use was less dramatic among all sexually active persons of ages 15-45. Nevertheless the reported increased use of condoms was evident in aggregate sales of condoms in drugstores. National sales figures indicated large gains in condom use during the period of the campaigns. Further evidence of increased condom use was observed in national STD rates. Although the rates of syphilis and gonorrhea had been declining already when the campaigns began, gonorrhea continued to decline, and syphilis rates leveled off before appearing to rise again.

The results of the campaigns in the Netherlands are one of the most complete documentation of the impact of mass media on safe sex practices. Although many factors other than media-based

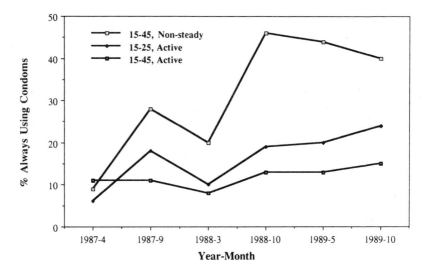

Figure 8.1. Reported Use of Condoms (Always) During the Past 6 Months Among Persons With Nonsteady Partners, Young People, and All Active Persons Between the Ages of 15 and 45

SOURCE: Data are from "AIDS in the Netherlands: The Effects of Several Years of Campaigning" by E. M. M. deVroome, M. E. M. Paalman, T. G. M. Sandfort, et al., 1990, *International Journal of STD & AIDS, 1.*

education could have produced the observed changes, additional analyses indicated that exposure to the campaign was an important contributor to the change. Furthermore evaluations of campaigns in Switzerland (DuBois-Arber, Lehmann, Hausser, Gutzwiller, & Zimmermann, 1988; Hausser, Zimmermann, Dubois-Arber, & Paccaud, 1991) and the United Kingdom (Kapila & Wellings, in press) also suggest that multimedia campaigns can have large effects on the behavior of general audiences, especially those more at risk of infection.

Barriers to the Use of Mass Media

The present examples of the use of mass media for HIV education and prevention suggest a promising opportunity to use these channels to an even greater degree in the United States. Test programs should be developed to explore the feasibility and cost-effectiveness of mass media as both an adjunct to personal communication programs and as a primary intervention to create appropriate meanings for safe sexual behavior, to increase the social acceptance of safe-sex practices, and to reduce misconceptions and fears about the illness.

It would be misleading to advocate the use of mass media without also acknowledging the barriers that exist in using the media for health education, especially for HIV disease. At this writing, it is not feasible to mount national television campaigns in the United States that advocate the use of condoms. Only a few local stations will permit such material to appear. Carter-Wallace, the major manufacturer of condoms in the United States, relies on the use of local radio advertising to market its brands. Radio, however, is an excellent channel to reach young people, and television may be an option in states where health departments are committed to large-scale HIV-education campaigns (as in the case of Michigan).

Another challenge to using media, especially television, is the sheer cost of purchasing time. Most public service campaigns depend on donated time for placing announcements on air. This solution, however, is often unsatisfactory as the sole source of media time. Donated placements tend to occupy time slots that are left unsold to commercial bidders, and these periods are not heavily watched. Earlier examples of the California smoking campaign and the HIV-education program in Michigan did not rely totally on donated time. Nevertheless the massive national campaign against drug use appears to have obtained quality placements on television and radio. Perhaps as HIV prevention becomes a more pressing concern for all audiences, more support will be given to sending HIV-prevention messages over the air.

Encouraging signs are appearing that television is acknowledging the threat of the HIV epidemic in its entertainment and public service programming. More shows are appearing with HIV-related themes, especially those aimed at young people (O'Connor, 1991). An entire episode of the popular show "A Different World" was dedicated to a story about an attractive female college student who was infected with HIV (this show appeared in April 1991). Public television stations, such as WNET in New York, have devoted entire days of programming to HIV education ("AIDS Awareness

Day"). As shows like this occur with more frequency, knowledge and understanding of HIV infection will grow. Until health educators begin to use mass media in a deliberate fashion, however, we will allow a potentially powerful and pervasive influence on young people, especially persons at risk of HIV infection, to go unused.

References

Alcalay, R., & Taplin, S. (1989). Community health campaigns: From theory to action. In R. E. Rice & C. K. Atkin (Eds.), *Public communication campaigns* (2nd ed.). (pp. 105-130). Newbury Park, CA: Sage.

Altman, D. G., Flora, J. A., Fortmann, S. P., & Farquhar, J. W. (1987). The cost-effectiveness of three smoking cessation programs. *American Journal of Public Health, 77*, 162-165.

American Association of Advertising Agencies. (1990). *What we've learned about advertising from the media-advertising partnership for a drug-free America.* New York: Author.

Anderson, R., Underhill, G., Kenny, C., Shah, N., Burnell, R., Jeffries, D. J., & Harris, J. R. (1987). AIDS publicity campaigns. *Lancet, 1*, 1429-1430.

Bauman, K. E., Brown, J. D., Bryan, E. S., Fisher, L. A., Padgett, C. A., & Sweeney, J. M. (1988). Three mass media campaigns to prevent adolescent cigarette smoking. *Preventive Medicine, 17*, 510-530.

Bauman, K. E., LaPrelle, J., Brown, J. D., Koch, G. G., & Padgett, C. A. (1991). The influence of three mass media campaigns on variables related to adolescent cigarette smoking: Results of a field experiment. *American Journal of Public Health, 81*, 597-604.

Black, G. S., DiPasquale, S., Bayer, L., Cirillo, P., & Palmerini, J. M. (1990). *The Partnership for a Drug Free America attitude tracking study: A summary of the fourth year results.* New York: American Association of Advertising Agencies.

Centers for Disease Control (CDC). (1990, June). *National AIDS Hotline: 1-800-342-AIDS.* Paper presented at VI International Conference on AIDS, San Francisco, CA.

Dalglish, P. (in press). "Survivors": A cartoon for street children on AIDS. In R. Berkens (Ed.), *Case studies in monitoring and evaluation.* Geneva, Switzerland: World Health Organization.

DeJong, W., & Winsten, J. A. (1989). *Recommendations for future mass media campaigns to prevent preteen and adolescent substance abuse.* Boston: Harvard School of Public Health.

deVroome, E. M. M., Paalman, M. E. M., Sandfort, T. G. M., Sleutjes, M., de Vries, K. J. M., & Tielman, R. A. P. (1990). AIDS in the Netherlands: The effects of several years of campaigning. *International Journal of STD & AIDS, 1*, 268-275.

Dubois-Arber, F., Lehmann, P., Hausser, D., Gutzwiller, F., & Zimmermann, E. (1989). *Evaluation of the Swiss preventive campaigns against AIDS: 2nd assessment report*. Lausanne, Switzerland: Institute Universitaire de Medecine Sociale et Preventive.

Fisher, J. D. (1988). Possible effects of reference group-based social influence on AIDS-risk behavior and AIDS prevention. *American Psychologist, 43*, 914-920.

Flay, B. R. (1987a). Mass media and smoking cessation: A critical review. *American Journal of Public Health, 77*, 153-160.

Flay, B. R. (1987b). *Selling the smokeless society*. Washington, DC: American Public Health Association.

Freimuth, V. S., Hammond, S. L., Edgar, T., & Monahan, J. L. (1989, May). *Reaching those at risk: A content analytic study of AIDS PSAs*. Paper presented at the annual meeting of the International Communication Association, San Francisco, CA.

Freudenberg, N. (1989). *Preventing AIDS*. Washington, DC: American Public Health Association.

Hausser, D., Zimmermann, E., Dubois-Arber, F., & Paccaud, F. (1991). *Evaluation of the AIDS prevention strategy in Switzerland: 3rd assessment report*. Lausanne, Switzerland: Institute Universitaire de Medecine Sociale et Preventive.

Hornik, R. C. (1989). Channel effectiveness in development communication programs. In R. E. Rice & C. K. Atkin (Eds.), *Public communication campaigns* (2nd ed.). (pp. 309-330). Newbury Park, CA: Sage.

Kapila, M., & Wellings, K. (in press). The UK public education campaign: Evaluation and evolution. In R. Berkens (Ed.), *Case studies in monitoring and evaluation*. Geneva, Switzerland: World Health Organization.

Katz, E. (1980). On conceptualizing media effects. *Studies in Communication, 1*, 119-141.

Kizer, K. W., & Honig, B. (1990). *Toward a tobacco-free California: A status report to the California Legislature on the first fifteen months of California's Tobacco Control Program*. Sacramento: California Department of Health Services.

Kotler, P., & Roberto, E. L. (1989). *Social marketing: Strategies for changing public behavior*. New York: Free Press.

Moore & Associates. (1990). *The 1989 Michigan AIDS prevention media campaign. An evaluation report*. Lansing: Michigan Department of Public Health.

Moran, J., Janes, H., Peterman, T., & Stone, K. (1990). Increase in condom sales following AIDS education and publicity, United States. *American Journal of Public Health, 80*(5), 607-608.

Nowak, A., Szamrej, J., & Latane, B. (1990). From private attitude to public opinion: A dynamic theory of social impact. *Psychological Review, 97*, 362-376.

Nutbeam, D., Aar, L., & Catford, J. (1989). Understanding children's health behavior: The implications for health promotion for young people. *Social Science and Medicine, 29*, 317-325.

O'Connor, J. J. (1991, April 11). Three shows about AIDS (straight AIDS, that is). *New York Times*, p. C15.

Office of Technology Assessment. (1988). *How effective is AIDS education?* Washington, DC: U.S. Congress.

Rogers, E. M. (1983). *Diffusion of innovations* (3rd ed.). New York: Free Press.

Singer, E., Rogers, T. F., & Glassman, M. B. (1991). Assessing an information campaign on AIDS. *Public Opinion Quarterly, 55*, 161-179.

Shikles, J. L. (1988). *AIDS education: Activities aimed at the general public implemented slowly* (GAO/HRD-89-21). Washington, DC: U.S. General Accounting Office.

Warner, K. E. (1987). Television and health education: Stay tuned. *American Journal of Public Health, 77,* 140-142.

Weinstein, M. C., Graham, J. D., Siegel, J. E., & Fineberg, H. V. (1989). Cost-effectiveness analysis of AIDS prevention programs: Concepts, complications, and illustrations. In C. F. Turner, H. G. Miller, & L. E. Moses (Eds.), *AIDS: Sexual behavior and intravenous drug use* (pp. 471-499). Washington, DC: National Academy.

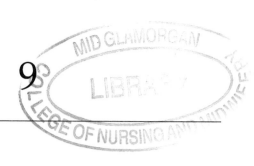

9

School-Based Prevention Programs: Design, Evaluation, and Effectiveness

DOUGLAS KIRBY

Introduction

By now, any person familiar with the prevention of HIV / AIDS has read one or more times that effective education leading to behavior change is currently the only method of reducing HIV transmission. For two reasons, school-based programs are an obvious focus of many HIV / AIDS-prevention efforts. First, the primary purpose of schools is education. Although our educational system has many critics, schools do increase the knowledge of our youth. Second, schools are the one institution in our society regularly attended by most young people: Nearly 95% of all children and youth are in elementary or secondary schools (Iverson & Kolbe, 1983). Moreover, virtually all youth are in schools before they initiate risk-taking behaviors that may expose them to HIV. Thus many people perceive schools as the public institution with the broadest opportunity for reducing HIV-risk-taking behaviors.

159

On the other hand, the case for school-based programs should not be exaggerated; adolescents at highest risk of transmitting HIV—youth with numerous sexual partners and IV drug users—are disproportionately likely to have dropped out of school. Consequently other institutions and the broader community also must develop programs. In addition, schools alone cannot dramatically reduce risk-taking behavior even among those youth in school; schools do need to be supported in a variety of ways by the broader community.

For almost a century, school-based programs have attempted to reduce unprotected sexual activity. As the threat of AIDS became more prominent in our society, some programs focused primarily on AIDS. In previous decades, however, other programs attempted to reduce sexual intercourse outside of marriage, unintended pregnancy, and sexually transmitted diseases other than AIDS. Because all of these efforts had the potential to affect those factors related to the transmission of HIV—the onset of sexual intercourse, the frequency of intercourse, the number of sexual partners, and the use of condoms—they are discussed in this chapter. Sex education is discussed in this chapter for an additional reason: Many health professionals believe that HIV/AIDS-education programs will be most effective if they are taught as part of more comprehensive sex education programs that attempt to teach skills and change norms. More recently some schools have attempted to improve access to contraceptives, including both oral contraceptives and condoms. Those efforts also are discussed in this chapter.

Support for Sexuality and HIV/AIDS Education

Sex education and HIV/AIDS education are widely supported in this country. Almost 50 years ago, in 1943, the Gallup poll asked whether adults approved of sex education in schools; 68% of adults did so (Gallup, 1972). By 1986, this approval had increased to 85% (Leo, Delaney, & Whitaker, 1986; Louis Harris & Associates, 1988). This support extends to subjects sometimes considered controversial: 77% believe sex education for 12-year-olds should include information on contraception, and almost two thirds believe it should include discussions of homosexuality and abortion (Quinley, 1986). Not surprisingly adolescents also strongly support sex education programs (Norman & Harris, 1981). Support for HIV/AIDS education is even higher. Ninety-four percent of parents think public schools should have an HIV/AIDS education program, and only 4% think they should not. More than 80% of parents want their children to be taught about safer sex as a way of preventing AIDS (Gallup, 1987).

Prevalence of Sex and HIV/AIDS Education and Barriers to More Comprehensive Programs

In light of this widespread support for sex education, it is not surprising that sex education and AIDS education programs exist in most communities (Forrest & Silverman, 1989). In a 1988 national survey of 4,241 teachers who might teach sexuality or HIV/AIDS education in grades 7-12, 93% said that their school offered sex education or AIDS education at one or more grade levels, and 77% said that they offered both (Forrest & Silverman, 1989). Sex education and AIDS education were most likely to be taught in the 9th and 10th grades; however, 35% of the teachers said that sex education was taught in the 7th grade, and 35% said it was taught in the 8th grade. Both sex education and AIDS education were most usually taught in other courses, especially health education. The vast majority of courses and teachers covered sexual decision making, abstinence, birth control methods, sexually transmitted diseases, how HIV is transmitted, symptoms of the disease, effects of the disease, abstinence as prevention, and condoms as prevention. More than three fourths of the teachers covered how to use condoms. Only two thirds covered specific sources of help for students, and only half discussed sources of contraception. According to the teachers, the three most important topics they taught were (a) exercising responsibility regarding sexual relationships and parenthood, (b) knowing the importance of abstinence and how to resist pressure to become sexually active, and (c) having correct information about AIDS and other STDs (Forrest & Silverman, 1989).

Among those schools teaching these topics, the amount of time spent on sex education and AIDS education increased from about 12 hours per academic year in the 7th grade to about 18 hours in the 12th grade. Among those schools that taught sex education or

AIDS education, 42 hours cumulatively in grades 7-12 were devoted to these topics; about 5 hours were spent on birth control methods, and 6 hours on STDs (Forrest & Silverman, 1989). Up to a third of the teachers indicated that they faced specific problems as sex education or AIDS education teachers.

Despite the widespread support for sex education and AIDS education, the single most common problem preventing sex education or AIDS education has been pressure from parents, the community, or the school administration. These results are consistent with those of an earlier study of barriers to sex education that revealed that the single most important barrier to sex education was not the opposition itself but rather unnecessary fear of the opposition (Scales & Kirby, 1983). Opponents were often vocal but small in number. Thus when controversies arose in communities, programs more commonly were strengthened than weakened after the controversy. It should be recognized that well-publicized controversies are not representative of most communities. In most communities, sex- and AIDS-education programs have been developed and taught with relatively little opposition. Of course, when opposition arose, so did publicity, and thus media coverage may have provided a biased impression.

When students (as opposed to teachers) were surveyed, far fewer reported receiving education about sexuality or AIDS. A 1986 poll revealed that only 60% of teenagers received at least some sex education, only 39% of 12- to 17-year-old youth had received instruction about different kinds of birth control, only 30% had received information about where to get contraception, and only 32% had received information about abortion (Quinley, 1986). Furthermore only a small percentage of students had participated in comprehensive programs, and only a small percentage had participated in K-12 programs (Sonenstein & Pittman, 1984). In addition, many topics were taught in high school after students had previously had sexual intercourse (Marsiglio & Mott, 1986).

The discrepancies between the 1988 teacher survey and the 1986 student survey can be explained partially by three factors: (a) The 1986 survey occurred prior to the development of numerous AIDS-education programs, (b) most schools may offer sex education or AIDS education, but not all students may actually receive that instruction, and (c) students who receive the instruction may be more likely to forget they received that instruction than are the teachers who taught the material.

In sum, the vast majority of states and school districts mandate or support sex education and HIV/AIDS education, most schools offer such education, and important topics are covered in most courses. Many students, however, are still not exposed to comprehensive programs, additional youth fail to receive instruction on sources of contraception or other important topics, and many do not receive this instruction in a timely manner. Thus there is considerable room for improvement.

The Generations of Sex and HIV/AIDS Education Curricula: How Effective?

Many sexuality education programs are concerned with a wide range of sexual issues and do not focus primarily on reducing unprotected intercourse. Since the mid-1970s, however, when this country became more concerned about teenage pregnancy, a search for and the development of sex education programs to reduce sexual behaviors that place youth at risk of pregnancy have been under way; since the mid-1980s when this country became more concerned about AIDS and HIV, a search for AIDS education programs that reduce behaviors that may transmit HIV has been under way.

Although the hundreds of curricula that have been developed contain activities or elements reflecting a wide variety of approaches, these curricula can be grouped loosely into five generations. Notably, these generations somewhat parallel the generations of curricula to reduce smoking and alcohol and illegal drug use.

The first generation of sex education curricula focused primarily on increasing knowledge and emphasizing the risk and consequences of pregnancy. They were based on the premise that if youth had greater knowledge about sexual intercourse, pregnancy, methods of birth control, the probability of pregnancy, and the consequences of childbearing, then they would rationally choose to avoid unprotected intercourse. This generation of curricula paralleled the first smoking and substance abuse curricula that described different drugs and emphasized the consequences of substance use (e.g., the long-term impact of smoking and its relationship to cancer).

The second generation of sex education curricula included considerable knowledge content but did not give as much emphasis to "the endless pursuit of the fallopian tubes." Instead they devoted much more emphasis to values clarification and skills, especially decision-making and communication skills. The values clarification exercises were designed to help the students become clearer about their basic values, as well as their values about sexual behavior. Teachers gave students dilemmas to solve and discuss but commonly did not emphasize that particular values were right or wrong. These curricula emphasized generic skills, such as the basic steps involved in making a decision and the basic components in communicating with one's partner (e.g., "I" messages, paraphrasing, and careful listening). When these skills and values were applied to sexual issues, curricula often spelled out the pros and cons of engaging in sexual intercourse and the pros and cons of using contraception but did not consistently and clearly emphasize that the students should not engage in unprotected sexual activity. Proponents of this approach believed that if students' values became clearer and their decision-making skills improved, then they would become more likely to decide to avoid risk-taking behavior and, if their communication skills improved, then they would be more likely to communicate effectively those decisions to their partners.

Numerous studies have measured the impact of these first two generations of programs on the knowledge of the students, and the findings from these studies are nearly unanimous: Instruction did increase knowledge of sexuality (Kirby, 1984). Findings have been similar for STD education programs (Yarber, 1986). It has been increasingly recognized, however, that knowledge about such sexual issues as contraception is very weakly related to behavior and that increasing knowledge may not produce much reduction in risk-taking behavior (Whitley & Schofield, 1985-1986).

A smaller number of studies examined the impact of different sex education programs on values and attitudes. Those studies indicate that when specific values were not given prominent emphasis in the course, little evidence was found that the courses had any measurable impact on the students' values. When several more liberal courses taught during the 1970s focused on increasing the students' acceptance of the sexual practices of other students, however, some change in that direction was noted (Hoch, 1971; Parcel & Luttman, 1980, 1981). Finally, during the early 1980s, when several courses focused on increasing the clarity of students' values, they succeeded in making the students slightly clearer (Kirby, 1984).

Whether these sex education courses measurably affected students' skills depended both on how the skills were taught and how they were measured. One curriculum used an intensive cognitive-behavioral approach that focused on teaching and practicing communication skills in the classroom through modeling, role playing, and rehearsal. When the evaluators measured these skills with vignettes and videotapes, they found a measurable impact (Schinke, Blythe, & Gilchrest, 1981). In contrast, a different study evaluated the impact of a variety of exemplary sex education programs on skills as they were practiced in everyday life and not in the classroom. That study did not find a measurable impact (Kirby, 1984).

Five major studies have examined the impact of sex education on the initiation of intercourse and the subsequent frequency of sexual intercourse. Four of these studies were based on surveys of large random samples of teenagers or young adults in this country and included questions about both participation in sex education programs and personal sexual experience. Thus those studies measured the impact of a cross section of sex education programs existing at that time. Two of these studies found that for older teens, participation in sex education was not associated with subsequently initiating intercourse, but for younger teens (e.g., 14 or 15 years old), participation in sex education was associated with subsequent initiation of intercourse (Dawson, 1986; Marsiglio & Mott, 1986). The third study found no statistical relationship between sex education and sexual experience (Zelnik & Kim, 1982), and the fourth found that sex education was associated with delayed initiation of intercourse (Furstenberg, Moore, & Peterson, 1985). The fifth study examined the impact of 14 specific sex education programs and had smaller sample sizes in each of the programs (Kirby, 1984). The study found that none of the programs increased or decreased sexual experience.

Four of these five studies examined the impact of sex education on the use of birth control; the first three also relied on national surveys of youth. Their results were mixed. The study with the most positive results found that having taken pregnancy and contraceptive education was positively related to use of birth control during first intercourse and to use of birth control ever. Pregnancy and contraceptive education were not, however, related to current use of contraception. Similarly, a second survey found weak relationships between having had sex education and use of contraception both during first intercourse and during any sexual activity, but these relationships were statistically significant only for blacks. A third study focused on current use of birth control and found inconsistent results that depended on how sex education was defined. Finally, in the study of 14 sex education courses, it was possible to measure the impact of 11 of the courses on contraceptive use; none of these courses had a measurable impact on use of contraception.

Three of these studies examined the relationship between sex education and pregnancy; none found a measurable and significant impact of sex education on pregnancy.

Although the results of these evaluations produced somewhat inconsistent results, they clearly demonstrated that these first two generations of sex education programs did not dramatically reduce sexual risk-taking behavior or measurably reduce teenage pregnancy; at best, they may have increased slightly the use of birth control among selected groups.

The third generation of programs did not evolve out of the first two generations but instead developed in reaction to the first two generations of sex education programs. Concerned that the first two generations of programs were "value free," a different group of educators developed the third generation of programs. They generated a moralistic and ideological fervor and consistently emphasized the message that youth should not engage in intercourse until marriage. To avoid any possibility of a "double message," these programs commonly did not discuss contraception.

Abstinence programs such as Teen Aid and Sex Respect have been evaluated, and the results indicate that the programs did affect a wide variety of attitudes regarding premarital intercourse (Donahue, 1987; Weed & Olsen, 1988). In all cases, attitudes became significantly less accepting of premarital intercourse in the short term. These effects, however, may have been produced partially by response biases, and the studies either did not measure long-term effects or alternatively they measured long-term effects and found that the effects had diminished greatly. Only a few studies have examined the impact on behavior of abstinence programs. The methods employed in those studies have been limited, but thus far those evaluations indicate that the programs did not delay intercourse or reduce frequency of intercourse (Christopher & Roosa, 1990).

The fourth generation of programs designed to change adolescent sexual behavior is the HIV/AIDS education programs. Many of these developed quite independently of the previous three generations of sex education programs and at least initially did not build on the successes and failures of sex education programs.

These programs typically had a variety of goals, including (a) reducing misinformation about HIV infection and transmission, and reducing unnecessary fears associated with the disease; (b) encouraging young people to delay premature sexual intercourse; (c) supporting safer sex by encouraging teenagers who are sexually active to use condoms every time they have any kind of intercourse or to practice only those sexual behaviors that do not place one at risk of HIV infection; (d) encouraging youth to avoid drug use; and (e) helping students develop compassion for people infected with HIV.

Many of the HIV/AIDS education curricula developed during the first few years relied heavily on didactic presentations and group discussions of information about HIV and AIDS. Partially because of the short length of most HIV/AIDS program units, rarely were serious attempts made to improve skills or to change norms. Thus like the early sex education programs, they either explicitly or implicitly assumed that correcting youth's myths about HIV and AIDS would change their behavior.

Recognizing that most youth knew few people who were infected with HIV and that consequently most youth would deny any personal vulnerability, some curricula also focused on personalizing the information by having a person with AIDS, especially a young person with AIDS, speak to students.

Early evaluations of these programs indicated that many of them did increase knowledge, some made youth more sensitive to the rights of people with AIDS, and some reduced unnecessary fear about getting HIV from such improbable sources as blood donations and mosquito bites (DiClemente et al, 1989; Hall, 1989;

Huszti, Clopton, & Mason, 1989; Miller & Downer, 1988; Rickert, Gottleib, & Jay, 1990). Few studies, however, rigorously measured the impact of these programs on sexual behaviors.

Although the impact of individual programs on behavior was not well evaluated, national surveys provide some evidence that school-based programs may have had some impact. First, numerous studies have indicated that teenagers are remarkably knowledgeable about the transmission of HIV. Second, a national survey conducted in 1988 of teenage males indicated large increases in the use of condoms among males; specifically, use more than doubled from 21% to 58% between 1979 and 1988 (Sonenstein, Pleck, & Ku, 1989). Although these data suggest that such programs might have contributed to greater knowledge and greater use of condoms, it is not possible to determine whether this increase was due to school-based AIDS education programs, the innumerable other AIDS education programs in communities and the media, or other extraneous factors.

A fifth generation of sex education and AIDS education programs and evaluation studies is now emerging. This generation differs from the previous generations in several ways: (a) its programs are based on theoretical approaches that have been demonstrated to be effective in other health areas, (b) they build on the successes and failures of previous programs, and (c) each program is far more carefully and validly evaluated.

One fifth-generation study was based primarily on the health belief model (HBM) but included elements of social learning theory. It was intended to "increase teenagers' awareness of the probability of personally becoming pregnant or causing a pregnancy; the serious negative personal consequences of teenage maternity and paternity; and the personal and interpersonal benefits of delayed sexual activity and consistent, effective contraceptive use" (Eisen, Zellman, & McAlister, 1990, p. 22). It used lectures, discussions, and role plays but did not strongly emphasize that students should avoid unprotected intercourse. The evaluation employed a true experimental design. The study also had a large sample size and tracked students for 1 year. Its results were mixed and varied by gender and sexual experience at pretest. In comparison with their counterparts in the control group, male students in the treatment group were less likely to initiate sex, but the female students were more likely to initiate sex (although not significantly so). Among those students who initiated intercourse after the baseline data were collected, both males and females in the treatment groups were less likely to use contraception than their control group counterparts, but this difference was only significant among females. Finally, among males and females who had initiated intercourse prior to the baseline data, both the treatment and control groups improved their contraceptive use by approximately equal amounts. Multivariate analyses that statistically controlled for several background variables and for immediate posttest variables produced similar but slightly different results.

A second fifth-generation program is Postponing Sexual Involvement (PSI) (Howard & McCabe, 1990). It was based on a social-influences approach to changing behavior. During this program, high school students were trained as peer educators and then presented a 5-session program to junior high school students. They emphasized that the junior high school students should delay having sex and employed a variety of exercises, including role playing, to establish and emphasize that norm. Although the evaluation did not employ an experimental design, the weight of the evaluation evidence suggests that the program delayed the onset of intercourse among students.

The third fifth-generation program is Reducing the Risk: Building Skills to Prevent Pregnancy (Barth, 1989). Like PSI, it also contained elements of a social-influences model, social learning theory, and a cognitive-behavioral model. It made extensive use of role-playing activities and clearly emphasized the norm that students should avoid unprotected sexual activity. It included more experiential activities, such as visiting a family planning clinic or pricing condoms at a drugstore. Like PSI, it did not have a significant impact on the behavior of those students who had already had sex, but it did significantly prevent unprotected sexual behavior among those who had not had intercourse prior to the program. Mostly it reduced unprotected sex by delaying the onset of sexual intercourse; to a slight extent, it also increased the use of contraception among those who initiated sex after the program (Kirby, Barth, Leland, & Fetro, 1991).

In sum, evaluations of the first four generations of school-based educational programs to change adolescent sexual behavior indicate that the second generation of programs may have slightly increased use of birth control and that AIDS education programs may have helped increase adolescents' knowledge about AIDS and thereby increased the use of condoms. None of the studies of the first four generations of programs, however, provide convincing evidence that one approach is more effective than another. Only three studies have well-evaluated, specific curricula, all three of which were fifth-generation curricula. They indicate that curricula based on the health belief model may be less effective at changing behavior and that those based on a social-influence approach may be more effective, at least in delaying the onset of sexual intercourse. Unfortunately none of these curricula appeared to increase significantly the use of condoms.

Schoolwide Educational Programs

Junior and senior high schools have developed a wide array of imaginative and creative schoolwide activities to educate students about HIV. These include peer counselors who discuss HIV/AIDS issues both in classrooms and individually with students; dramatic and powerful theatrical presentations, such as SECRETS, that vividly portray the risks of HIV; school assemblies or school health fairs with presentations about HIV/AIDS or presentations by young people who are HIV positive; weekly discussion sessions on sexual issues; surveys of condom availability and ease of purchase at nearby community sources; and health columns on AIDS in the school newspaper.

Few studies have measured the impact on behavior of these schoolwide programs, partly because it is always extremely difficult to measure the impact of schoolwide programs that may reach many youth but are likely to have only a small impact on each youth.

Process assessments have indicated considerable variation in the quality and probable impact of these schoolwide programs. For example, some theatrical presentations, such as SECRETS, are rated very positively by students and clearly have at least a short-term impact on their perceptions of the risks and consequences of HIV/AIDS, while other theatrical presentations have been neither liked nor understood by the targeted students.

On the one hand, because these schoolwide programs may reach numerous youth, they may be a cost-effective method of reaching youth. On the other hand, because they are so short, they are not likely to have a major impact on behavior; at best, they may reinforce messages and norms developed in more intensive class-room programs.

School-Based Programs to Improve Access to Contraceptives

As the problems of unintended teenage pregnancy and AIDS have gained greater prominence in our society, some schools have developed programs to directly improve access to contraceptives. The first such efforts were school-based clinics. These are health clinics located on school campuses that provide youth with a wide range of medical and counseling services, including primary health care, physical examinations, laboratory tests, diagnosis and treatment of illness and minor injuries, immunizations, gynecological exams, birth control information and referral, pregnancy testing and counseling, nutrition education, weight reduction programs, and counseling for substance abuse. Some of them prescribe and dispense contraceptives. The first clinics opened in 1970; the first clinics to prescribe or dispense contraceptives did so in 1973. In 1990, more than 178 school-based clinics were open, and the number is continuing to increase (Hyche-Williams, 1990).

Relatively little research has been done on the clinics' impact on student sexual behaviors, partly because most of the growth in school-based clinics has occurred in the last few years. A few studies, however, provide mixed evidence for the impact of clinics.

The most widely quoted findings are those based on the St. Paul clinics. The findings describe substantial percentages of students using the clinics for reproductive health services and large decreases in birth rates (Edwards, Steinman, Arnold, & Hakanson, 1980), but subsequent analyses of improved birth rate data indicate the clinics did not reduce birth rates (Kirby et al., in press).

Additional evidence for the effectiveness of school-linked services was found in a study examining an experimental pregnancy-prevention program that combined classroom presentations and counseling in two inner-city Baltimore schools with reproductive health services provided to the students at a nearby clinic. Younger students at the experimental schools were more likely than those in the control schools to use contraception (Zabin, Hirsh, Smith, Street, & Hardy, 1986).

A more recent study of the impact of school-based clinics revealed that the clinics studied did not increase sexual activity and had varying effects on contraceptive use (Kirby, Waszak, & Ziegler, 1991). In one site at which the clinic school focused on high-risk youth, emphasized pregnancy prevention, and dispensed birth control pills, the use of birth control pills among females was significantly greater than in the comparison school. Unfortunately no increase occurred in use of condoms. In two other sites that dispensed both condoms and oral contraceptives, no significant differences were found in the student use of condoms between the clinic schools and the comparison schools.

Because of the increasing threat of AIDS in some communities (e.g., New York City), schools are dispensing condoms even if they do not have school-based clinics. Because these programs are just beginning, little evidence of their impact has been seen. In general, the experience of the school-based clinics distributing condoms suggests that simply distributing condoms through the schools does not substantially increase the use of condoms. This finding, given that condoms are readily available in drugstores and convenience stores in most communities, is not terribly surprising. Although youth may be embarrassed by purchasing condoms in those stores, they may be equally embarrassed obtaining them at their own school, where they are known by school staff. Recognizing this, some schools are considering making condoms available at very low cost through condom dispensing machines in the students' bathrooms.

Comprehensive School-Based Programs

These research findings suggest that no single approach is likely to produce a dramatic impact. Multiple components in a single school, however, may have either an additive or synergistic effect. Few studies have evaluated such programs. A San Francisco high school, however, implemented a variety of components and was evaluated (Kirby, Waszok, & Ziegler, 1991). In particular, it introduced a widely recognized educational component called the *WEDGE*, which included both information about HIV/AIDS and presentations in each class by a young person with AIDS. After-school group sessions were held that dealt with sexual issues, and a variety of schoolwide activities heightened student consciousness about AIDS. Finally, the school opened a school-based clinic that did not dispense condoms but did emphasize condoms and did provide students with a prescription that enabled them to get condoms anonymously and free of charge at a nearby community health clinic. Of course, all of this took place in a community where AIDS became very prominent and where many media and community activities were presented to reduce unprotected sexual activity. Over a 2-year period, the percentage of males in the school who used condoms the last time they had sex increased substantially. Although it is impossible to distinguish the impact of the school activities from community activities, it seems likely that the school activities contributed to the change.

Discussion

In combination with other sources of information, especially the media, AIDS education programs have increased significantly adolescents' knowledge about AIDS and have reduced the prevalence of commonly held myths. This important role should not be minimized, because it appears likely that all sources of information in combination contributed to the substantial increase in condom use among teenage males.

Most adolescents, however, now know the basic facts about the transmission of HIV (Anderson & Christenson, 1991; Dawson, Cynamon, & Fitti, 1987; United Press International, 1989). In fact, if anything, youth overestimate the chances of contracting HIV from such nonsources as mosquitos, public toilets, and donating blood (Miller & Downer, 1988). Thus the belief is growing that knowledge about HIV/AIDS is no longer related to risk-taking behavior (DiClemente, Forrest, & Mickler, 1990; Stevenson & DeBord, 1988) or only weakly related to risk-taking behaviors (Anderson et al., 1990) and that AIDS educational programs are not likely to produce greater reductions in risk-taking behavior unless they do substantially more than increase knowledge (Greico, 1987; Keeling, 1987). For example, a survey of San Francisco adolescents found that sexually experienced adolescents knew that condoms prevented

STD and thought it was important to protect against STD, yet they did not intend to use condoms (Kegeles, Adler, & Irwin, 1988). Somehow AIDS education programs must produce greater motivation to avoid unprotected sexual activity.

Innumerable suggestions appear in the AIDS education literature for improving the effectiveness of AIDS education programs; for example, developing curricula that are developmentally appropriate, reaching youth early enough, accepting the teenagers' sexual behavior, discussing contraception in a straightforward manner, providing explicit education about safe sex, giving more emphasis to the risks of unprotected intercourse, providing complete information about HIV testing, involving parents in the instruction, and providing counseling. Some of these changes may or may not improve the effectiveness of AIDS education programs. For example, it appears logical that giving greater emphasis to the risks of unprotected sex might reduce unprotected sex. Different studies, however, have produced conflicting findings on the relationship between perceived risk and unprotected sexual behavior; some have found a relationship (DiClemente et al., 1990), while others have not (Kegeles et al., 1988). Some of these suggestions have been incorporated already into sexuality education programs, without apparent effect on behavior. Because it is costly to implement all of these ideas, the rationale for implementing particular approaches must be compelling.

At least three potentially effective approaches exist to determine which of these and other ideas may be most effective. First, program designers can address the reasons that adolescents provide for having unprotected sex. In numerous studies (Kirby, Waszak, & Ziegler, 1991; Whitley & Schofield, 1985-1986), youth have cited most frequently two reasons for having sex without birth control. One, they did not expect to have intercourse—"it just happened." To counter this reasoning, effective programs must reduce the frequency of unexpected sex by either reducing the frequency of intercourse or increasing the expectedness of and the planning for intercourse. Two, they did not think pregnancy would occur— they felt invulnerable. Numerous people have written about and/or documented this general perception of invulnerability on the part of teenagers, and others have documented that most young people do not feel at risk of AIDS (Freimuth, Edgar, & Hammond, 1987; O'Donnell & Kodama, 1987). According to the National Health

Interview Survey, 91% of the 18-29-year-olds thought their chances of getting the AIDS virus were low or none (Dawson, 1986).

A very real problem for AIDS education is that for most teenagers the probability of having sex with someone infected with the HIV virus is quite small, and the probability of their actually contracting the HIV virus from that person is smaller still. Because teenagers, like adults, have difficulty making decisions when probabilities are very small, they are less likely to change their behavior even when they have been given accurate information. This is especially true given that many young people *overestimate* the number of cases of AIDS in this country and *overestimate* the chances of getting AIDS from a single unprotected act of heterosexual intercourse (Freimuth et al., 1987). Thus exposure to more correct estimates may logically reduce their concern, not increase it. In addition, numerous studies in psychology and health education have demonstrated that people are less likely to avoid a risk when the negative consequences are remote—both unlikely and in the distant future (U.S. General Accounting Office, 1988).

This problem may be overcome partially by providing more certain and more immediate positive rewards for avoiding unprotected sex. These rewards probably need to be symbolic in the form of social approval for avoiding risks. Such rewards require changing peer norms.

Reducing both the frequency of unplanned intercourse and perceptions of invulnerability is a challenging task; nevertheless these goals should provide new direction for AIDS education programs.

A second potentially effective means for determining which programmatic ideas may be effective is to employ a risk factor approach. The history of implementing risk factor approaches indicates that this approach has been effective in other adolescent risk-taking areas. For example, neither smoking education nor drug education was effective when knowledge was emphasized, but when programs focused on those factors that were both related to the smoking and drug behaviors and amenable to change, programs became substantially more effective.

An important risk factor amenable to change is perceived referent-group norms for use of condoms and unprotected sex (Fisher, 1988). Everyone is affected by his or her perceptions of peer norms, perhaps adolescents even more so than adults. If so, then changing peer norms through school surveys or classroom activities that demonstrate that most youth believe it is important to avoid unprotected sex and to use condoms if having sex may be an effective strategy.

A third potentially effective method of enhancing the effectiveness of AIDS education programs is to examine and adapt those theoretical approaches that have reduced effectively other risk-taking behaviors, such as substance abuse. Here the research is clear: Those curricula that focused on cognitive approaches were effective in changing knowledge but not behavior, while those curricula that employed a social-influence approach or social learning theory also changed behavior. These latter curricula identified external factors that affected behavior, taught skills to resist pressures, and established more positive and more accurate norms about risk-taking behavior. Although major differences occur in the etiology of substance abuse behaviors and sexual behaviors, at least the potential exists for these theoretical approaches to reduce unprotected intercourse, especially when sex education programs that employed these approaches reduced unprotected intercourse.

These types of changes require that AIDS education be embedded in sex education programs that have far more than 4 hours of instruction and that thereby provide greater opportunity to change norms and skills. Even 15 hours of instruction will not dramatically change behavior; many schoolwide activities undoubtedly will be necessary to change schoolwide norms about unprotected sexual intercourse and actual behavior.

In the past, people and institutions concerned with HIV transmission have not joined forces with those concerned with pregnancy prevention. This independence has had at least two negative consequences. First, AIDS education has not properly benefitted from the mistakes made in sex education. Second, at least two studies have demonstrated that the large majority of students who use condoms do so primarily to prevent pregnancy and not to prevent HIV transmission. Thus by failing to emphasize the role of condoms in pregnancy prevention, AIDS education programs may have diminished their effectiveness in increasing condom use.

Conclusions

Despite the limited research on the impact of HIV / AIDS education programs on actual sexual behavior, a number of conclusions can be reached:

1. Schools are a promising institution through which to reach youth and to reduce risk-taking behavior.
2. No known programs currently exist that dramatically reduce sexual risk-taking behavior.
3. Given that most youth now know most of the basic facts about HIV transmission, further increases in knowledge are not likely to have a major impact on sexual behaviors.
4. The typical AIDS education program lasting about 4 hours has insufficient time to change behavior substantially; thus programs must be either lengthened or integrated into sex education programs.
5. According to the limited evaluation studies, programs that use a social-influences approach and that model and provide practice in important skills and norms may be more effective than other programs in reducing unprotected intercourse.
6. Implementing a variety of classroom and schoolwide activities that consistently emphasize that students should avoid unprotected sex might change school norms and thereby reduce unprotected sex.
7. Simply distributing condoms on campus is not likely to increase their use substantially, although condom distribution might reinforce school norms against unprotected sex and thus might be more effective as part of a larger, more comprehensive program to reduce unprotected sex.
8. A great need remains both for the development of more effective programs and for rigorous research on the impact on behavior of these programs.

References

Anderson, J. E., Kann, L., Holtzman, D., Arday, S., Truman, B., & Kolbe, L. (1990). HIV / AIDS knowledge and sexual behavior among high school students. *Family Planning Perspectives, 22,* 252-255.

Anderson, M. D., & Christenson, G. M. (1991). Ethnic breakdown of AIDS related knowledge and attitudes from the National Adolescent Student Health Survey. *Journal of Health Education, 22,* 30-34.

Barth, R. (1989). *Reducing the risk: Building skills to prevent pregnancy.* Santa Cruz, CA: Network.

Barth, R., Leland, N., Kirby, D., & Fetro, J. (1992). Enhancing social and cognitive skills to prevent adolescent pregnancy. In B. Miller, J. Card, R. Paikoff, & J. Peterson (Eds.), *Preventing adolescent pregnancy: Model programs and evaluations* (pp. 53-82). Newbury Park, CA: Sage.

Christopher, S., & Roosa, M. (1990). An evaluation of an adolescent pregnancy prevention program: Is "Just Say No" enough? *Family Relations, 39,* 68-72.

Dawson, D. (1986). The effects of sex education on adolescent behavior. *Family Planning Perspectives, 18,* 162-170.

Dawson, D. A., Cynamon, M., & Fitti, J. E. (1987). AIDS knowledge and attitudes. Provisional data from the National Health Interview Survey, August, 1987. National Center for Health Statistics. *Advance Data, 146,* 1-11.

DiClemente, R. J., Forrest, K., & Mickler, S. (1990). College students' knowledge and attitudes about HIV and changes in HIV-preventive behaviors. *Journal of AIDS Education & Prevention, 2,* 201-212.

DiClemente, R. J., Pies, C., Stoller, E., Straits, K., Oliva, G., Haskin, J., & Rutherford, G. (1989). Evaluation of school-based AIDS curricula in San Francisco. *Journal of Sex Research, 26,* 188-198.

Donahue, M. (1987). *Technical report of the national demonstration project field test of human sexuality: Values and choices.* Minneapolis: Search Institute.

Edwards, L., Steinman, M., Arnold, K., & Hakanson, E. (1980). Adolescent pregnancy prevention services in high school clinics. *Family Planning Perspectives, 12*(1), 6-14.

Eisen, M., Zellman, G. L., & McAlister, A. L. (1990). Evaluating the impact of a theory-based sexuality and contraceptive education program. *Family Planning Perspectives, 22,* 262.

Fisher, J. (1988). Possible effects of reference group-based social influence on AIDS-risk behavior and AIDS prevention. *American Psychologist, 43,* 914-920.

Forrest, J. D., & Silverman, J. (1989). What public school teachers teach about preventing pregnancy, AIDS and sexually transmitted diseases. *Family Planning Perspectives, 21,* 65-72.

Freimuth, V., Edgar, T., & Hammond, S. (1987). College students' awareness and interpretation of the AIDS risk. *Science, Technology and Human Values, 12.*

Furstenberg, F., Moore, K., & Peterson, J. (1985). Sex education and sexual experience among adolescents. *American Journal of Public Health, 75,* 1331-1332.

Gallup, A. (1987). *The 19th annual Gallup polls of the public's attitudes toward the public school.* Princeton, NJ: Author.

Gallup, G. (1972). *Gallup poll public opinion 1935-1971.* New York: Random House.

Greico, G. (1987). Cutting the risks for STDs. *Medical Aspects of Human Sexuality, 21,* 70-84.

Hall, J. (1989). *A local school district implemented state mandated instructional program on AIDS prevention.* Paper presented at the Annual Meeting of the American Educational Research Association, San Francisco, CA.

Hoch, L. (1971). Attitude change as a result of sex education. *Journal of Research in Science Teaching, 8,* 363-367.

Howard, M., & McCabe, J. (1990). Helping teenagers postpone sexual involvement. *Family Planning Perspectives, 22,* 21-26.

Huszti, H. C., Clopton, J. R., & Mason, P. G. (1989). Effects of an AIDS educational program on adolescents' knowledge and attitudes. *Pediatrics, 84*, 986-991.

Hyche-Williams, H. (1990). *School-based clinics: Update 1990.* Washington, DC: Center for Population Options.

Iverson, D. C., & Kolbe, L. J. (1983). Evaluation of the national disease prevention and health promotion strategy: Establishing a role for the schools. *Journal of School Health, 53*, 294-302.

Keeling, R. P. (1987). Effects of AIDS on young Americans. *Medical Aspects of Human Sexuality, 21*, 22-33.

Kegeles, S., Adler, N., & Irwin, C. (1988). Sexually active adolescents and condoms: Changes over one year in knowledge, attitudes and use. *American Journal of Public Health, 78*, 460-461.

Kirby, D. (1984). *Sexuality education: An evaluation of programs and their effects.* Santa Cruz, CA: Network.

Kirby, D., Barth, R., Leland, N., & Fetro, V. (1992). Reducing the risk: Impact of a new curriculum on sexual risk-taking. *Family Planning Perspectives, 23*, 253.

Kirby, D., Resnik M. D., Downes B., Kocher T., Gunderson P., & Blum R. W. (in press). The effects of school-based health clinics in St. Paul upon school-wide birth rates. *Family Planning Perspectives.*

Kirby, D., Waszak, C., & Ziegler, J. (1991). Six school-based clinics: Their reproductive health services and impact on sexual behavior. *Family Planning Perspectives, 23*, 6-16.

Leo, J., Delaney, P., & Whitaker, L. (1986, November 24). Sex and schools. *Time.*

Louis Harris and Associates. (1988). *Public attitudes toward teenage pregnancy, sex education and birth control.* Poll conducted for the Planned Parenthood Federation of America. New York: Planned Parenthood.

Marsiglio, W., & Mott, F. (1986). The impact of sex education on sexual activity, contraceptive use and premarital pregnancy among American teenagers. *Family Planning Perspectives, 18*, 151-162.

Miller, L. & Downer, A. (1988). AIDS: What you and your friends need to know-A lesson plan for adolescents. *Journal of School Health, 58*, 137-141.

Norman, J., & Harris, M. (1981). *The private life of the American teenager.* New York: Rawson Wade.

O'Donnell, M., & Kodama, C. (1987). *AIDS and the college campus: A model prevention program.* Paper presented at III Intentional Conference on AIDS, Washington DC.

Parcel, G., & Luttman, D. (1980). Effects of sex education on sexual attitudes. *Journal of Current Adolescent Medicine, 2*, 38-46.

Parcel, G., & Luttman, D. (1981). Evaluation of a sex education course for young adolescents. *Family Relations, 30*, 55-60.

Quinley, H. (1986, November 17). [Memorandum to all data users regarding *Time/Yankelovich Clancy Shulman* poll findings on sex education].

Rickert, V., Gottleib, A., & Jay, M. (1990). A comparison of three clinic-based AIDS education programs on female adolescents' knowledge, attitudes, and behavior. *Journal of Adolescent Health Care, 11*, 298-303.

Scales, P., & Kirby, D. (1983). Important barriers to sex education: A survey of professionals. *Journal of Sex Research. 30*, 229-237.

Schinke, S., Blythe, B., & Gilchrest, L. (1981). Cognitive-behavioral prevention of adolescent pregnancy. *Journal of Counseling Psychology, 28*, 451-454.

Sonenstein, F., & Pittman, K. (1984). The availability of sex education in large city school districts. *Family Planning Perspectives, 16,* 19-25.

Sonenstein, F. L., Pleck, J. H., & Ku, L. C. (1989). Sexual activity, condom use and AIDS awareness among adolescent males. *Family Planning Perspectives, 21,* 152-158.

Stevenson, M. R., & DeBord, K. (1988). *AIDS awareness: Will knowledge of the facts change behavior?* Paper presented at the meetings of the Society for the Scientific Study of Sex, Chicago, IL.

United Press International. (1989, January 29). Teens: We have sex, don't use condoms. *San Francisco Chronicle.*

U.S. General Accounting Office. (1988). *AIDS education: Reaching populations at higher risk.* Washington, DC: Author.

Weed, S., & Olsen, J. (1988). *Evaluation of the Sex Respect program: Results for the 1987-88 school year.* Salt Lake City: Institute for Research and Evaluation.

Whitley, B. E., Jr., & Schofield, J. W. (1985-1986). Meta-analysis of research on adolescent contraceptive use. *Population and Environment, 8,* 173-203.

Yarber, W. (1986). *Pilot testing and evaluation of the CDC-sponsored STD curriculum.* Bloomington: Indiana University, Center for Health and Safety Studies.

Zabin, L. S., Hirsh, M. B., Smith, E. A., Street, R., & Hardy, J. B. (1986). Evaluation of a pregnancy prevention program for urban teenagers. *Family Planning Perspectives, 18*(3), 119-126.

Zelnik, M., & Kim, Y. (1982). Sex education and its association with teenage sexual activity, pregnancy, and contraceptive use. *Family Planning Perspectives, 16,* 117-126.

10

Innovative Approaches to Interpersonal Skills
Training for Minority Adolescents

STEVEN P. SCHINKE

ADAM N. GORDON

Introduction

The disproportionate spread of AIDS and HIV infection among
African-American and Hispanic-American adolescents (DiClemente,
in press) requires responsive interventions that are culturally sensitive, idiomatically relevant, and age appropriate to be directed
at minority youth. Early intervention efforts to prevent social and
health problems relied on providing the targeted audience with
simple information. Health educators believed that if individuals
were provided with facts about the consequences of health-compro-
mising behaviors, they would alter their behaviors as a result of

AUTHORS' NOTE: Research reported in this chapter was supported by the National
Institute on Drug Abuse (DA05321) under the auspices of an AIDS Prevention
Research Center.

this knowledge. The results of information-based interventions, however, were disappointing. Various reviews of the literature on information-based interventions show that increased knowledge does not result in behavior change (Bandura, 1990; Evans & Raines, 1982; Green, 1984; Thompson, 1978). Indeed, informational prevention programs have been associated with increased experimentation (Gordon & McAlister, 1982).

With respect to AIDS, other studies have shown that while adolescents are fairly knowledgeable about AIDS, few have initiated behavior change in response to AIDS (Office of Technology Assessment, 1988). For example, even when sexually active adolescents have been made aware that condom use reduces AIDS risk, actual condom use and intention to use condoms remain low (Kegeles, Adler, & Irwin, 1988; Strunin & Hingson, 1987).

The need for a skills-based approach to prepare adolescents to cope with the pressures, demands, and exigencies of modern life has been underscored by Petersen (1982) who notes:

> Preparation for experiences may be the best way to reduce stress and anxiety and to increase the likelihood of good outcomes for adolescents. . . . We know that adolescents have ample opportunity and, in many cases, pressure to experiment with such behaviors as smoking, drug use, and sex. Without preparation for these experiences, it is as if they were permitted to drive a car without skills or training. (p. 68)

Behavioral risks associated with HIV infection, such as intravenous drug use and unsafe sexual practices, are preventable (Centers for Disease Control, 1988a, 1988b; Day, Houston-Hamilton, Deslondes, & Nelson, 1988). Yet rigorously evaluated interventions do not exist for youth at highest risk for HIV infection (Brooks-Gunn, Boyer, & Hein, 1988; DiClemente, Boyer, & Morales, 1988; Flora & Thoresen, 1988). Because these youth are disproportionately African-American and Hispanic, interventions to help African-American and Hispanic adolescents prevent HIV infection by reducing their risks for drug use and unsafe sexual activity are justified. One theoretical model that has been demonstrably effective in its application across a variety of adolescent problem behaviors is social learning theory (cf. Bandura, this volume).

Interventions grounded in social learning theory have shown promising results in influencing youth's risk-reduction behavior

(Bandura, 1990; Bobo, Snow, Gilchrist, & Schinke, 1985; Schinke, Moncher, & Holden, 1989; Schinke, Orlandi et al., 1990). Social learning theory offers a social-systems approach that is rich and flexible yet also sufficiently detailed and prescriptive to suggest assessment and intervention procedures for many kinds of presenting problems, including unwanted pregnancies, drug and alcohol use, and cigarette use.

AIDS-Prevention Interventions

In the following section, we describe the development of two AIDS-prevention interventions. Grounded in social learning theory and cognitive-behavioral approaches, and personalized to communicate culturally specific AIDS prevention information, these two AIDS-prevention interventions are a self-instructional "rap style" comic book and a computer-based AIDS-prevention software program.

The comic book is a culturally sensitive and idiomatically relevant illustrated booklet that includes a companion trainer's manual. Emphasized in the comic book are effective strategies for youth to manage interpersonal situations and personal behaviors in order to reduce their risk of HIV infection. Informed by the results of focus studies, we developed a prototypical curriculum that incorporates a variety of skills-intervention components. Using a 5-stage problem-solving model with the acronym SODAS, the skills-intervention curriculum integrates major elements of problem solving, coping, and communication skills, including refusal, avoidance, awareness, and escape skills.

As a prologue to learning these skills, essential AIDS knowledge and facts are taught with optimum use of illustrations and simplified text. The comic book is designed in a contemporary, colorful style intended to make the material more accessible to minority youth and to simplify communication of AIDS information. The engaging and fun style of presentation tempers potentially fear-inducing and anxiety-arousing material that might otherwise block learning. A cartoon character drawn to mirror participants' age and ethnic-racial backgrounds serves to guide youth through the text.

Using rap music verse, the character describes how adolescents can contract AIDS and how they can avoid it through behavior

change. The guide devotes attention to risks associated with intravenous drug use, including needle sharing, sexual contact with
partners who inject drugs, and decisions and steps that could lead
to intravenous drug use.

Brief vignettes at the beginning of each new work page introduce the reader to a variety of high-risk situations that provide
several opportunities for learning and practicing the SODAS model.
The reader indicates responses and decisions by filling in the
speech balloons above the characters' heads. Each character prompts
the reader for a response, reinforces use of the SODAS model, and
encourages the reader to proceed to the next high-risk situation.

The comic book is divided into two sections. The first section,
HIV Facts, is organized into five learning modules: (a) AIDS definition, (b) HIV transmission, (c) high-risk behaviors, (d) symptoms,
and (e) prevention. After explaining the behavioral risks of AIDS
and ways to avoid these risks, the guide introduces participants
to the cognitive problem-solving model, SODAS. This sequence
uses a game format that asks youth to make hypothetical decisions
about situations involving drug use and AIDS risks ("This game
is called SODAS; but you don't exactly drink it. . . . In order to
play it, you gotta *think* it!"). The steps in the sequence are (a) Stop,
(b) Options, (c) Decide, (d) Act, and (e) Self-Praise.

In the first step—Stop—participants learn that they should pause
and give themselves time to consider their choices and the consequences of their choices when facing drug use and other risk-taking
situations. ("Really stop and *think* what these choices could *really*
mean for you, today, tomorrow . . . for *years* to follow").

The second step—Options—instructs youth to brainstorm a variety of possible solutions for solving the identified problem. To graph-
ically show participants how to consider their options, the guide
depicts a scale on which various outcomes from decisions are
weighed. ("The *best* way to choose your option is to think of a scale
that measures how much you gain and how much you would fail.")

The third step—Decide—shows participants how to choose the
best solution from their options. The Decide step helps youth
evaluate the positive and negative consequences of each possible
solution and the feasibility of each option before selecting the best
alternative for a given situation.

Integral to the decision-making process are elements of situational
perception training. Situational perception training teaches youth

how to use a given skill at the appropriate time and place relative to the person with whom they are interacting. Emphasizing that appropriate responses will vary, depending on the problem, the guide recommends that participants base their decisions on an informed assessment of the problem. The guide teaches participants to consider whether a solution to a problem situation might involve danger, rejection, or other risk taking ("Before you take action, don't jump right on in—first draw an arrow to the situation you find yourself in"). Participants then note the decision that was best for them.

Situational perception training is increasingly necessary as greater numbers of young people become the victims of violence and intimidation. In such a climate, such facile responses as "just say no" are unrealistic and naive. Instead, what is needed are tailored approaches that young people, particularly inner-city youth, can use with confidence. The development of effective survival strategies requires that young people are taught how to make the appropriate responses and to take the appropriate actions in ways that will best ensure their safety. Successful coping outcomes for youth are based on facility with three Rs: resilience, resistance, and resourcefulness.

The fourth step—Act—helps youth plan and rehearse their best response to a problem situation. In this step, youth consider five possible types of verbal responses to peer pressure situations: (a) "I" statements, (b) delay statements, (c) refusal statements, (d) alternative suggestions, and (e) blunt and blur statements.

In the second section of the self-instructional comic book, participants are presented with five problem situations and are asked to apply the problem-solving model, SODAS. These problem situations are referred to as *puzzles* ("Now move on to my puzzles. Let me see how you do. You heard enough from me. I wanna hear from you!"). For each puzzle, participants are asked to solve the problem situation for a cartoon character.

At the end of each problem-solving puzzle, participants are reinforced for work completed and are encouraged to move on to the next problem ("Good answer! Now you've got the hang of it, so keep on goin'. Try the next one on your own."). This reinforcement constitutes the fifth and final step—Self-Praise—of the problem-solving model.

A randomized clinical field trial of the self-instructional comic was conducted during the summer of 1989. Participants were 60 adolescents enrolled in an urban job-training program. The 34 females (56.7%) and 26 males (43.3%) had a mean age of 16.01 years. Participants were from African-American (36.7%), Hispanic (26.6%), and Caribbean-black (15%) backgrounds, with the remaining participants from other minority groups (11.7%) and nonminority groups (10%). Youth were invited to participate in the study as an adjunct to job-training program activities. In an initial session, youth learned about study procedures and risks. Then participants and their parents were given passive consent forms. No youth or parents passively declined study participation.

Participants completed a pretest battery coded to ensure confidentiality and to enhance the accuracy of self-reports. The battery contained scales on demographic items, drug use and sexual activity, and HIV-infection knowledge, attitudes, and risks. Overall alpha reliability for the self-report battery was .89. Test-retest reliability for the measure from responses to expectedly stable questions over two assessment occasions averaged .97.

Subjects were assigned to one of three groups: the self-instruction comic book plus small group intervention, the self-instruction comic book alone, and an information only control condition. Our findings revealed that 60% of the participants approved highly of the intervention and that only 6% of the participants said they already knew the intervention content. Subjects who received the self-instruction intervention improved from pretest to posttest on their ratings of the value of AIDS education. Participants in the self-instruction guide plus small group intervention decreased their permissiveness toward IV drug use, whereas participants in the control condition increased their permissiveness toward IV drug use. After exposure to the intervention, participants in the self-instruction plus small group intervention were more likely to talk with friends about sexual matters.

Computer-Based AIDS-Prevention Intervention

A second intervention also designed to personalize AIDS-prevention information for inner-city minority-culture youth resulted in software for a computer-based AIDS-prevention intervention. Designed as a computer game and based on the AIDS-prevention comic book, the computer program presents general information about the AIDS virus, including a definition of the A-I-D-S acronym, symptoms of AIDS, and how AIDS is and is not transmitted.

Two beliefs guided our development of the computer-based AIDS-prevention intervention. First, we believe that many contemporary American youth are put off by traditional pedagogical methods of instruction. To reach these youth, interventions that focus on preventing or reducing problem behaviors require strategies that are syntonic with young people's cultural preferences. Second, we believe that the ethnic-racial diversity of American youth requires interventions that are tailored to their cultural heterogeneity.

The instructional goals of the computer-based AIDS-prevention program were threefold: (a) to provide youth with simple information about AIDS, (b) to introduce youth to a cognitive-behavioral skills model for reducing behavioral risks associated with acquiring AIDS, and (c) to provide youth with the opportunity to practice skills for confronting AIDS-related risk situations.

Written in Hypertalk 1.2 for the Apple Macintosh, the computer-based AIDS-prevention program presumes no special knowledge of computer use. The program merely requires basic reading skills and the ability to comprehend simple verbal and written instructions.

Animation in the computer-based intervention increases youth's interest in AIDS information; youth's sustained interest increases the probability of greater learning outcomes. In addition, animation allowed us to elaborate on ideas in ways that the linear format of the comic book could not accomplish.

Preliminary testing of the AIDS computer-based intervention was conducted with primarily African-American (61.7%), Hispanic (20.0%), Caribbean-black (10%), and other minority groups (6.7%) who attended an after-school tutoring program in Harlem. A questionnaire with items on attitudes and behavioral risks related to HIV transmission was delivered in face-to-face interviews to 60 adolescents. The 32 females (53.3%) and 28 males (46.7%) had a mean age of 16.27 years ($SD = 1.27$).

Participants completed a confidential and anonymous pretest and posttest questionnaire. The pretest and posttest questionnaire, administered on the same day, consisted of 29 items that assessed youth's attitudes and intentions with respect to substance and alcohol use, sexual behaviors, and condom use, as well as specific questions regarding frequency of substance use, alcohol use, sexual intercourse, and condom use. Participants also completed a brief evaluation of their level of satisfaction with the computer-based AIDS-prevention intervention. The computer intervention itself also contained 10 questions related to HIV-infection knowledge and risks. Test-retest reliability for the measure from responses to expectedly stable questions over two assessment occasions averaged .98.

After completing the pretest battery, participants interacted with the 20-minute computer-based AIDS-prevention intervention. Using animation, original music, menu-driven screens, and peer- and age-relevant characters, the computer-based intervention presented HIV facts, including (a) AIDS definition, (b) HIV transmission, (c) high-risk behaviors, (d) symptoms, and (e) prevention (Schinke, Gordon, & Weston, 1990). Immediately following intervention, participants completed a 14-item evaluation of their experience with the computer program, and a posttest questionnaire.

Dependent t tests revealed pretest and posttest differences after exposure to the AIDS-prevention computer-based intervention, as well as differences based on self-reported sexual activity among the adolescents surveyed. The percentages of correct responses to the computer-based AIDS knowledge questions ranged from 83% to 97% correct.

After participants interactively used the AIDS-prevention computer-based intervention, their posttest scores were significantly different from their pretest scores with respect to their receptivity to using condoms ($t(59) = -2.68$, $p<.009$), their disapproval of occasional drug use ($t(59) = -2.56$, $p<.013$), their disapproval of hanging out with same-age peers who get high ($t(59) = -2.01$, $p<.049$), and their perceived harmfulness of occasionally having alcoholic drinks ($t(59) = -3.40$, $p<.001$).

Among the 30% ($n = 18$) of the sample reporting sexual intercourse during the 4 weeks prior to the survey, 39% were females, 78% were African-American, and 17% were Hispanic-American. Youth who did not report having sexual intercourse in the 4 weeks prior to testing were 16.09 ($SD = 1.34$) years of age, whereas youngsters who reported having sexual intercourse were 16.67 ($SD = 1.03$) years of age. Among youth who had sexual intercourse, 55% ($n = 10$) reported using condoms on each occasion, and 27% ($n = 5$) did not use condoms on any occasion.

Youth who did not report having sexual intercourse during the 4 weeks prior to testing significantly improved between pretest and posttest on the same items as youth who reported having sexual intercourse. In addition, youth who reported not having sexual intercourse significantly improved at posttest from pretest assessments in their perceived harmfulness of using marijuana ($t = -2.47$, $p<.018$). Youth who reported having sexual intercourse showed significant improvement at posttest on their disapproval of spending time with same-age peers who got high ($t = -2.38$, $p<.029$) and their perceived harmfulness of occasionally having alcoholic beverages ($t = -2.68$, $p<.016$).

Despite the limitations of the study, which include small sample size, lack of a control group, and possible confounding effects, microcomputer interventions hold promise for reducing the risk of HIV infection among minority-culture youth.

Conclusions

Traditional interventions based on a disease model have proven costly, lengthy, and of arguable effect. As an empirically based approach to prevention, cognitive-behavioral interventions represent a viable alternative to traditional psychosocial approaches toward preventing the spread of AIDS among adolescents.

One advantage to employing a model that uses learning theory to explain problem behaviors is that the approach avoids labeling and stigmatization, while emphasizing proactive behaviors. Learning theory places control within the individual, creating positive expectations for change and simultaneously stressing that maladaptive behaviors can be unlearned and replaced by health-promoting behaviors. Further, cognitive-behavioral approaches reject causal explanations based on intrapsychic processes and instead focus on overt target behaviors and on methodologies for measuring outcomes. Because the focus is on overt, measurable behaviors, cognitive-behavioral interventions lend themselves to controlled research and hypothesis testing.

Cognitive-behavioral approaches are also modular and portable. A repertoire of cognitive-behavioral interventions can be built into one comprehensive program that addresses such issues as decision-making, problem solving, seeking positive role models, escape-avoidance and self-defense skills, social-skills training, communications skills, coping skills, and assertiveness training. Because these modules are adaptable to a variety of formats and presentations, they can be tailored easily for culturally and racially diverse groups.

The adaptability of cognitive-behavioral interventions to such media as games, comic books, novellas, or computers is testimony to the flexibility and creativity of cognitive-behavioral approaches for preventing HIV infection. The computer's added technological flexibility makes software a promising yet untapped mode of delivery for effective AIDS-prevention messages.

The study findings reported earlier suggest that computer-based interventions can influence attitudes and intentions toward drug use, peer influence, and sexual behaviors with minority-culture youth. Future research should include the development and testing of a comprehensive AIDS-prevention software program that incorporates information about AIDS transmission along with skills training to teach youth to regulate their behavior. Our findings suggest that timing the interventions to coincide with specific developmental stages may be critical for effective AIDS-intervention outcomes. Obviously the onset of adolescent sexual activity is an important developmental marker for interventions with AIDS-information content.

AIDS-prevention interventions designed for the microcomputer can be portable, reliable, and inexpensive. The interactive capacity of these interventions can attract and hold adolescents' interest. Via custom software, youth can elicit facts and skills in areas of concern to them. Powerful microprocessors allow computer programs to personalize youth's learning, permit flexibility, enhance youth's involvement, and provide immediate feedback (Gustafson, Bosworth, Chewning, Hawkins, & Van Koningsveld, 1987; Levin, 1983).

Results from computer-based instruction indicate that computers can be more effective than traditional interventions; computer learning requires less time than conventional learning; computer learning generates positive attitudes toward subject material and toward computers themselves; and computer instruction may be especially effective with disadvantaged youth (Condry & Keith, 1983). Additionally computer interventions can provide automatic and accurate measurement of subjects' progress, provide information for instructional improvement, allow for personal control and freedom to explore the learning environment, and support self-paced learning. Further, computer formats can give youth confidential access to information about HIV transmission and risks. Confidentiality is essential if young people are to relate AIDS behavioral risks to life-style practices. Reliable information is crucial if young people are to separate truth from myth. By interacting with computer software, adolescents can learn a repertoire of AIDS-prevention skills and gain the confidence to apply that learning. For adolescents from lower socioeconomic and disadvantaged backgrounds, computer interventions appear especially beneficial (Becker, 1988; Jamison, Suppes, & Wells, 1974; Johnson & Mihal, 1973; Saracho, 1983; Shurdak, 1967; Suppes & Morningstar, 1969). Still, before the potential for developing relevant computer-based interventions can be realized, market forces must adjust to the needs of inner-city youth for access to utilitarian hardware and responsive software.

The interactive computer has the capacity to allow youth to control their rate of learning. Computer interventions with disadvantaged youth show considerable promise because of the computer's ability to provide in vitro practice, to concretize abstract concepts, to be relatively self-instructional, to integrate behavioral procedures, to provide intrinsic motivation and reward, and, through the use of enhanced graphics and voice simulation, to minimize the need for reading skills.

In the absence of a cure for AIDS, continued efforts to develop and test innovative, culturally sensitive interventions remain our best hope for preventing the spread of HIV infection among minority youth. Computer-based interventions that are theory-driven hold promise for tailoring interventions to address specific ethnic groups, developmental stages, and geographic locations.

References

Bandura, A. (1990). Perceived self-efficacy in the exercise of control over AIDS infection. *Evaluation and Program Planning, 13*, 9-17.

Becker, H. J. (1988). Using computers for instruction. *BYTE, 12*, 149-162.

Bobo, J. K., Snow, W. H., Gilchrist, L. D., & Schinke, S. P. (1985). Assessment of refusal skills in minority youth. *Psychological Reports, 57*, 1187-1191.

Brooks-Gunn, J., Boyer, C. B., & Hein, K. (1988). Preventing HIV infection and AIDS in children and adolescents: Behavioral research and intervention strategies. *American Psychologist, 43,* 958-964.

Centers for Disease Control. (1988a). HIV-related beliefs knowledge and behaviors among high school students. *Morbidity and Mortality Weekly Report, 37,* 717-721.

Centers for Disease Control. (1988b). Number of sex partners and potential risk of sexual exposure to human immunodeficiency virus. *Morbidity and Mortality Weekly Report, 37,* 566-568.

Condry, J., & Keith, D. (1983). Educational and recreational uses of computer technology: Computer instruction and video games. *Youth and Society, 15,* 87-112.

Day, N. A., Houston-Hamilton, A., Deslondes, J., & Nelson M. (1988). Potential for HIV dissemination by a cohort of black intravenous drug users. *Journal of Psychoactive Drugs, 20,* 179-182.

DiClemente, R. J. (in press). Epidemiology of AIDS, HIV seroprevalence and HIV incidence among adolescents. *Journal of School Health.*

DiClemente, R. J., Boyer, C. B., & Morales, E. S. (1988). Minorities and AIDS: Knowledge, attitudes and misconceptions among black and Latino adolescents. *American Journal of Public Health, 78,* 55-57.

Evans, R. I., & Raines, B. E. (1982). Control and prevention of smoking in adolescents: A psychosocial perspective. In T. J. Coates, A. C. Petersen, & C. Perry (Eds.), *Promoting adolescent health: A dialogue on research and practice* (pp. 225-249). New York: Academic Press.

Flora, J. A., & Thoresen, C. E. (1988). Reducing the risk of AIDS in adolescents. *American Psychologist, 43,* 965-970.

Gordon, N. A., & McAlister, A. L. (1982). Adolescent drinking: Issues and research. In T. J. Coates, A. C. Petersen, & C. Perry (Eds.), *Promoting adolescent health: A dialogue on research and practice* (pp. 201-223). New York: Academic Press.

Green, L. (1984). Health education models. In J. D. Matarazzo, S. M. Weiss, J. A. Herd, N. E. Miller, & S. M. Weiss (Eds.), *Behavioral health: A handbook of health enhancement and disease prevention* (pp. 181-199). New York: John Wiley.

Gustafson, D. H., Bosworth, K., Chewning, B., Hawkins, R. P., & Van Koningsveld, R. (1987). *Final survey evaluation report: Barn project.* Madison, WI: Center for Health Systems Research and Analysis.

Jamison, D., Suppes, P., & Wells, S. (1974). The effectiveness of alternative instructional media: A survey. *Review of Educational Research, 44,* 1-61.

Johnson, D. F., & Mihal, W. L. (1973). Performance of blacks and whites in computerized versus manual testing environments. *American Psychologist, 6,* 694-699.

Kegeles, S. M., Adler, N. E., & Irwin, C. E. (1988). Sexually active adolescents and condoms: Changes over one year in knowledge, attitudes, and use. *American Journal of Public Health, 78,* 460-461.

Levin, W. (1983). Interactive video: The state-of-the-art teaching machine. *Computing Teacher, 2,* 11-17.

Office of Technology Assessment. (1988). *How effective is AIDS education?* Washington, DC: Government Printing Office.

Petersen, A. C. (1982). Developmental issues in adolescent health. In T. J. Coates, A. C. Petersen, & C. Perry (Eds.), *Promoting adolescent health: A dialogue on research and practice* (pp. 251-270). New York: Academic Press.

Saracho, O. N. (1983). The effects of a computer-assisted instruction program on basic skills achievement and attitudes toward instruction of Spanish-speaking immigrant children. *American Educational Journal, 19,* 201-219.

Schinke, S. P., Gordon, A. N., & Weston, R. E. (1990). Self-instruction to prevent HIV infection among African-American and Hispanic adolescents. *Journal of Consulting and Clinical Psychology, 58,* 432-436.

Schinke, S. P., Moncher, M. S., & Holden, G. W. (1989). Preventing HIV infection among black and Hispanic adolescents. *Journal of Social Work and Human Sexuality, 8,* 63-73.

Schinke, S. P., Orlandi, M. A., Gordon, A. N., Weston, R. E., Moncher, M. S., & Parms, C. A. (1990). AIDS prevention via computer-based intervention. *Computers in Human Service, 5,* 147-156.

Shurdak, J. J. (1967). An approach to the use of computers in the instructional process and an evaluation. *American Educational Research Journal, 4,* 59-73.

Strunin, L., & Hingson, R. (1987). Acquired immunodeficiency syndrome and adolescents: Knowledge, beliefs, attitudes, and behaviors. *Pediatrics, 79,* 825-828.

Suppes, P., & Morningstar, M. (1969). Computer-assisted instruction. *Science, 166,* 343-350.

Thompson, E. I. (1978). Smoking education programs 1960-1976. *American Journal of Public Health, 68,* 250-257.

11

Community-Based HIV-Prevention Programs
for Adolescents

BENJAMIN P. BOWSER

GINA M. WINGOOD

Introduction

Adolescence is the most social and risk taking of the psychological developmental stages (Kett, 1977). Anyone who has ever tried parenting teenagers knows the extent to which teens belong to their peers and the media. For adolescents, what is "in" either in their perception or in fact among their peers becomes almost totally self-defining. To not conform threatens the adolescent's social acceptance and sense of self and is literally cause for existential embarrassment. But along with slavish conformity with their peers comes a need to become independent of parents and other socializing adults. It becomes important to be able to make one's own decisions and to act independently. It is also important now to test oneself in the adult world, where one has been a dependent and a child for so long. The challenge, the freedom to act, and new experiences are so exciting that the risks seem minimal. Risk taking and the sense that they can and will live forever regardless of what they do are part of this developmental period. This is why neighborhood and community are so important to the rearing of adolescents. Parents of young children know that eventually their generally compliant youngsters will become adolescents. When that happens, the community and the places where their adolescents will act out their transition to adulthood are equally if not more important than what goes on in their homes.

The social and risk-taking nature of adolescents also characterizes adolescent sexuality. Our public culture, official history, religious ideals, and laws do not acknowledge adolescent sexuality (Hernton, 1965). But the reality is that adolescents are sexual, and since 1960, increasing proportions are sexually active (Henshaw & Fort 1989). Sex is one of the many things adolescents are curious about, want to experience, feel that they must know about in order to be adults, and are willing to take risk over. In this sense, *adolescence* is not narrowly defined as 13- to 19-year-olds. Many young adults who successfully put off initial sexual experimentation are still adolescent in their sexuality well into their 20s and beyond. Still other adults never make the transition to adult sexuality. They are experimenting, testing, and trying to find themselves well into middle age.

Adolescents and HIV

The extraordinary challenge and difficulty that the public health community has in getting adults to change their HIV high-risk behaviors are only magnified with adolescents. It is difficult for sexually experienced adults to plan rationally and execute their sexual and emotive lives in such a way that they absolutely minimize their risks of becoming HIV infected. Whenever one experiences adolescent sexuality, it is without prior experience, without prior trial and error in planning and negotiating sexual relations, and without skill in managing strong emotions that motivate sexual risk taking. Beginning adolescent sexuality also occurs without a compelling perspective on one's very real vulnerabilities, in which case, being an adolescent is itself a high-HIV-risk condition. As HIV continues to spread, even at a very slow rate, the likelihood that sexually active adolescents will be exposed and infected with HIV increases and could exceed the statistical risks of becoming HIV infected among sexually active adults outside of high-risk groups. This high risk level is indicated by increasing rates of STDs among some adolescents (O'Reilly & Aral, 1985).

The potential for the HIV epidemic to collide with adolescent sexuality and to challenge our already limited attempts at prevention is already on us. Especially high-risk groups among sexually active adolescents are homosexual teens (Stall, Coates, & Hoff, 1988); homeless teens who trade sex for drugs and money; and socially isolated and economically disadvantaged African-American (Miller, Turner, & Moses, 1990), Puerto Rican, and Native-American adolescents (Centers for Disease Control, 1990). What all of these adolescents have in common is that their social and sexual networks run in and out of networks of adults at high risk of being HIV infected—primarily gay and bisexual men and injection drug users. The folklore of teens limiting their sexual experimentation with other teens is simply not the case for these groups. The sex partners of teen homosexuals, as well as minority adolescent females, may very well be older males. What we do not know is the extent to which adolescents in the general low-risk majority have sexual partners who are adults.

In light of the nature of adolescents to peer-conform, to seek independence from adults, to experiment, and to take risks, it would seem that HIV prevention might be very difficult. Subgroups of adolescents who are at greatest risk have the additional difficulty of being socially isolated and distinct in subculture. HIV prevention now may seem virtually impossible. But an important point is not immediately apparent: HIV prevention may in fact be easier among adolescents precisely because they are such conformists and are so heavily influenced by peer (perceived and actual) influences and social norms. This point may not be apparent on the individual level, where people are abstracted out of their social and community context. Once the community context is made apparent, however, possible strategies to begin AIDS prevention among the diversity of adolescents becomes apparent.

The Problem of Levels of Analysis

The community context of adolescents and other high-risk groups is not well known. An important reason is that HIV-prevention research focuses foremost on the individual as the unit of analysis and objective for intervention (Coates, 1990). This is very appropriate for medical doctor-to-patient or counselor-to-client, one-on-one interventions. But we must acknowledge the influence of the community on individuals' behavior. Recognition is increasing that peers, shared norms, and "culture" shape the individual's response to his or her sexuality and how he or she perceives the HIV threat and HIV-prevention information. Cultures and aspects of cultures that might reinforce HIV-risk behaviors among adolescents are not changed by focusing on individuals. Let us assume that one is successful in changing an adolescent's risk behaviors. The effect will not automatically be multiplied to others.

Culture is a group, not individual, concept. *Culture* describes the norms, agreements, arrangement of systems of meanings, and expectations of groups of people (Kroeber & Kluckholm, 1963). The most important characteristics of individuals are their group memberships and identities (Cooley, 1964). Group identities are what make individuals human and social—most like other individuals with the same range of group memberships and identities. While sexual and needle-sharing risk behaviors occur between individuals, the interaction between needle sharers is social in nature. What this means is that what is good sex, bad sex, risky sex, or safe sex is socially or group defined, reinforced, or negatively sanctioned. Even charismatic leaders do not have the power to define group norms as individuals. They must act within their group-defined role as "leader." Individuals voluntarily elect what groups they will consciously identify with, but the social nature of individual behavior more than suggests that the group is a crucial unit of analysis in HIV prevention and the level where the greatest impact can be made on large numbers of individuals.

As it is with individuals, groups and group identities are multidimensional. The social identity that may shape an individual's sexual behavior and HIV risks cannot simply be defined and abstracted. We have to understand the group's social context—the conditions that shape its members' social experiences. The success of any effort to make widespread change in human behaviors is dependent on knowing the social context of the behaviors targeted for change. To miss the social context is to miss the meaning of the behavior whether it is for adolescents or adults (Leech, 1974). To illustrate, ask an individual under what circumstance he or she might engage in some high- or low-risk sexual behavior. You will get one answer. Pose the same question to a small group in which that individual is a participant. If you keep the discussion focused on the question, you will get not only a different answer from this same individual, you also will get a sense of what he or she might do under a variety of circumstances. Both responses were valid, but the second response was closer to what may happen in social context (Gregory & Carroll, 1978).

Once our unit of analysis—the social group rather than the individual—is clear, then we can approach the challenge of understanding and changing some aspect of a group's culture. More specifically, we have to understand the conditions that shape adolescent sexual culture. *Sexual culture* is defined as "the systems of meaning, of knowledge, beliefs and practices, that structure sexuality in different social context" (Parker, Herdt, & Carballo, 1991, p. 79). When intervention is sought at the most appropriate level of human organization—the group—the HIV-risk-reduction message will have a greater likelihood of acceptance and impact. This is why social movements first seek to change group norms and beliefs in order to gain widespread support. In the same way, HIV low-risk behaviors can be achieved and multiplied across large numbers of individuals in the group. The precondition is that the adolescent systems of meanings and norms of what is to be emulated or shunned must be consistent with and supportive of low-risk ideals—abstinence, and safer sex negotiated relations.

Community and Adolescent AIDS Prevention

If HIV prevention is to succeed at all for any group, it must do so at the community level. The success of gay communities in HIV epicenters in reducing their HIV-risk behaviors is one of the clearest examples. Once the nature of the HIV threat was realized, the community mobilized and used classic social movement tactics to change social norms to favor low-risk behaviors (McKusick, Conant, & Coates, 1985). From a perspective of historic social change, three factors were important in this success. First, the gay community was organized and functioning as a self-identified, politically present, and physically bound community. Second, the AIDS-prevention movement came from within the gay community. Third, the gay community had the resources, both human and financial, to mobilize and support a general social movement. But if we look more closely at the AIDS-prevention success of the gay community, we see that the success was in fact bound or limited in scope. As with all other groups, there is no one gay community. The HIV-prevention success occurred primarily in the white, middle-class, gay community. Gay men of color, gay working and lower-class men, and gay men outside of the HIV epicenters have yet to achieve the low-risk norms of their middle-class white peers. There is a lesson in this example for adolescent AIDS prevention.

The first thing to be learned from the limited community-based success of gay men in HIV prevention is that there is no one adolescent community. Even within the same race and culture, adolescents' social networks, norms, and value systems vary by social class. While adolescents may be self-identified, they do not have a political presence, and all of their communities are not necessarily physically bound. The HIV-prevention message will not initially come from among adolescents, yet the message must be indigenous in order to be accepted and acted on. Finally, adolescents do not have the resources or the organization to sustain a general social movement among themselves to change HIV high-risk behaviors. Clearly, a strategy that worked for one group may not necessarily work in the same way for another. The main reason why adolescents will have to be approached differently is not because they are adolescents but because they are as diverse as the parent communities in which they reside. In which case, any attempt at AIDS prevention among adolescents must first define which group of adolescents one wants to target, what the group's community is, and how that community is structured and organized.

Community Diversity

Because adolescence is the most social of all the psychosocial developmental stages, variations in the character of adolescents and the extent to which they are sexually active and engage in HIV-related risk behaviors vary by the nature and organization of their communities; that is, the very character of adolescence will vary by the quality and character of community. Based on community research since the 1920s, physically bound residential neighborhoods have life cycles (Choldin, 1985). The social context of the community varies by stages within a neighborhood's life cycle. The first three stages show transition from initial development through full maturity: (a) rural, (b) developmental, and (c) full occupancy. This constitutes the first 30-40 years. In stage two—developmental—neighboring has not yet developed. By inference, adolescents are isolated from one another, social networks have yet to develop, and socialization is close to adult norms. In stage three—full occupancy—neighboring develops; a critical mass of adolescents forms initial social groups, but their activities are still largely defined by their parents and organized activities. Adolescence in stages two and three is defined largely by parent norms and is fairly uniform and enforced throughout the neighborhood. We can infer that adolescent HIV risks in early stage neighbors will be minimal and individual. In such neighborhoods, one-to-one, directed, HIV-risk-reduction counseling may be utilized effectively for adolescents.

If the nature of adolescence subtlety changes as the community changes, the challenge is when adolescent parent communities reach stages four through five. From stage four on, the neighborhood begins its slow aging and decline. In stage four, the informal social agreements that were used to rear successfully the first generation of adolescents from the neighborhood begin to break down. Single family homes are subdivided, and renters become a visible proportion of residents. "Community parenting" ceases (Mitchell, 1991). In stage five, buildings deteriorate. Those who can, move. The social bonds that have defined the community become more and more fragmented. What had been the community becomes the old people who were left behind or who chose to stay. In stages four and five, the neighborhood becomes a patchwork of unrelated and fragmented social networks. Residents who might have been middle or working class in the earlier stages of the neighborhood's life cycle are now reduced to being part of the economic lower and underclass. It is in these latter stages that adolescents form gangs for social support, are not under the control and shading influences of "community parents" or adult norms, and become sexually active in their early teens.

As a community declines, the behavior of adolescents in that community reflects the declining social structure of the neighborhood. The neighborhood becomes increasingly transient, economically marginal, home for multiproblem and troubled individuals and households. In this setting, adolescents who are part of the public life in the community also change. Social bonds shift from family to peers, both financial and emotional independence are sought earlier, and there is greater isolation and anomie. Fewer and fewer young people are connected to school, to home, or to a future. This is the adolescent social context in which HIV prevention becomes more difficult. It is more difficult because the adolescent community and social networks are self-defined and self-contained along boundaries that may or may not conform to the adult's definition and boundary of *community*.

The factor of *community diversity* suggests that adolescence varies across three dimensions. First is the dimension of *community life cycle*, already discussed. Second is the dimension of *social context*. Young people who depend on street-based peers and social networks are our first identified social context. They are the specific HIV high-risk group we are concerned with because they are usually sexually active earlier, have more partners, use condoms less frequently, are more isolated from information about HIV, are less likely to believe what they do hear, and are more likely to take risks. Yet another social context exists—adolescents who are restricted from the streets and who are home based. We know a lot less about these young people and how their families manage to keep them from street influence. Finally are the adolescents whose social context is their extended family network. They socialize exclusively within their extended family. We know even less about these young people. It is possible that HIV-risk behaviors vary radically across these social contexts, as well as the way in which risk taking is initiated and the way in which one would have to access young people in each social context.

Then there is the third dimension by which adolescents and community can vary. The research on communities and neighboring has long debated the extent to which it is appropriate to define *community* in terms of geographically bound physical areas. Evidence suggests that "urbanization permits people to have communities of intimate relationships that branch out well beyond the neighborhood" (Connerly, 1985, p. 538). This evidence is in contrast to the more traditional view that interpersonal neighboring is bound by proximity. What this tells us is that there may be subpopulations of adolescents whose communities may or may not be physically bound. Their community may be physically diffused across a number of locations, and their community boundaries may conditionally shift every so often (Unger & Wandersman, 1985). In this case, their social and sexual risk-taking network may not conform to their physically bound neighborhood. This means that any attempt at AIDS prevention among adolescents or any other high-risk group first must determine "the form of social linkage between individuals, and only then inquire into the degree to which these networks form social solidarities concentrated in neighborhoods" (Connerly, 1985, pp. 537-538). It may very well be that the highest risk takers in declining communities may not be directly accessible through what may appear to be their physically bound neighborhood. They may cross into other communities.

We can no longer assume that an individual's or group's social networks and social participation are physically bound by the immediate neighborhood in which they live. Public health officials define communities by their political boundaries and favor mass communications techniques. The billboards, fliers, and public service radio and television spots are salient for people who participate in mass society. But lower class and underclass HIV high-risk adolescents are outsiders to mass society and take an outsider's view of its media and messages. Those messages are dismissed, reinterpreted, or viewed with suspicion. More often, adults and people in community organizations see community as physically bound—where they live or their service area. The adolescents' social and sexual networks may run across several physically bound communities and may be highly mobile and conditional. Where these young people live is an important AIDS-risk factor. The location of their primary social identity within these communities, however, is even more important.

Behavior change interventions may be more effective by knowing what level of social organization is being targeted (individual or group norms), who specifically among those at risk are the high-risk takers, and how community is perceived and organized among high-risk takers. In HIV-prevention research, what constitutes the community for those who are at risk and for those who take risks cannot be assumed. If these points are overlooked or not taken into consideration, an intervention may be targeted at the wrong subgroup within the community and may be directed in an

Table 11.1   Levels of Community Diversity

Life Cycle of the Community			
Residential Development	Full Occupancy	Down-Grading	Thinning Out

Social Context of Adolescent Community		
Street Based	Home Based	Extended Family

Community Scope			
Physically Diffuse	Physically Bound	Conditionally Bound	Mass Society

inappropriate manner. Either way, the intervention is less likely to be effective. Table 11.1 reviews the dimensions of community that must be considered in developing HIV-prevention research and interventions for adolescents.

Any combination of these qualities of community structure results in a very different social context for adolescents. The qualities also structure a difference in sexual cultures for adolescents. Clearly, HIV risk-taking behaviors will vary, depending on the combination of community qualities. Minority adolescents who are high-risk takers have an adolescence that is structured by socialization in declining urban neighborhoods, have a street-based social context, and may have social and sexual networks diffused across a number of physically bound communities. In this case, even visual and radio media appeals that are culturally sensitive will have a limited impact because these communications tools are seen as an extension of mass society. In contrast, the information that is important to street-based adolescents with diffused social networks comes word-of-mouth from other peers on the streets. In the same way, a community-based organization may have an important role to play in disseminating HIV-prevention information and in fostering HIV-preventive behaviors within indigenous populations in its community. But the organization's perception of community may not correspond to that of high-risk adolescents whose sense of community may be diffused across a number of communities. The adolescent for whom an HIV-prevention program is intended may not "hang out" in the neighborhood or be available for the program. If adolescents' social network is diffuse, they might not even identify with the organization or its activity in their behalf, and therefore they have to be reached directly by word of mouth from persons in their own network based in a variety of locations.

Community-Based Adolescent HIV Prevention

In the United States, sex education usually is considered to be the domain of parents. By extension, HIV-prevention education also is the role of parents. The increasing levels of sexual activity among adolescents suggest that parents are having some difficulty fulfilling this role. Furthermore the increasing prevalence of sexually transmitted diseases and pregnancy among some adolescents in declining communities suggests that some parents in these settings have very little impact on their adolescent's sexuality. Some evidence exists that adolescents are in fact emulating the example of parents. In these cases, schools and community-based organizations are called on to be the frontline of intervention. While sex education has been conducted in schools for some time, HIV-prevention education is relatively new. It is questionable, however, whether school-based HIV-prevention education will effectively reach and dispose high-risk adolescents to change their behavior. For one thing, the highest risk takers among minority adolescents probably have dropped out of school by the time these programs are implemented (usually in the 10th grade or higher) or are marginal and suspicious of school-based information. This leaves community-based organizations as having the greatest potential to reach those young people.

In comparison with school-based AIDS prevention and other potential intervention agents, community-based organizations (CBOs) have the potential to be more aware of the social contexts to which adolescents are responsive. CBOs are culturally specific and are perceived as more credible sources of information and thus have a greater potential to be trusted by their clients. CBOs have access to the young people and their peers through community youth centers and direct street outreach. They have access to parents in their homes through direct outreach. While offering a number of avenues of access to hard-to-reach adolescent populations, CBOs do have limitations. They have limited fiscal resources; as such, staffs are more often poorly trained, overworked, and limited in size. They are called on often to do far more than they can reasonably manage. The following are examples of three community-based adolescent AIDS-prevention efforts. These project are not unique; however, they are highly regarded as being very successful. These examples provide an opportunity to look at the "state of the art" in terms of community-based HIV intervention efforts, as well as affording an opportunity to see how these programs might be improved and evaluated, given our greater sensitivity to the variations in community and in adolescents.

The Bayview-Hunter's Point Foundation

The Bayview-Hunter's Point Foundation is located in the largest working class, African-American sector of the city of San Francisco—the Bayview-Hunter's Point area. This community is struggling through its downgrading stage in the community life cycle. In this struggle, the foundation provides a broad spectrum of city-supported social and health services. For adolescents, peer counseling, a home detention monitoring project for youthful offenders paroled to home, and an African-American gang task force are available. The foundation's efforts toward AIDS prevention among adolescents began with a teen rap contest. Since then, the use of rap music has been formalized to produce rap public service announcements for radio and television. In addition, adolescents from the community have been trained as peer counselors. Elements of their peer education include African-American pride, AIDS education, communications skills, assertiveness training, behavioral self-management, and improving coping strategies. Clearly, these services are directed appropriately at street-based adolescents. It is assumed that the young people's sense of the community is physically bound, as is the foundation's service area.

While the foundation's specific efforts have not been evaluated, a similar effort has been evaluated by Gilchrist and Schinke (1983). These investigators found that African-American adolescents who participated in a multicomponent cognitive-behavioral treatment (providing information; teaching problem-solving, modeling, and communications skills) were more knowledgeable about sex and contraception. Project participants had more favorable attitudes and intentions regarding contraception. They also had better sexual communication skills and sexual self-efficacy. But we do not know two very important things from this evaluation: First, from what social context did these adolescents come? Second, what was their sense of community scope? Without this information, we are limited in knowing for which group of adolescents these research findings are most applicable.

Teenage Father's Responsibility and Support Program

African-American males are central to a host of social problems, including rapidly increasing rates of sexually transmitted diseases (STDs) and teen pregnancies. Community-based organizations have begun to target limited program resources on this subgroup. The Teen Father's Responsibility and Support Program in San Francisco began in 1987 as a collaborative effort with three community centers aimed at developing a model program for African-American adolescent fathers (ages 14-17). The program objectives are to reduce the incidence of sexually transmitted disease, including HIV infections, and teen pregnancies. A number of program participants have several children, and the prevalence of STDs is substantial. Program clients are drawn from the most economically depressed African-American community in San Francisco and the most advanced in its decline—the Western Addition.

The program uses focus groups and case management as its primary intervention tools. Case management includes client outreach, individual assessment, and identifying jobs, scholarships, and legal services. It also links clients to health services. In individual counseling with a case manager, each program client receives HIV education and access to condoms, continuing education, and vocational rehabilitation. In attempting to improve each client's skills, the program strives to combat the low self-esteem and high unemployment that is the social context for early sexuality (Bowser, Fullilove, & Fullilove, 1990; Fullilove et al., 1990). Again, we do not know the client's social context or sense of community. For this reason, it is difficult to assess to what extent the Teen Father's Responsibility and Support Program represents an efficacious and generalizable community-based model for HIV prevention. For one thing, if HIV enters the social and sexual networks of these young people, effective prevention will have to be implemented before they become sexually active or parents.

Blacks Educating Blacks
About Sexual Health Issues (BEBASHI)

BEBASHI began in Philadelphia in 1985 as a response to the increasing number of African-Americans being seen in the infectious disease unit at Albert Einstein Medical Center. In 1989, the project began conducting HIV counseling, anonymous and confidential HIV testing, and syphilis screening. Program clients are African-American women, gay and bisexual men, and low-income housing project residents.

For adolescents, BEBASHI conducts basic information classes in schools, in inpatient and outpatient substance abuse clinics, and in juvenile detention facilities. Skills training is provided through peer educators who focus on the risk of HIV infection and through a street outreach effort to adolescents that distributes condoms and HIV-education literature. The peer educators work with youth wherever they find them—in schools, churches, buses, locker rooms, rest rooms, and other informal and formal settings. Finally, BEBASHI offers classes in human sexuality, sexual communication, and sexual relationships. This approach has not been evaluated, and we do not know the social context or community scope of BEBASHI program clients. But of the three cases outlined, this one might have potential to be the best AIDS-prevention model. It is mobile and crosses across physical communities and settings to reach young high-risk takers. It also connects with and informs the social networks of potential high-risk takers with street-based peer outreach. BEBASHI comes closest to affecting the social norms of highly mobile adolescent risk takers and therefore multiplies its impact beyond immediate program clients.

Program Evaluation and Improvements

These programs are first generation. They bring to HIV-prevention activities all of the advantages of being community based. The culture of the community and the specific subculture of adolescents are intrinsic to their efforts and are not "tacked on" to strategies that have not been proven effective in African-American communities. In addition the ways in which minority CBOs approach their clients and hope to attain their goals are based in a long history of direct action and the use of education for social change. These were the tactics used to achieve general education and literacy among African-Americans at the turn of the century. The same tactics were used to mobilize support for civil rights reforms and legislation at the turn of the century, during the late 1940s, and again in the 1950s. Whatever the crisis, African-Americans use direct action and general education. The question to be answered in the coming decade is, Will these tactics, as reflected above, be sufficient to change the HIV-related drug and sexual behaviors of underclass African-American adolescents?

A rapid increase in sexually transmitted diseases continues among African-Americans in communities served by these organizations. Rising STD rates are not an isolated phenomenon particular to San Francisco and Philadelphia. This epidemic of STDs reflects a broad national phenomenon among underclass African-American youth. This phenomenon suggest two potential problems. First, current programs are not extensive enough to reach a large enough proportion of adolescents to make a difference in aggregate STD statistics. Second, the programs themselves are traditional and, although well intentioned, may not be maximally effective. Without sufficient evaluation research, it is difficult to answer either problem. A provisional guess is that the limited scale and effectiveness of these programs are problems that will have to be addressed.

Three things will have to happen before the issues of scale and effectiveness of community-based AIDS prevention are addressed. First, minority communities have to recognize that HIV is a major health issue. Then they will have to mobilize a general social movement to extract financial and technical resources from fiscally conservative and hard-pressed governments to support large-scale prevention efforts. Second, the movement will have to generate a large enough scale of awareness in the community to challenge group norms that reinforce HIV high-risk behaviors. For the moment, African-Americans view HIV as just one more crisis among the many more immediate problems plaguing their communities. In addition homophobia and antidrug use feelings are strong enough to engender indifference to a disease that appears to be attacking only gay, bisexual men and injection drug users. As the increasing incidence of HIV infections among African-American adolescents is recognized, it will become clear that this epidemic will not stop with groups considered to be marginal to the African-American community. Third, once action is demanded and taken, program efforts will have to be evaluated.

Lives will be dependent not simply on having extensive HIV-prevention programs but, as important, on whether these programs are effective in motivating the adoption and maintenance of low-risk behaviors. Compare the diversity of African-American communities and the resultant quality of adolescence with the prevention strategies of the first generation of adolescent HIV-prevention programs outlined above. From such a comparison, the following concerns will have to be addressed in program development and evaluation:

1. While individual behavior change may be the objective of any AIDS-prevention program, changing group social norms is the most efficient and effective way to change the behaviors of large numbers of individuals.

2. Adolescent HIV-prevention efforts in ethnic communities cannot assume that all youth in their communities have similar HIV-risk profiles because the youth are from the same subculture or live under the same economic and social conditions. New programs have to be very specific in determining who is at highest risk and in targeting the social norms of those youth for intervention.

3. It is very important to understand how HIV risk-taking adolescents define themselves. Are they a community unto themselves? Do they know, interact, and take risks with one another? How do they differ from their lower risk-taking peers in the community? If they are a community, can they be reached as a community? If they are distinct in some way from others in their immediate community, then one has to determine how they will be reached. The worst scenario is that they are not a group but are randomly dispersed and isolated individuals. Whatever the answers, this is essential information in order to devise the most efficient intervention strategy.

4. If high-risk takers are in a series of even loosely defined subcommunities, one's effort should aim specifically at the social networks of these high-risk takers. One cannot assume that a community fair, public access program, or posters will reach, be salient to, or be credible for the highest risk individuals.

5. Programs have to be designed not only to affect the social norms of specific high-risk adolescents in the community but also to fit the specific community and even neighborhood. Even low-income ethnic communities vary in their stage in the community life cycle and in the extent that adults control public space and adolescent social norms. If a community is very tightly knit, the most effective way to affect adolescents at high risk is to target high-risk adults who serve as role models.

6. In communities at the end of their life cycle, peer and street-based strategies have to be emphasized. Adolescence in these communities is qualitatively different—more isolated, marginal to adult influence, and mistrustful of mainstream media. For communities in any of the earlier stages of their life cycle, school-based programs may be sufficient to reach adolescents at high risk.

References

Bowser, B., Fullilove, M. T., & Fullilove, R. T. (1990). African-American youth and AIDS high-risk behavior: The social context and barriers to prevention. *Youth and Society, 22*(1), 54-66.

Centers for Disease Control. (1990). *HIV surveillance report, Table 4, May 10, 1990.* Atlanta: Author.

Choldin, H. (1985). *Cities and suburbs.* New York: McGraw-Hill.

Coates, T. (1990). Strategies for modifying sexual behavior for primary and secondary prevention of HIV disease. *Journal of Counseling and Clinical Psychology, 58*(1), 57-69.

Connerly, C. (1985). The community question: An extension of Wellman and Leighton. *Urban Affairs Quarterly, 20*(4), 537-556.

Cooley, C. (1964). *Human nature and the social order.* New York: Schocken.

Fullilove, M., Weinstein, M., Fullilove, R., Crayton, E., Goodjoin, R., Bowser, B., & Gross, S. (1990). Race/gender issues in the sexual transmission of AIDS. In P. Volberding & M. Jacobson (Eds.), *AIDS clinical review* (pp. 25-62). New York: Marcel Dekker.

Gilchrist, L. & Schinke, S. (1983). Coping with contraception: Cognitive and behavioral methods with adolescents. *Cognitive Therapy and Research, 6,* 379-388.

Gregory, M., & Carroll, S. (1978). *Language and situation: Language varieties and their social contexts.* London: Routledge and Kegan Paul.

Henshaw, S., & Fort, J. (1989). Teenage abortion, birth and pregnancy statistics. *Family Planning Perspectives, 21*(2), 85-89.

Hernton, C. (1965). *Sex and racism in America.* New York: Grove.

Kett, J. (1977). *Rites of passage: Adolescence in America, 1790 to the present.* New York: Basic Books.

Kroeber, A., & Kluckholm, C. (1963). *Culture: A critical review of concepts and definitions.* New York: Random House.

Leech, G. (1974). *Semantics*. Baltimore: Penguin.

McKusick, L., Conant, M., & Coates, T. (1985). The AIDS epidemic: A model for developing intervention strategies for reducing high risk behavior in gay men. *Sexually Transmitted Diseases, 12*, 229-234.

Miller, H. G., Turner, C. F., & Moses, L. E. (Eds.). (1990). *AIDS: The second decade*. Washington, DC: National Academy.

Mitchell, L. (1991). We are the children of everyone: Community co-parenting—A biographic note. In B. Bowser (Ed.), *Black male adolescents: Parenting and education in community context* (pp. 160-179). Lanham, MD: University Press of America.

O'Reilly, K., & Aral, S. (1985). Adolescents and sexual behavior: Trends and implications for STD. *Journal of Adolescent Health Care, 6*, 262-270.

Parker, R., Herdt, G., & Carballo, M. (1991). Sexual culture, HIV transmission, and AIDS research. *The Journal of Sex Research, 28*(1), 77-98.

Stall, R., Coates, T., & Hoff, C. (1988). Behavioral risk reduction for HIV infection among gay and bisexual men: A comparison of published results from the U.S. *American Psychologist, 43*, 859-864.

Unger, D., & Wandersman, A. (1985). The importance of neighbors: The social, cognitive, and affective components of neighboring. *American Journal of Community Psychology, 13*(2), 139-163.

12

Developmentally Tailoring Prevention
Programs: Matching Strategies to
Adolescents' Serostatus

MARY JANE ROTHERAM-BORUS

CHERYL KOOPMAN

MARGARET ROSARIO

Introduction

While the absolute number of adolescent AIDS cases is still relatively low (Centers for Disease Control, 1991), it is estimated that more than 60,000 HIV-positive adolescents are in the United States today (Rotheram-Borus, Koopman, & Ehrhardt, 1991). While few of these HIV-positive youth are aware of their serostatus, increasing numbers will be identified as HIV testing is adopted as a

AUTHORS' NOTE: This work was supported in part by center grant 5-P50-MH43520 from the National Institute of Mental Health and the National Institute on Drug Abuse (Anke A. Ehrhardt, Ph.D., Principal Investigator).

prevention strategy (Kutchinsky, 1988) and as youth gain access to prophylactic treatments (Knox & Clark, 1991). Preventing the spread of HIV by youth who are infected is critical to reduce long-term negative public health and economic consequences of the AIDS epidemic. In addition, it is important in halting progression of the disease to each new age cohort. Therefore it is critical to understand the special needs of HIV-positive youth.

Secondary Prevention
for HIV-Positive Adolescents

To prevent the spread of HIV, we must institute secondary prevention programs for those already infected. Such programs are particularly critical because HIV-positive adolescents often experiment with sexual behavior, alcohol, and drugs (Brooks-Gunn, Boyer, & Hein, 1988), are likely to be sexually active for many years before becoming symptomatic (Hein, 1989), and thus may infect many persons over their lifetimes if their risk acts continue. In addition, these youth often do not have access to ongoing health care, nor do they adhere to medical regimens if treated. The health care costs of treating these youth will be contained only if programs are mounted to help youth adopt consistent, positive health care habits. Given these concerns, the purpose of this chapter is to examine how a modification of the AIDS risk reduction model can be tailored to a youth's risk status to best prevent the spread of HIV through sexual and drug-use risk acts and to extend the youth's life with adoption of health care practices. This process entails three goals: (a) identification of risk acts, (b) adherence to appropriate health care regimens, and (c) booster sessions to maintain support for new skills and safe behavior.

The AIDS Risk Reduction Model

The *AIDS risk reduction model* (ARRM) is a stage model that was developed specifically for HIV-related risk acts, although it was not specifically designed to be used with adolescents. The AIDS risk reduction model appears to be useful and appropriate as a general risk-reduction theory. Developed from work with adult gay men (Catania, Kegeles, & Coates, 1990), the ARRM describes three prerequisite stages for reducing HIV-risk acts: (a) HIV-risk acts must be perceived as a problem, (b) persons must become motivated to act safely, and (c) skills to implement safe acts (sexual and substance use behaviors that pose no risk of HIV transmission) must be acquired and practiced. This model is general enough to serve as a framework for understanding and classifying other prevention efforts.

The ARRM builds on earlier theoretical models and therefore self-efficacy theory, the theory of reasoned action, and the health belief model are applicable to specific stages of the ARRM. For example, *self-efficacy,* a belief that one is competent in a specific activity (Bandura, 1977), is related to motivation for health-enhancing behavior, Stage 2 of the ARRM. Similarly the *theory of reasoned action* (Ajzen & Fishbein, 1980) focuses on the acquisition of motivation for HIV-safe acts. In contrast, the *health belief model* (Becker, 1974) details factors relevant to each of the three stages of the ARRM. Stage 1, the perception of HIV as a problem, is related to two factors within the health belief model—perceived threat of HIV, and susceptibility and severity of HIV. Stage 2 of the ARRM, motivation to engage in safe acts, is related to the perceptions of benefits and barriers. Finally, Stage 3, implementing safe acts, is related to identifying cues to action, another aspect of the health belief model.

Use of a theoretical framework such as the ARRM is an important starting point for designing HIV-prevention programs. Use of such a framework, however, requires further specification of the characteristics of the targeted population and the particular problems it faces. Adolescents have in common certain characteristics that distinguish them from adults and children and that must be considered in developing effective HIV-prevention programs.

The AARM is not well suited for the specific developmental problems of adolescent HIV prevention. Before adolescents can begin to integrate the HIV-transmission information they receive, they must be able to understand how this knowledge might affect their lives. For example, before youth can perceive HIV as a problem, they must be aware of their own reactions in situations that involve drugs and sex. Adolescents must know themselves better before they can imagine accurately the circumstances that place them at risk.

Anticipatory Awareness in HIV-Prevention
Programs for Adolescents

Adolescents endorse teenage sexuality (Association for the Advancement of Health Education, 1988) and do not uniformly report socially desirable responses. Therefore the gap between adolescents' intentions and behaviors cannot emerge solely from denial or trying to create a favorable impression. Rather, we attribute inconsistencies between adolescents' risk behaviors and their reportedly high self-efficacy or intentions to adolescents' lack of anticipatory awareness across risk situations. Situations vary in the level of risk behavior they are likely to elicit, and adolescents lack experience. Developmentally adolescents are in situations involving sex and drugs for the first time.

Adolescents do not know themselves well enough to anticipate accurately their likely reactions to the kinds of situations that are most likely to elicit high-risk behavior from youth—sexual, romantic, and pleasure-oriented activities (e.g., drinking parties) with others. They do not anticipate accurately their emotions, thoughts, or behaviors in such situations. For example, an adolescent male attending a party at which a pornography film will be shown might not anticipate his emotions, thoughts, and behaviors in response to viewing such a film. Given their lack of experience, combined with their biological arousal patterns, adolescents do not anticipate that in such situations they are likely to experience intense sexual excitement, romantic feelings, or fear of rejection by peers. They neither anticipate these feelings nor identify and label these feelings when they occur.

Also adolescents do not anticipate having thoughts that are dysfunctional in supporting safe behavior in high-risk situations, for example, "I'm in love so I don't have to worry about condoms." Finally adolescents do not anticipate the negative future consequences that may follow from high-risk situations that occur in the present. These situations often offer immediate emotional rewards for high-risk behaviors, and adolescents have little experience in exerting self-control in the face of such tempting rewards. For example, an HIV-positive youth may be coaxed by a friend to attend a social gathering that turns out to be a party at which everyone is sharing a hypodermic syringe to inject cocaine. To behave responsibly in order to prevent the transmission of HIV, this youth must exert self-control despite peer pressure and being presented with an opportunity to get high. Youth who have not developed the anticipatory awareness to recognize their likely feelings, thoughts, and behavior in such a situation are more likely to share the syringe than they would if they had already developed this anticipatory awareness. In these situations, adolescents have competing goals: They want to say no, and they want to keep their friends. Achieving both these goals requires certain social skills. For example, an adolescent who wants to avoid using cocaine at a party can say that something is wrong with his or her nose and so does not want to snort this time. Each time, the adolescent can present a different excuse so that friends do not reject him or her, and yet the youth does not have to use cocaine.

Of course, substantial individual differences exist in the degree of arousal and risk presented by specific situations. A situation that will elicit intense emotional flooding leading to unsafe behavior in one youth will present no temptation to behave unsafely to another adolescent. Therefore a youth's development of anticipatory awareness requires the adolescent to understand the personal risk posed by different situations. Adolescents need to become aware of the characteristics of high-risk situations for themselves. For example, many adolescents feel "onstage" in social situations and need to recognize that placing great importance on the impression they make is likely to increase the risk of acting unsafely in social situations. They also need to become aware of their likely bodily and emotional reactions to being touched or to using drugs or alcohol.

If an adolescent lacks such anticipatory awareness, he or she will have no perception of HIV as a problem, the necessary first step in the AIDS risk reduction model. Therefore in working with adolescents, the development of anticipatory awareness is a crucial precursor for recognition of HIV as a problem. An adolescent may have cognitive knowledge of the means of HIV transmission but will not internalize that information in a way that affects behavior until he or she can imagine the situation and emotions that might elicit such behavior in him- or herself. Without accurately being able to anticipate the emotions, thoughts, and behaviors that a high-risk situation is likely to elicit, adolescents fail to perceive the problem that they face in that situation. If they do not perceive the problem, they are unlikely to be able to live up to their best intentions to behave safely or, more importantly, to enact safe behaviors.

While the development of anticipatory awareness is relevant to HIV-prevention efforts across adolescent populations, some important differences among adolescents must be considered in designing maximally effective prevention programs. Foremost is the youth's serostatus. Preliminary evidence suggests that primary prevention programs have been mounted that can effectively reduce adolescents' high-risk behavior; however, HIV-positive youth are likely to have additional needs not typically addressed by such programs that must be considered by secondary prevention programs. Therefore, below we discuss primary prevention programs that have been developed to stop youth from becoming infected. Our goal is to modify existing prevention programs for youth of unknown serostatus for the particular benefit of HIV-positive youth.

Primary Prevention Programs Can Change Adolescents' HIV-Risk Behaviors

Although adolescents are relatively well informed abut AIDS and have positive attitudes toward safe acts (DiClemente, 1990; Hingson, Strunin, & Berlin, 1990; Koopman, Rotheram-Borus, Henderson, Bradley, & Hunter, 1990; Sonenstein, Pleck, & Ku, 1989), this knowledge has not translated into changing risk behaviors (Kegeles, Adler, & Irwin, 1988; Strunin & Hingson, 1987; Vermund, Hein, Cary, Drucker, & Reuben, 1988). There is reason to expect, however, that adolescents may change their HIV-risk acts. Nationally adolescents are using condoms more frequently (Mosher, 1990; Sonenstein et al., 1989). More important, reductions in high-risk acts have been demonstrated with middle-class gay adult males (Kelly, St. Lawrence, Hood, & Brasfield, 1989), drug users (Watters et al., 1990), adults in methadone maintenance (Schilling, El-Bassel, Schinke, Gordon, & Nichols, 1991), runaways (Rotheram-Borus, Koopman, Haignere, & Davies, 1991) and gay youth (Rotheram-Borus, Meyer-Bahlburg et al., in press). These programs have demonstrated that prevention programs can work, similar to prevention of adolescent substance abuse (Botvin & Tortu, 1988).

Successful programs have been described by the following characteristics: (a) Each consists of multiple intervention sessions; (b) a major component of the training is assertiveness and coping skills training, as well as ensuring acquisition of knowledge and positive attitudes toward safe acts; (c) the individual's personal risk behaviors are identified, ranked in order of risk, and systematically addressed; and (d) ongoing support for behavior change is structured actively (e.g., through group meetings to enhance peer support and social norms for safe acts). While minor differences exist in these programs, the implementation is structured in a similar manner, consistent with the principles of social learning theory. Social rewards, positive role models, active rehearsal, problem solving, and brainstorming among members of a small group characterize each program. The goals in all groups remain the same: Identify risk acts, encourage health care adherence, and support maintenance of safe behavior.

Each of the components addressed in these programs can also be conceptualized within the framework of the AIDS risk reduction model (Catania et al., 1990). From this perspective, in Stage 1, participants must come to see their risk acts as a problem. This involves having realistic expectations about transmission. The adolescents must know that if they engage in risky behavior, they may contract the virus. This requires knowledge about HIV infection itself. The participants must know that risky acts include sharing needles and engaging in unprotected sexual intercourse. Based on adult models, perception of HIV/AIDS as a problem emerges when knowledge about AIDS is acquired and positive attitudes toward safe acts are developed to enhance adolescents' general concern regarding HIV/AIDS. Rather than through didactic lectures, however, AIDS information is best transmitted through video workshops, activities with an art or drama therapist (e.g., criticizing the artistic quality of three or four HIV-prevention videos, rap contests about HIV), and adolescent theater groups. Basic to adolescents' increased knowledge of HIV is increased knowledge about sexuality and substance use. A question box in which adolescents can anonymously ask embarrassing questions that get answered in group discussion can effectively teach HIV information related to definitions, outcomes of HIV infection, means of transmission, means of prevention, relative risk of sexual behaviors, and HIV testing.

Another aspect of Stage 1, perceiving HIV as a problem, involves developing anticipatory awareness. Adolescents must become aware of the links between risk situations and their own affective, cognitive, and behavioral reactions. This is a cornerstone of skills training programs. Rotheram-Borus, Miller, Koopman, Haignere, and Selfridge (1992) use a "feeling thermometer" as an initial means of providing adolescents with a vocabulary to discuss their feelings and to begin to be aware of the intensity of various emotional states, to describe and monitor the intensity of their feelings, and to manage and self-control highly charged emotional reactions (Rotheram, Armstrong, & Booraem, 1982). Each youth identifies social situations in which his or her feeling thermometer, similar to a thermometer for measuring the temperature of the atmosphere, is 20, 40, 60, 80, 100. The feeling thermometer typically is used to indicate a dimension of comfort (temperature of 0) to discomfort (temperature of 100); however, recognition of feelings of sexual excitement and identification of an individual's threshold for self-controlling emotional responses can also be useful. The youth identifies past high-risk behaviors and links the situations, thoughts, and feelings associated with those risk acts. Having built a personal-risk hierarchy, the youth now has prevention activities tailored for him or her.

Motivation to act safely, Stage 2 of the ARRM, is likely to be based on desires for self-preservation and acceptance from peers and romantic partners. Motivation must encompass elements of self-preservation, self-efficacy, and the desire to protect others. Adolescents must have a sense of their own positive futures as employed, productive members of society and must recognize that this goal is threatened if they contract HIV. They must believe also that they have the ability to act in ways that protect their health. Finally they must be motivated to protect others. One of the most effective ways to instill this concern is to have the adolescents recognize that their own behavior may put their own children at risk. Developmental features associated with adolescence often make it difficult to mobilize these motivations. First, adolescence is characterized by a sense of invulnerability (Strunin, 1991), as well as norms that downplay the negative consequences of death through AIDS. For example, one gay youth minimized the potential negative impact of HIV with the phrase, "Die young, stay pretty!" Particularly among inner-city minority youth whose lives are chronically stressed and among youth engaging in multiple problem behaviors, HIV is only one potential problem against the reality of being killed in a drug deal or ending up in prison.

Within such a context, motivation to adopt safe behavior patterns is most likely to emerge only within a supportive peer group and neighborhood. Successful programs have targeted both the community (e.g., Kelly & St. Lawrence, 1990) and institutional settings (e.g., Rotheram-Borus et al., 1991). A cohesive atmosphere in which social norms that endorse safe acts are established within a social support network maximizes individual youth's motivation. Within such a group, youth can be provided with accurate information about peers' behavior to dispel myths. Additional activities are designed to motivate youth to act safely. For example, Walter (1991) found that 80% of adolescents believed that their peers were engaging in sexual intercourse, while in reality only 50% were sexually active. Youth who were not sexually active felt atypical and stigmatized rather than perceiving themselves as normative. Finally, motivations for protecting others can be elicited by having youth visit orphanages for HIV-positive babies and attending presentations by HIV-positive young adult role models.

Stage 3, the implementation of safe acts, is based on skills training (interpersonal problem-solving ability, social skills) and access to comprehensive care. Implementation requires the acquisition of interpersonal skills, appropriate self-talk, and access to the resources required to maintain a healthy life-style. *Interpersonal problem solving* refers to youth's ability to set goals, to generate alternatives to solve these goals, and to evaluate the *means* required to implement various alternatives, the *selection* of one alternative, and the *evaluation* of the success of one's efforts (Spivack, Platt, & Shure, 1976). The training helps youth to identify and analyze an interpersonal problem in terms of the risks, costs, and opportunities that it offers in relation to one's needs (e.g., "This is the kind of situation that could easily lead to unsafe sex") and to consider and evaluate alternative ways of handling the situation (e.g., evaluating the pros and cons of trying to abstain from sex). Three behavioral skills are targeted: (a) clear requests, (b) refusals, and (c) coping with criticism. The specific content of the behavioral training will be based on the identification of risk situations when building the risk hierarchy. Access to health care, mental health care, and condoms is necessary to maintaining safe acts and is provided at each site. This is particularly critical because an adolescent who has no place to sleep and does not know where the next meal is coming from has little time or energy to worry about a distant reality such as HIV infection.

Modifying HIV-Prevention Programs for HIV-Positive Youth

The goals of an HIV-prevention project shift with HIV-positive youth. With HIV-negative adolescents or those of unknown serostatus, the primary goal is to lower each person's probability of contracting HIV. With HIV-positive youth, the goals are different. In particular, an HIV-positive adolescent must achieve two goals: (a) prevent spreading the virus to others, and (b) obtain appropriate health care. Accomplishing these goals minimizes health care costs, as well as prolongs the adolescent's life.

Before adolescents can begin to address these public and personal health care concerns, however, they first must deal with the reality of their own serostatus. A recent case referred to our office reflects the problems associated with current pretest and posttest HIV counseling with adolescents:

A 19-year-old female learned on a Thursday that her 20-year-old boyfriend was HIV-positive, the father of her 15-month and 6-month-old children. She simultaneously learned that he had another sexual partner. On Friday morning, she was tested for HIV and given an appointment in 3 weeks to learn the results. While she had asked about getting an HIV test for her children, she was unclear whether the children should be tested, and the children had not been tested that morning. She arrived at our office Friday afternoon, suicidal and lacking condoms. Her boyfriend, who accompanied her to a research interview, had been seen at the HIV-testing clinic twice in the previous two days but had not received a doctor. He had an abscess on his finger that had also gone untreated despite two visits to a hospital-based HIV-testing site. Both youths were treated in an emergency room. The HIV-positive boyfriend was too embarrassed to tell the doctor in the emergency room of his serostatus; however, the research assistant that accompanied him willingly disclosed for the youth, with the youth's consent. The girl was hospitalized for suicidality and released in two days; her boyfriend watched the children.

This case illustrates a number of the problems that result from testing alone. First, this woman was not provided with a health care liaison to help her negotiate the medical system or to explain to her the relative merits of testing her children. She was not given condoms and thus had no immediately available means of risk reduction at her disposal. Second, neither she nor her boyfriend received adequate or timely health care services. Such scenarios appear common among HIV-positive youth. HIV testing alone, without appropriate health care and risk-reduction counseling, simply identifies the problem. Without appropriate support, an adolescent has no way of knowing what his or her serostatus means for his or her health or for the danger he or she presents to others. These problems highlight the need for developmentally tailoring prevention programs to youth's serostatus.

In addition to risk of spreading HIV infection to others, learning one's serostatus may be associated with increased depression, conduct problems, and extreme anxiety. HIV-positive youth must cope with feelings of denial, of anger, and about death (Stuber, 1991). These responses have been documented among adult gay men (Stern, Singer, Leserman, Silva, & Evans, 1991) even many years after being informed of their diagnosis (e.g., Rabkin & Remien, 1991). Clinicians working with adolescents report that youth often demonstrate erratic behavior, long periods of denial, self-destructive behavior, and angry actions intended to harm others. In other words, knowledge of serostatus alone often leads to an intensified negative emotional state. Among 24 youth testing HIV-positive, suicidal ideation was common, but no suicide attempts occurred (Futterman, 1991). However, 21% of New York City high school students spontaneously reported they would commit suicide if they were HIV-positive (Goodman & Cohall, 1989). Rotheram-Borus, Koopman, and Dobbs (1991) also found that many youth reported that they would attempt suicide and/or "take many people with them" by having unprotected sexual intercourse with others if they were HIV-positive. The very limited and sketchy data available indicate the importance of stopping secondary spread of HIV infection and promoting positive health care regimens among HIV-positive youth.

At this stage, the goal is not merely to acknowledge the problem intellectually but to deal with the associated emotions. In HIV-negative youth, it was assumed that adolescents do not know their own feelings and responses and need to learn more about them before they can perceive themselves to be at risk. In contrast, HIV-positive youth must cope with their emotions of denial and anger before they are assaulted with new knowledge and information about how not to infect others.

Because of these concerns, recruiting HIV-positive youth into secondary prevention programs must begin at posttest counseling to provide follow-up services and support for coping with denial and anger. Community-based programs report that it is often difficult to recruit youth and that few model programs have been identified. A variety of activities has been developed that appears to hold adolescents' attention while helping them cope with denial, anger, and other reactions to the stress of learning their HIV-positive status. For example, youth can plan how they would like the newspaper and/or friends to remember them.

While the ARRM identifies the components of successful prevention programs, applications of the model to secondary prevention with HIV-positive youth require that each stage be modified. With HIV-positive adolescents, the first step of a Stage 1 awareness of HIV as a problem involves dealing with the affective component of positive serostatus. The adolescent must first acknowledge his or her serostatus. Once this is done, the youth must recognize that he or she presents a risk to others. The adolescent must learn also to deal in appropriate ways with the negative emotions that inevitably follow such an acknowledgment. As with HIV-negative youth, adolescents' scripts about themselves rarely coincide with their behavior, and they are rarely aware of the inconsistences. Just as HIV-negative youth need to perceive themselves to be at risk before they can see HIV as a problem, HIV-positive adolescents often need to acknowledge their anger and denial before they are willing to recognize themselves as a risk to others. Thus adolescents need to be educated about who they are and what their behavior pattern is before they can be taught more intellectually based knowledge about AIDS. Without this foundation, adolescents may be too emotionally unstable and distraught to be able to understand and integrate whatever information they receive.

Stage 1, acknowledging that HIV is a problem, involves a health care component as well. Infected adolescents must learn to take care of themselves. This involves obtaining consistent medical care, gaining knowledge about the course of HIV infection, and learning to understand medical information about themselves. Taking care of themselves may also necessitate developing drug-free social support networks, as well as dealing with the emotional reactions to stopping drug use or to changing sexual behavior.

The strategies to accomplish Stage 2 goals of motivating safe behavior shift with HIV-positive youth as well. The youth must learn to value others' health and to protect others from being infected. Changing risk acts at this stage is motivated by altruism, as a youth must now be concerned with transmitting, rather than contracting, the virus. To accomplish this goal, adolescents participate in discussions with adult HIV-positive and ex-substance abusers who serve as role models for safe behavior.

Among HIV-positive youth, motivation for self-preservation shifts to adherence of health care regimens (Stiffman, Earls, Robins, & Jung, 1988). Their motivation derives from a desire to live as long and healthy a life as possible. The ambition to maintain health will be fostered by generating peer support and developing strong peer norms that endorse routine health habits. In addition, altruism and responsibility to others must be mobilized to motivate HIV-positive youth to act safely. This is quite different from the perspective of primary prevention with HIV-negative youth.

Finally new and different behaviors need to be implemented by HIV-positive youth in Stage 3—disclosure of serostatus to present and past sexual and needle sharing partners, and avoiding and coping with discrimination and stigmatization. Disclosure and avoiding discrimination are directly linked, as avoiding disclosure is an obvious strategy for avoiding discrimination. Disclosure of serostatus to present and past partners, however, is a critical public health strategy to stop the spread of infection. On the one hand, disclosure of serostatus by HIV-positive youth is likely to lessen risk of HIV infection among partners. On the other hand, HIV-positive youth who disclose their serostatus are likely to experience discrimination. In a study of 150 self-identified gay youth, 55% had experienced gay bashing (Rotheram-Borus, Rosario, & Koopman, 1991). It is likely that a higher percentage will need to cope with prejudice and discrimination. Scripts that help HIV-positive youth selectively disclose their serostatus and strategies for avoiding or controlling potentially violent or other negative reactions from others must be a cornerstone of the social skills training.

In contrast to HIV-negative youth, the implementation of safe behavior for HIV-positive adolescents will require consistent and rigorous adherence to appropriate health care regimens. This adherence will necessitate access to health care, mental health care, and condoms.

The primary method proposed to help increase youth's concern and practice of consistent health habits is a beeper system. The use of a beeper and a diary to monitor youth's health care habits and to help them develop new habits such as taking a dose of zidovudine (AZT) once every 4 hours is proposed by Futterman (1991) as one method of maintaining good health. These techniques have been used by community psychologists to assess children's social networks. Youth wearing a beeper can be contacted also by research and clinical staff. Having youth make self-confrontational videos is a technique used in substance abuse prevention research that may be useful with HIV-positive youth. Youth are asked to talk about their drug use or sexual risk behaviors on videotape and to play these tapes back for the individuals. Also a case manager must be available to HIV-positive youth to facilitate and coordinate their access to health, mental health, and social services.

To maintain safe behaviors effectively among HIV-positive youth, it is critical to anticipate relapse and to design programs to prevent it (Becker & Joseph, 1988; Stall, Ekstrand, Pollack, McKusick, & Coates, 1990). It is likely to be many years before HIV-positive youth are symptomatic; thus, preventing the HIV-positive youth from infecting others requires long-term maintenance of behavior change. Evidence exists among adult gay men (Ekstrand & Coates, 1990; Kelly & St. Lawrence, 1990) that relapse of high-risk sexual behavior is common. Among gay men, relapse was especially likely among the younger males (Kelly & St. Lawrence, 1990), suggesting it may be an even greater problem among adolescents.

Relapse prevention would address the three stages of the ARRM through the booster module of the proposed intensive intervention condition: (a) helping HIV-positive youth identify high-risk problem situations; (b) strengthening their motivation to avoid high-risk behavior; and (c) further developing their behavioral coping skills, particularly the coping with dysfunctional thoughts.

Relapse prevention typically consists of follow-up meetings at a minimum of five 3-hour workshops over a 6-month period offered once every 2 weeks. HIV-positive youth must develop a social support network that encourages consistently safe behavior and in which rewards can be delivered for maintaining safe acts on an ongoing basis. To maintain and enhance motivation, a youth's social network or small group meeting needs to share success experiences in acting safely. Situations in which it was difficult to maintain safe acts may be identified on an ongoing basis to allow further specification of risk factors as new social encounters arise. In a small group, youth brainstorm, problem-solve, and rehearse alternative actions to acting unsafely. The discussion of problem situations will not be limited to a discussion of AIDS issues but may include a variety of issues.

HIV-positive youth must receive rewards for acting safely and attending to their health on a daily basis in order for these behaviors to be maintained. Therefore boosters focus on self-rewards, group compliments, and planning pleasurable activities that are safe as a means of increasing motivation.

Tailoring Programs to Individual Youth

The AIDS surveillance data for adolescents and young adults indicate that HIV-positive youth are a heterogenous group, varying by gender, ethnicity/race, and risk factors for HIV infection; the latter refers primarily to differences in sexual orientation and drug use. The potential effect of each one of these factors on the effectiveness of prevention programs for HIV-positive youth must be considered during the design, delivery, and evaluation of such programs. In addition, the impact of the youth's symptomatology or pathology will affect any preventive intervention in numerous and possibly surprising ways. We found, for instance, that gay and bisexual male youth who were in therapy reported the highest prevalence of risky sexual behaviors and voluntarily attended many more HIV-prevention sessions than those who were not in therapy.

Conclusion

A substantial gap exists between (a) the current practices in primary and secondary prevention programs and HIV testing of youth and (b) the theoretical sophistication of prevention theories and model programs. A challenge exists to replicate the model programs, while maintaining excellence in the implementation of these programs. The challenge for prevention researchers is to document the effectiveness of their theories and programs. The problem is transferred then to legislators who must prioritize these efforts in contrast to other national concerns.

References

Ajzen, I., & Fishbein, M. (1980). *Understanding attitudes and predicting social behavior.* Englewood Cliffs, NJ: Prentice-Hall.

Association for the Advancement of Health Education. (1988). *National adolescent student health survey.* Reston, VA: Author.

Bandura, A. (1977). *Social learning theory.* Englewood Cliffs, NJ: Prentice-Hall.

Becker, M. H. (Ed.). (1974). The health belief model and personal health behavior. *Health Education Monographs, 2,* 324-508.

Becker, M. H., & Joseph, J. G. (1988). AIDS and behavioral change to reduce risk: A review. *American Journal of Public Health, 78,* 394-410.

Botvin. G. J., & Tortu, S. (1988). Preventing adolescent substance abuse through life-skills training. In R. H. Price, E. L. Cowen, R. P. Lorion, & J. Ramos-McKay (Eds.), *Fourteen ounces of prevention: A casebook for practitioners* (pp. 98-110). Washington, DC: American Psychological Association.

Brooks-Gunn, J., Boyer, C. B., & Hein, K. (1988). Preventing HIV infection and AIDS in children and adolescents: Behavioral research and prevention strategies. *American Psychologist, 43,* 958-964.

Catania, J. A., Kegeles, S. M., & Coates, T. J. (1990). Towards an understanding of risk behavior: An AIDS risk reduction model (ARRM). *Health Education Quarterly, 17,* 53-72.

Centers for Disease Control (CDC). (March 1991). *HIV/AIDS surveillance report.* Atlanta: Author.

DiClemente, R. J. (1990). Adolescents and AIDS: Current research, prevention strategies and public policy. In L. Temoshok and A. Baum (Eds.), *Psychological aspects of AIDS and HIV disease* (pp. 52-64). Hillsdale, NJ: Lawrence Erlbaum.

Ekstrand, M. L., & Coates, T. J. (1990). Maintenance of safer sexual behaviors and predictors of risky sex: The San Francisco men's health study. *American Journal of Public Health, 80,* 973-976.

Futterman, D. (1991, January). *Medical issues with HIV-infected adolescents.* Paper presented at the National Pediatric Conference on AIDS, Washington, DC.

Goodman, E., & Cohall, A. T. (1989). Acquired immunodeficiency syndrome and adolescents: Knowledge, attitudes, beliefs, and behaviors in a New York City adolescent minority population. *Pediatrics, 84,* 36-42.

Hein, K. (1989). AIDS in adolescence: Exploring the challenge. *Journal of Adolescent Health Care, 10,* 10S-35S.

Hingson, R., Strunin, L., & Berlin, B. (1990). Acquired immunodeficiency syndrome transmission: Changes in knowledge and behaviors among teenagers, Massachusetts statewide surveys, 1986 to 1988. *Pediatrics, 85,* 24-29.

Kegeles, S. M., Adler, N. E., & Irwin, Jr., C. E. (1988). Sexually active adolescents and condoms: Changes over one year in knowledge, attitudes, and use. *American Journal of Public Health, 78,* 460-461.

Kelly, J. A., St. Lawrence, J. S., Hood, H. V., & Brasfield, T. L. (1989). Behavioral intervention to reduce AIDS risk activities. *Journal of Consulting and Clinical Psychology, 57,* 60-67.

Kelly, J. A., St. Lawrence, J. S., Betts, R., Brasfield, T., & Hood, H. V. (1990). A skills-training group intervention model to assist persons in reducing risk behaviors for HIV infection. *AIDS Education and Prevention, 2*(1), 24-35.

Knox, M., & Clark, ?. (1991). Early HIV detection: A common health role. *Journal of Mental Health Administration, 18,* 21-35.

Koopman, C., Rotheram-Borus, M. J., Henderson, R., Bradley, J., & Hunter, J. (1990). Assessment of knowledge of AIDS and beliefs about AIDS prevention among adolescents. *AIDS Education and Prevention, 2,*(1), 58-70.

Kutchinsky, B. (1988). *The role of HIV testing in AIDS prevention.* Copenhagen, Denmark: University of Copenhagen.

Mosher, W. D. (1990). Contraceptive practice in the United States, 1982-1988. *Family Planning Perspectives, 22,* 198-205.

Rabkin, J., & Remien, R. (1991, May). *Depression, stress, and immune status in two HIV positive cohorts & psychological outlook and suicidality in AIDS long-term survivors.* Paper presented at the HIV Center, Columbia University, New York, NY.

Rotheram, M. J., Armstrong, M., & Booraem, C. (1982). Assertiveness training with elementary school children. *American Journal of Community Psychology, 10,* 567-582.

Rotheram-Borus, M. J., Koopman, C., & Dobbs, L., (1991, May). *HIV testing of adolescents: Policy implications of a survey of runaway and gay youth.* Presentation at the annual meeting of the American Psychiatric Association, New Orleans, LA.

Rotheram-Borus, M. J., Koopman, C., & Ehrhardt, A. A. (1991). Homeless youths and HIV infection. *American Psychologist, 46*(1), 1188-1197.

Rotheram-Borus, M. J., Koopman, C., Haignere, C., & Davies, M. (1991). Reducing HIV sexual risk behaviors among runaway adolescents. *Journal of the American Medical Association, 266,* 1237-1241.

Rotheram-Borus, M. J., Meyer-Bahlburg, H. F. L., Koopman, C., Rosario, M., Exner, T. M., Henderson, R., Matthieu, M., & Gruen, R. (in press). Lifetime sexual behaviors among runaway males and females. *Journal of Sex Research.*

Rotheram-Borus, M. J., Miller, S., Koopman, C., Haignere, C. S., & Selfridge, C. (1992). *Adolescents living safely: AIDS awareness, attitudes and action.* New York: HIV Center for Clinical and Behavioral Studies.

Rotheram-Borus, M. J., Rosario, M., & Koopman, C. (1991). Minority youths at high risk: Gay males and runaways. In S. Gore & M. E. Colten (Eds.), *Adolescence stress: Causes and consequences* (pp. 181-200). Hawthorne, NY: Aldine de Gruyer.

Schilling, R. F., El-Bassel, N., Schinke, S. P., Gordon, K., & Nichols, S. (1991). Building skills in recovering drug users to reduce heterosexual AIDS transmission. *Public Health Reports, 106,* 297-304.

Sonenstein, F. L., Pleck, J. H., & Ku, L. C. (1989). Sexual activity, condom use and AIDS awareness among adolescent males. *Family Planning Perspectives, 21,* 152-158.

Spivack, G., Platt, G., & Shure, M. (1976). *A problem solving approach to adjustment.* San Francisco: Jossey-Bass.

Stall, R., Ekstrand, M., Pollack, L., McKusick, L., & Coates, T. J. (1990). Relapse from safer sex: The next challenge for AIDS prevention efforts. *Journal of Acquired Immune Deficiency Syndromes, 3,* 1181-1187.

Stern, R., Singer, N., Leserman, J., Silva, S., & Evans, D. (1991, September). *Denial in self-report of cognitive functioning in HIV.* Paper presented at the Annual Meeting of the American Psychiatric Association, New Orleans, LA.

Stiffman, A. R., Earls, F., Robins, L. N., & Jung, K. G. (1988). Problems and help seeking in high-risk adolescent patients of health clinics. *Journal of Adolescent Health Care, 9,* 305-309.

Strunin, L. (1991). Adolescents' perceptions of risk for HIV infection: Implications for future research. *Social Science & Medicine, 2,* 221-228.

Strunin, L., & Hingson, R. (1987). Acquired immunodeficiency syndrome and adolescents: Knowledge, beliefs, attitudes and behaviors. *Pediatrics, 79,* 825-828.

Stuber, M. (Ed.). (1991). *Children and AIDS.* Washington, DC: American Psychiatric Press.

Vermund, S., Hein, K., Cary, J., Drucker, E., & Reuben, N. (1988). Heterosexually acquired AIDS in New York City adolescents. *Pediatric Research, 23,* 207A.

Walter, H. (1991, February). *AIDS prevention with high school students.* Presentation, Grand Rounds, New York State Psychiatric Institute, New York, NY.

Watters, J. K., Cheng, Y., Segal, M., Lorvick, J., Case, P. K., & Carlson, J. (1990). Epidemiology and prevention of HIV in intravenous drug users in San Francisco, 1986-1989. In *Abstracts: IV International Conference on AIDS* (p. 116). San Francisco: University of California.

PART III

Policy and Legal Perspectives

13

Public Policy Perspectives
on HIV Education

JAMES A. WELLS

Introduction

Public policy is the applied science of governmental behavior. It is concerned with how governments recognize and formulate problems, how they devise and implement solutions, and how they judge which are feasible, effective, and affordable. In this chapter, the role of public policy in shaping HIV education directed toward adolescents will be discussed. Although this topic is of global interest and significance, the discussion in this chapter will confine itself to affairs in the United States. This chapter in the United States context, however, will define HIV education most broadly. Although many discussions of HIV education policy concern themselves only with school-based education, this discussion will also address HIV education directed toward out-of-school adolescents. I will not specifically discuss policies of HIV education directed toward students in colleges or universities.

I will adopt a broad and somewhat imprecise definition of *adolescence* that includes persons in the teenage years, ages 11-19. With regard to schooling, this covers approximately the period starting with junior high (seventh grade). Clearly this overlaps developmentally with the initiation of puberty, which may begin later for some teens than for others and occasionally before the teen years. At the other end of this span, the boundaries of adolescence are even less precise. Some individuals will adopt the obligations of work, marriage, and parenthood before they are out of their teens. Others, college students in particular, will extend their education and dependence on parents into their early 20s.

Certainly the scope of adolescence is intrinsically problematic for policymakers. It is a period of life that begins in childhood but ends in adulthood. Policies for young adolescents contend with the prerogatives of the family, while policies for older adolescents are policies for persons with the legal and social status of adults (Elkin & Handel, 1978; Kerckhoff, 1972). Likewise it is a problematic span of ages for educators because the assumptions made about the background and experience of young adolescents are quite different from those made for older adolescents and young adults. Conversely it is the period in which many of the behaviors are initiated that are most likely to place adolescents at risk of HIV infection, namely sexual behavior for the majority, and drug use for a smaller number (DiClemente, 1990b; Fraser & Mitchell, 1988; Miller, Turner, & Moses, 1990).

This changeable mix of factors makes adolescence a particularly suitable time of life in which to educate for the prevention of HIV infection. But adolescents remain a difficult audience to reach and a problem in terms of promulgating policies that affect the health education of youth in an appropriate way (General Accounting Office, 1991). Adolescents are targeted with messages about the prevention of HIV infection for a number of reasons, which are explicitly treated in other chapters of this volume (e.g., see Hein; Sondheimer; Morris et al.; Rotheram-Borus et al.).

Policy as a process consists of the formulation of goals and strategies, their implementation, and the evaluation of their outcomes. *Evaluation* may be concerned with whether the stated goals were achieved, as well as with evaluating the process of implementation itself, emphasizing potential barriers to success.

In the case of HIV education for adolescents, policy is made primarily at the state and local level. It often is forgotten that schools are governmental entities subject to fiscal constraints and political forces, as are other governing bodies. School board members as elected officials must be responsive to the electorate. Most boards have a broad mandate to determine school policies, with some constraints on budget or scope exercised by state governments and in some cases county or local governments as well. Other governmental entities, such as county boards or health departments, also may provide HIV education for adolescents. Although the federal government does not directly provide education or determine its content locally, many jurisdictions rely on guidelines and materials developed or approved by the Centers for Disease Control or other federal agencies.

Elements of HIV Educational Policy

The prime ingredient in the development of public policy is the clarity of policy goals. Pertaining to AIDS education, it is important to define the scope of the epidemic and how it affects adolescents. For example, should HIV education address the current risks of adolescents, or should it prepare them for a set of risks they will encounter in the future? Should all adolescents be educated about AIDS/HIV infection, or should only high-risk adolescents? And is the purpose of educating adolescents about HIV to increase their knowledge, to change their attitudes, to alter their behavior, or a combination of these?

Although nearly all adolescents are or will be at some risk either now or in the future, an important policy decision is that regarding the breadth or depth of HIV education. This is a matter of distinguishing high- from moderate- or low-risk segments of the adolescent population. The policy issue is quite straightforward. Given limited resources, we would want to use them in a way that would maximize their impact. One problem with such a calculation is that we really know very little about either the short-term or the long-term impact of HIV education for adolescents, certainly too little to decide easily whether more HIV infections would be avoided by broad-based education versus highly specific targeting. An additional consideration that further complicates this picture is the problem of educating adolescents before the emergence of adult behavioral patterns. Thus education of individuals in early adolescence may precede the development of sexual identity and sexual or drug-injecting behaviors that might place adolescents at a higher risk of HIV infection. In the absence of an ability to target those individuals who may become injection drug users or who may engage in unsafe sexual practices, we are left by default with the single option of educating all adolescents. One advantage of this approach is that it may serve in the long run to create a set of community norms that promote preventive behaviors across various segments of the adolescent population. Conversely this approach requires that explicit instruction in HIV prevention be provided to all adolescents, even to those who ultimately would not have engaged in high-risk behavior.

A further impediment to precise targeting is the difficulty in reaching some individuals at highest risk of HIV infection. These include out-of-school, homeless, runaway, and throwaway youth. These individuals are often beyond the immediate and casual reach of such conventional institutions as the schools. Thus extraordinary measures are necessary to reach these adolescents. At the same time, they form a particularly high-risk segment of the adolescent population by being more sexually precocious, more likely to use drugs, and more likely to trade sex for money.

A number of approaches to HIV education are possible. Fraser and Mitchell (1988) offer a list of topics and approaches that hold promise for behavior change; these include comprehensive health education, community support and involvement, peer-mediated programs, psychosocial models, and targeting youth who have dropped out of schools. In addition, messages should be factual and devoid of moralizing and should be sensitive to the special characteristics of the target population (Center for Population Options, 1989).

Comprehensive health education is recommended by most organizations involved in HIV education (e.g., World Health Organization, 1989a). The rationale is that the behaviors related to HIV infection are integrated into a personal life-style and are situated in a cultural context. Reinforced and socially supported behaviors are unlikely to be changed without understanding the full social context or appealing to health promotion for the individual on all levels.

Community support and involvement in health education are crucial for the success of educational programs both inside and outside the schools. This is both because education works best when integrated with community values and institutions and because community opposition can stop a program from being effective. Community support for school-based education includes defining sources of support, resolving such key questions as what will be included in the curriculum and the grades in which it will be presented, involving parents, involving teenagers, stating the values of the program, and recognizing that HIV education has political dimensions (Freudenberg, 1989; Haffner, 1988). Under these conditions, community support is possible because most parents feel they have responsibility for sexuality education of their youngsters, but few actually offer adequate information, most would like help, and most support sexuality education in the schools (Alan Guttmacher Institute, 1981; Metropolitan Life Foundation, 1988; Roberts, Kline, & Gagnon, 1981; Taylor, Genevie, & Zhao, 1988).

Ultimately, prevention of the spread of HIV infection requires behavior change on an enormous scale, and in many ways the challenge of educating adolescents is little different from the challenge of educating adults. Sexual behavior and drug use among adolescents are private acts, just as they are among adults, although they are private acts with social consequences (Bayer, 1989). Yet adults through exhortation and moral suasion already have attempted to channel these private acts of adolescents with what must be considered limited success (Nichols, 1989).

Certainly birth out of wedlock to teenagers has been perceived as a serious social problem. Yet over many years, their number has continued to grow (Haffner, 1989). Similarly, growth has occurred in sexually transmitted diseases and the use and abuse of such substances as alcohol and drugs (Center for Population Options, 1989; DiClemente, 1988; 1990b; Fraser & Mitchell, 1988).

Given this intractable nature of private behaviors, one might think that it would conjure an all-out effort to understand how to intervene in meaningful and productive ways. A rational policy might promote a line of attack that would address research on effective educational interventions with the same rigor with which we address pharmaceutical interventions. A rational approach would provide a basis for programs predicated on interventions that have been shown to be effective. Taking a broad view, however, it is quite clear that policy pertaining to educating adolescents about HIV does not have such a look.

The shape that public policy finally assumes is a function of political, as well as analytic, processes. What is known to be efficacious is not always an acceptable solution to all parties to the problem. Thus in an epidemic in which unprotected sex between men is a risk, educational materials produced with federal funds may not portray sex between men and may not give the appearance of promoting homosexuality. Furthermore, while adolescence is recognized as an important time for HIV educational intervention, the major vehicle for ascertaining HIV knowledge in the United States population surveys only persons 18 years or older (Hardy, 1990). Additionally Presidents Reagan and Bush have blocked efforts of the Public Health Service to undertake national surveys of sexual risk behaviors in adults and adolescents.

The status of knowledge and policy may be summarized as follows: No magic bullet exists for inducing behavior change. Both precocious sexual behavior and substance abuse are quite resistant behaviors. Barriers to changing these behaviors exist not only in the unwillingness of individuals to change but also in the lack of confidence for change, in resistant beliefs and values, and in cultural and social institutions supporting resistant beliefs and values.

Knowledge about HIV transmission can be changed and has increased steadily in all segments of the population (Hardy, 1990; 1991). Among adolescents, knowledge is perhaps even greater than among adults. Increases in knowledge, however, are not necessarily or even incidentally correlated with reductions in behavior (Wells & Sell, 1990). Some reductions in behavior are occurring, and they are more likely to occur among younger and unmarried individuals. It is not easy, however, to attribute these changes to any specific intervention or to any type of intervention (Wells & Sell, 1990).

Most public policies are strong on dictating the goal of increasing knowledge and are relatively weak, to the point of nonexistence in many cases, on addressing the goal of behavior change. Furthermore, some policies are actually resistant to interventions that program for behavior change, such as the adoption of the use of condoms.

HIV Education in Schools

One way to determine how implementation of school-based education is progressing is to survey adolescents to determine how knowledgeable they are about HIV prevention and how actively they participate in prevention activities. This approach monitors the goal of school-based education but does not ensure that schools are responsible for the changes that have occurred. Another approach is to survey schools, teachers, and school organizations to determine the scope of implementation of school-based AIDS/HIV education. I am aware of six recent surveys that speak to this issue (Council of Chief State School Officers, 1990; Forrest & Silverman, 1989; GAO, 1990a; Kenney, Guardado, & Brown, 1989; National School Boards Association [NSBA], 1990; Schumacher, 1989).

Because the information in these surveys has a short shelf life, any summary must be qualified. The overall results, however, are indicative of the state of implementation efforts in the period of roughly 1988 to 1990. Doubtless the trends observed then will have continued in a similar fashion in the short intervening period. The Council of Chief State School Officers (CCSSO, 1990) reports that in mid-1988, 41 states had AIDS/HIV education laws or policies. Of these states, 18 required AIDS/HIV education and 23 encouraged it (Kenney et al., 1989). By May of 1989, Schumacher (1989) reports, 29 states mandated AIDS/HIV education in schools. Thus a clear majority of state governing bodies had by legislative or executive action undertaken to initiate AIDS/HIV education in schools. Also, in the spring of 1990, the National School Boards Association surveyed 332 school districts nationwide. Of these districts, 79% required HIV education in schools; four fifths of the districts did so under mandate of law.

Most of the HIV education efforts were undertaken within a comprehensive health education program, family life education, or a communicable disease requirement (CCSSO, 1990; Kenney et al., 1989; NSBA, 1990; Schumacher, 1989). Among the mandated programs, more than half required education to begin in grades K-5; however, only three states required it to be taught annually (Schumacher, 1989). The General Accounting Office (1990a) found that in the junior and senior high school years, the number of school districts providing instruction declined, especially in grades 11 and 12. It also found the median number of class periods spent on HIV education was 5; 20% required 10 or more, while 25% required 3 or fewer class periods.

In addition to time spent in instruction, the kind of topics addressed is also important. Among 45 state curricula or curriculum guides, 96% included discussion of abstinence, condom use was mentioned in 87%, safer sex in 78%, and sharing needles in 84%; only 76% discussed having intercourse with an infected partner, and only 67% mentioned unprotected anal intercourse as a risk for HIV infection (CCSSO, 1990). The Centers for Disease Control reviewed curricula of 43 secondary school teaching guides (GAO, 1990a) and found that teaching guides often mentioned topics but that details were lacking. For example, 93% covered abstinence from sex, and 91% abstinence from drugs. Only 37%, however, covered peer resistance and refusal skills, and 44% covered enhancement of self-esteem, both considered essential for negotiating safer sex or maintaining abstinence. Although 93% of curriculum guides mentioned condoms, 79% noted that condoms reduce risk of exposure to HIV, but only 42% noted the additional protection provided by spermicide, 37% that condoms should be used properly from start to finish of a sexual act, and 16% provided any instruction or demonstration on condom use. Regarding drug use, only 12% mentioned cleaning works, and 23% encouraged the seeking of treatment if addicted. Kenney et al. (1989) report similar results for the 203 largest school districts in the country, with several interesting additions. Although 91% of curriculum guides mentioned abstinence as the best alternative, only 9% mentioned it as the only alternative. Additionally all topics received less treatment in grades 11-12 than in grades 7-10. Finally, explanation of how to use birth control methods (including condoms) was included in 74%, but information on specific clinics or physicians to go to for birth control was covered by only 41%.

In contrast to the curriculum guides, school nurses and teachers of health education, physical education, biology, and home economics reported relatively constant levels of coverage over grades 7-12 (Forrest & Silverman, 1989). Additionally the class time spent on HIV education remained higher in grades 11-12 than in grades K-8 (NSBA, 1990). Thus the lower coverage in later grades is a matter of course selection rather than of changes in level of effort within the classroom. According to NSBA, in the lower grades most HIV education is part of a health education curriculum and is taught by the classroom teacher. After grade 7, HIV education is taught in other classes and as a stand-alone curriculum with most of the teaching being done by a health teacher or school nurse with significant help from public health specialists, community agency staff, and physicians.

Teachers, however, reported very low levels of coverage of such topics as safer sex or sources of birth control. Moreover, of an average 38.7 hours devoted to sex education, only 5 hours are devoted to birth control, and only 5.9 hours are devoted to sexually transmitted diseases, including AIDS/HIV. Curiously, teachers tend to promote abstinence, condoms, and monogamy for the prevention of HIV more often than for other sexually transmitted disease, a result also reflected in curriculum guides (Kenney et al., 1989). Finally, teachers' opinions varied substantially from curriculum guidelines. Most teachers felt that some topics not always covered in the guidelines should be covered and that other topics should be covered at an earlier age. Instructive are the topics of homosexuality and safer sex. About 60% of school districts covered the topics, with fewer than half of those doing so by the end of grade 7. In contrast, 90% of the teachers felt that these topics should be covered, and more than half of those felt that the topics should be covered by the end of grade 7.

About 1 in 10 teachers of sex education reported that one of the biggest problems with teaching sex education was that they lacked adequate training (Forest & Silverman, 1989). GAO (1990a) estimates that 83% of HIV teachers receive training. Although a minimum of 12 hours of training is recommended, teachers in 67% of districts received fewer than 10, and in 32% of districts teachers received fewer than 4 hours of training. In more than half of the districts, such topics as the use of condoms to prevent the spread of HIV, multiple sex partners as risky behavior, and unprotected intercourse (homosexual or heterosexual) as risky behavior received fewer than 15 minutes of coverage. Between 30-50% of districts spent fewer than 15 minutes training teachers about legal and school district policies, community resources to deal with HIV issues, IV drug use as risky behavior, how to handle embarrassing questions, student self-esteem, and how to communicate sensitive subjects.

Another big problem for teachers is the availability of educational materials. Some 29% of teachers of sex education reported that one of their biggest problems is that materials are inadequate, unavailable, out of date, uninteresting or difficult to read, or difficult to get approved for use (Forrest & Silverman, 1989). Staff at the Centers for Disease Control, through the National AIDS Clearinghouse, have undertaken the evaluation of educational materials of all types. In the summer of 1990, teams of health education experts reviewed 1,313 brochures, posters, other print materials such as curricula, and videos (Ruscavage et al., 1991). Three reviewers rated each item on a 15-point scale, with scores lower than 6 indicating that the materials were not recommended because of inadequacies in content, design, technical production, translation if applicable, and cultural sensitivity. The reviewers could not recommend more than one in five (21%) of the items. In contrast, 27% were rated higher than 10, and the remaining 52% between 6 and 10.

These figures do not explicitly separate materials targeted to adolescents, but we may assume that a substantial proportion of those are also substandard. Another study explored the readability grade levels of written educational materials (Wells & Sell, 1991). This study found a median readability level of grade 11.4 in 136 brochures, pamphlets, comics, and monographs. Materials aimed at adolescents aged 16-20 and college students had a median readability of grade 8.9. In comparing the educational levels of these individuals to the readability of materials targeting them, the study found that 3.8% of 850,000 individuals would fall below the median reading grade of HIV educational materials. Moreover, this study included only adolescents above age 15 and included college students over age 20 as well, whose reading skills would be better than average. Clearly there is room for improvement in the quality of HIV education materials prepared for adolescents.

A Case Study of Policy-Making

These studies of policy-making at the general level give an indication that HIV education is widespread in American schools. The results also show, however, that a number of important issues may not be receiving appropriate emphasis, especially negotiation skills and use of condoms. A case study of attempts in New York City to make condoms available through schools may illustrate the kinds of problems that can result when schools try to address these important issues.

In late September of 1990, New York City schools Chancellor Joseph Fernandez proposed to distribute condoms through clinics in some New York City schools ("Chancellor has plan," 1990). This policy initiative was based on several considerations, including that New York has more adolescent cases of HIV than any other metropolitan area, that sexually transmitted disease and unwanted pregnancy rates were rising among adolescents, that school-based education emphasizing abstinence neglected the needs of sexually active students, and that sexually active students have little access to condoms. As finally proposed in December of 1990, the commissioner planned to have condoms distributed in all 120 high schools in New York, even those without health clinics ("New York school chief," 1990). The distribution would be done by faculty volunteers, and distribution would not require counseling or parental permission. Counseling would be unnecessary because classroom instruction on HIV prevention would be required in all grades.

Implementation of the program required approval of the 7-member central school board and passed in February 1991 by a 4-3 vote ("School board approves," 1991). An 11th-hour compromise proposal would have allowed parents to bar their children from receiving condoms. One member of the board voted for the program but vowed to introduce later an amendment allowing parents to opt out of the program. Some analysts have argued strongly that such options weaken and vitiate behavior change programs (DiClemente, 1988; 1990a). In New York, parents may bar their children from receiving selected services from school health clinics, but according to the director of one such clinic, only about 5% do so ("Clinic visit," 1991). In September 1991, however, an amendment to allow parents to opt out of the program was defeated by the school board ("Key to condom vote," 1991). The program began making condoms available to students in November of 1991. The Aaron Diamond Foundation of New York provided $450,000 to train volunteers who will distribute the condoms ("Foundation to help," 1991).

Opposition to condom availability in the schools was strong and was led in part by the Catholic Diocese of New York. Opponents argued that parents do not want the schools to take over this function and that abstinence is preferable to condom distribution. A Roper poll, however, indicated that 64% of a random sample of adults favored condom distribution in high schools, and 47% supported it in junior highs (Kerr, 1991). Although evidence exists from a study of inner-city youth that an abstinence-based program can postpone sexual initiation relative to controls (Howard & McCabe, 1990), the same study found that 24% of those in the program were sexually active in ninth grade. Thus educational programs must plan also for the time, at whatever age, when sexual activity will begin. Conversely, evaluation of sexuality education programs provides no evidence that the availability of contraceptives and counseling increases the likelihood of sexual initiation (Stout & Rivara, 1989). Availability of contraceptives does increase the likelihood of their use (Berger, Perez, Kyman et al., 1987; Dryfoos, 1988), and that is the hope of programs, such as New York's, that make condoms available.

Adolescents Out of School

While we rely on schools to educate most adolescents, another group of adolescents is inaccessible by these institutions: the out-of-school youth. This segment of adolescents may consist of adolescents with varying life circumstances, including homeless, runaway, or throwaway youth, street kids, and incarcerated youth (Woodworth, 1988). Additionally they may have varying levels of HIV risk, depending on their participation in sexual behavior, drug injection, or prostitution. These youth are not particularly hard to find and often may be located through programs designed for high-risk adults. They are hard to reach, however, because they lack trust in helping systems, they may not perceive themselves to be at risk, they have low self-esteem and feelings of self-efficacy, and lack a long-term perspective because their survival is often a day-to-day affair (Woodworth, 1988; World Health Organization, 1989b). Annually the United States has between 1.3 and 2 million homeless and runaway youth, about 100,000 to 300,000 of these being long-term runaways, that is, street kids (GAO, 1990b).

Education for youth in schools in funded primarily by local governments. Although some direct funding is provided, the federal role is primarily advisory; for example, the Centers for Disease Control issues guidelines for HIV educational curricula. Programming for out-of-school youth, in contrast, is more often supported directly by federal agencies. The most frequent providers of HIV education to out-of-school youth are staff at runaway shelters, runaway referral centers, and drop-in centers (GAO, 1990b). These

are funded by local public health departments, private foundations, and such federal agencies as the National Institute of Mental
Health, the National Institute on Drug Abuse, the Health Resources and Services Administration, the Job Corps, and the Office
of Juvenile Justice and Delinquency Prevention. The Centers for
Disease Control has funded several national agencies that direct
funds and programs toward youth service agencies and commu-
nity- based organizations.

Conclusion

It is accepted generally among health educators that educating
adolescents about HIV infection and AIDS is an important step in
preventing the spread of HIV. This recognition, however, has been
slow to diffuse among all segments of educational policy-making.
Most but not all school districts now require or suggest that HIV
education be included in the curriculum. The content of this
education, however, varies widely. The lack of universally mandated education and standardized curricula limits HIV-prevention
education. Students in areas of low HIV prevalence need the same
education as students in high-prevalence areas if the prevalence
in their communities is to remain low. Moreover, teacher training
and the commitment of classroom time and resources are also
essential but neglected ingredients of a successful HIV-prevention
campaign. Additionally it is disconcerting that the intensity of
HIV education falls off in the upper high school grades, just when
students may be most vulnerable to infection through sexual or
drug-injecting behavior. HIV education should be offered in every
grade and should not be made optional or available only to students electing certain courses in the upper grades.
Educational programs for adolescents also need to catch up
with current emphases on behavior change. Survey findings show
that AIDS/HIV curricula generally neglect behavior change strategies, sexual negotiation skills, and use of condoms, all essential
ingredients to the maintenance of either abstinence or safer sex
during sexual acts. The case of the proposed distribution of condoms in New York City schools illustrates the difficulty in providing real rather than spurious barriers between students and the
human immunodeficiency virus. Community resistance will

continue, however, and it is well to anticipate the objections that religious and community leaders may have to aggressive HIV prevention.

At the same time, the health education community must be reflective about HIV-prevention programs in the schools. Relatively few resources have gone into evaluating school HIV-education programs, and little consensus exists about how best to effect behavior change through education either in-school or out. Sooner or later, the costs of HIV education will be judged in a rational way, and concerns about costs may compromise prevention if more is not quickly learned about the benefits of HIV educational interventions (Birch & Stoddart, 1990).

Nonetheless an aggressive approach should be taken toward HIV. It is clearly a growing threat to adolescent health. To take the present generation of adolescents out of jeopardy will require continued and creative educational efforts.

References

Alan Guttmacher Institute. (1981). *Teenage pregnancy: The problem that hasn't gone away*. New York: Author.

Bayer, R. (1989). *Private acts, social consequences: AIDS and the politics of public health*. New York: Free Press.

Berger, D. K., Perez, G., Kyman, W. et al. (1987). Influence of family planning counseling in an adolescent clinic on sexual activity and contraceptive use. *Journal of Adolescent Health Care, 8*, 436-440.

Birch, S., & Stoddart, G. (1990). Promoting healthy behavior: The importance of economic analysis in policy formulation for AIDS prevention. *Health Policy, 16*, 187-197.

Center for Population Options. (1989). *Adolescents, AIDS and HIV: A community-wide responsibility*. Washington, DC: Author.

Chancellor has plan to distribute condoms to students in New York. (1990, September 26). *New York Times*, pp. A1, A16.

Clinic visit. (1991, February 21). *New York Times*, p. A21.

Council of Chief State School Officers (CCSSO). (1990). *Profile of state HIV/AIDS education survey results: 1988-1989*. Washington, DC: Council of Chief State School Officers, Resource Center on Education Equity.

DiClemente, R. J. (1988). Policy perspectives on the implementation and development of school-based AIDS prevention education programs in the United States. *AIDS & Public Policy Journal, 3*, 14-16.

DiClemente, R. J. (1990a). Adolescents and AIDS: Current research, prevention strategies, and policy implications. In L. Temoshok & A. Baum (Eds.), *Psychosocial perspectives on AIDS* (pp. 52-64). Hillsdale, NJ: Lawrence Erlbaum.

DiClemente, R. J. (1990b). The emergence of adolescents as a risk group for human immunodeficiency virus infection. *Journal of Adolescent Research, 5*, 7-17.

Dryfoos, J. G. (1988). School-based health clinics: Three years of experience. *Family Planning Perspectives, 20*, 193-200.

Elkin, F., & Handel, G. (1978). *The child and society: The process of socialization.* New York: Random House.

Forrest, J. D., & Silverman, J. (1989). What public school teachers teach about preventing pregnancy, AIDS and sexually transmitted diseases. *Family Planning Perspectives, 21*, 65-72.

Foundation to help distribute condoms in schools. (1991, June 18). *New York Times*, p. B3.

Fraser, K., & Mitchell, P. (1988). *Effective AIDS education: A policymaker's guide.* Alexandria, VA: National Association of State Boards of Education.

Freudenberg, N. (1989). Social and political obstacles to AIDS education. *SIECUS Report* (August/September), 1-6.

General Accounting Office (GAO). (1990a). *AIDS education: Public school programs require more student information and teacher training* (GAO/HRD-90-103). Washington, DC: Author.

General Accounting Office. (1990b). *AIDS education: Programs for out-of-school youth slowly evolving* (GAO/HRD-90-111). Washington, DC: Author.

General Accounting Office. (1991). *AIDS-prevention programs: High-risk groups still prove hard to reach* (GAO/HRD-91-52). Washington, DC: Author.

Haffner, D. W. (1988). Developing community support for school-based AIDS education. In M. Quackenbush, M. Nelson, & K. Clark (Eds.), *The AIDS challenge: Prevention education for young people* (pp. 185-193). Santa Cruz, CA: Network.

Haffner, D. W. (1989). AIDS education: What can be learned from teenage pregnancy prevention programs. *SIECUS Report* (August/September), 7-10.

Hardy, A. M. (1990). National health interview survey data on adult knowledge of AIDS in the United States. *Public Health Reports, 105*(6), 629-634.

Hardy, A. M. (1991, July). AIDS knowledge and attitudes for October-December 1990: Provisional data from the National Health Interview Survey. *AdvanceData, 204*, 1-8.

Howard, M., & McCabe, J. B. (1990). Helping teenagers postpone sexual involvement. *Family Planning Perspectives, 22*, 21-26.

Kenney, A. M., Guardado, S., & Brown, L. (1989). Sex education and AIDS education in the schools: What states and large school districts are doing. *Family Planning Perspectives, 21*, 56-64.

Kerckhoff, A. C. (1972). *Socialization and social class.* Englewood Cliffs, NJ: Prentice-Hall.

Kerr, D. (1991). Condom availability in New York City schools. *Journal of School Health, 61*, 279-280.

Key to condom vote: Dinkins power grasp. (1991, September 13). *New York Times*, pp. B1, B3.

Metropolitan Life Foundation. (1988). *Health you've got to be taught: An evaluation of comprehensive health education in American public schools.* New York: Author.

Miller, H. G., Turner, C. F., & Moses, L. E. (Eds.). (1990). *AIDS: The second decade.* Washington, DC: National Academy.

National School Boards Association (NSBA). (1990). *HIV prevention education in the nation's public schools.* Alexandria, VA: Author.

New York school chief to offer plan for distributing condoms. (1990, December 4). *New York Times,* pp. A1, B12.

Nichols, E. K. (1989). *Mobilizing against AIDS.* Cambridge, MA: Harvard University Press.

Roberts, E. S., Kline, D., & Gagnon, J. (1981). *Family life and sexual learning of children* (Vol. 1). Cambridge, MA: Population Education.

Ruscavage, D., Halleron, T., Bond, K. N., Wells, J. A., Wells, B. R., Cauthen, N., & Sennock, P. (1991, November). *Evaluation of HIV and AIDS educational materials.* Paper presented at the Annual Meeting of the American Public Health Association, Atlanta, GA.

School board approves plan for condoms. (1991, February 27). *New York Times,* pp. B1, B4.

Schumacher, M. (1989). *HIV/AIDS education survey: Profiles of state policy action.* Alexandria, VA: National Association of State Boards of Education.

Stout, J. W., & Rivara, F. P. (1989). Schools and sex education: Does it work? *Pediatrics, 83,* 375-379.

Taylor, H., Genevie, L., & Zhao, X. (1988). *Public attitudes toward teenage pregnancy, sex education and birth control.* New York: Louis Harris and Associates.

Wells, J. A., & Sell, R. L. (1990). *Project HOPE's international survey of AIDS educational messages and behavior change: France, the United Kingdom, and the United States.* Chevy Chase, MD: Project HOPE Center for Health Affairs.

Wells, J. A., & Sell, R. L. (1991). *Learning AIDS: A special report on readability, literacy, and the HIV epidemic.* New York: American Foundation for AIDS Research.

Woodworth, R. S. (1988). Runaways, homeless and incarcerated youth. In M. Quackenbush, M. Nelson, & K. Clark (Eds.), *The AIDS challenge: Prevention education for young people* (pp. 365-378). Santa Cruz, CA: Network.

World Health Organization. (1989a). *AIDS education in schools: Report on a European workshop.* Copenhagen: World Health Organization, Regional Office for Europe.

World Health Organization. (1989b). *AIDS prevention for the hard-to-reach: Report on a WHO consultation.* Copenhagen: World Health Organization, Regional Office for Europe.

14

Public Policy, HIV Disease, and Adolescents

LAWRENCE J. D'ANGELO

Introduction

How society views and treats adolescents is an important concern for teenagers and for their parents, health care providers, and advocates as well. Despite years of debate, major issues surrounding the legal status of adolescents, their rights with regard to confidentiality, and their ability to consent for the provision of health services continue to be discussed and debated. Elsewhere in this volume, both the role of public policy in determining educational programs, as well as legal issues surrounding adolescents and HIV infection, are reviewed (see Wells and English, respectively). More general questions, however, deserve to be discussed. These more fundamental issues include how adolescents are viewed by society with regard to human immunodeficiency virus (HIV) infection, how these views have been translated into "public policy," and how these policies have impacted on adolescents' ability to receive care, particularly care related to HIV infection.

At the outset, it is important to realize that many different policies dealing with HIV infection and potentially pertaining to adolescents have their origins in federal, state, and local legislative and planning bodies. These policies often overlap and frequently are in conflict with one another. For instance, the educational programs for AIDS and HIV infection suggested by several federal programs are subject to review and censorship by state and local school boards. This process, while part of the evolution of public policy, often results in programs quite different from the ones originally suggested. Similarly local laws governing consent and confidentiality have a dramatic impact on the type and availability of services for adolescents. Seemingly routine determinations of whether an illness is sexually transmitted may make the ultimate difference in whether an adolescent can receive care for concerns related to HIV infection. For instance, in states in which HIV has been declared a sexually transmitted disease, it is often much easier for adolescents to access care than in states in which HIV has been defined in another manner, because virtually all states allow adolescents to seek care for sexually transmitted diseases without parental consent (Ginzburg, 1991). While such potential differences in policy will exist surrounding any issue for which different jurisdictions see that they have specific interests, those in which differences are determined by age seem all the more arbitrary.

Ideally, the formulation of any public policy commences with the establishment of objectives meant to be achieved by the policy, a reasoned approach as to how to achieve those objectives, and a way of assessing whether those objectives actually have been achieved. Unfortunately this sequence has rarely if ever taken place for those policies that relate to adolescent health issues. A notable exception is the health promotion and disease prevention objectives for adolescents that are incorporated into the Healthy People 2000 objectives (AMA, 1990). Unfortunately those specifically related to HIV infection and adolescents are confined to recommendations for condom use and do not address other fundamental issues of HIV prevention.

The immediate impression one is left with when examining the nature of public policy surrounding HIV infection in adolescents is that it is fragmentary, frequently contradictory, and often heavily influenced by forces that have little to do with health concerns per se and that are dictated by political agendas. This impression is not surprising, in light of the evolution of most policies surrounding HIV infection, but it is disappointing. The remainder of this chapter will discuss how this lack of a coordinated policy evolved and the steps that should be done to address these shortcomings.

HIV Infection in Adolescents: Missing the Problem, Missing the Point

Early public policy concerning AIDS was driven by the mounting numbers of cases in clearly defined "risk groups." If a particular segment of the population was spared the end stages of HIV infection, it was also denied the attention of those responsible for setting priorities and allocating funds. With few cases early on, adolescents did not qualify as a group that garnered much attention.

Some health officials were alert to this dilemma, however, and by the late 1980s the problem of potential HIV spread in adolescents had been outlined (Hein, 1987; Vermund et al., 1989). At the same time, it became clear that the educational efforts of the mid-1980s had improved the overall knowledge level of adolescents (DiClemente, 1990; Steiner, Sorokin, Schiedmayer, & Van Susteren, 1990; Strunin & Hingson, 1987). Educational programs that were centered around the basics of retrovirology became part of public policy, but it became almost immediately clear that the increased knowledge that adolescents were acquiring was not convincing them to change their behavior (Kegeles, Adler, & Irwin, 1988). It also became clear that the biology of the virus was assisting us in our attempts to ignore the impact of HIV infection in adolescents. The long latency from infection to symptomatic disease made it virtually certain that few adolescents would develop AIDS until their 20s.

At the same time, it became clear that some adolescents would develop AIDS and that the need to evaluate their responses to newly emerging therapeutic agents would be necessary. Attempts were made to incorporate adolescents into existing AIDS Clinical Trials Group (ACTG) protocols, but initially no protocols allowed adolescents to be subjects. The age for the "adult" protocols commenced at age 18, and the pediatric protocols did not enroll anyone over age 12. Even when this omission was corrected, adolescents had little opportunity of being enrolled in clinical trials. Neither adult physicians nor pediatricians saw adolescents as an important source of patients for the evaluation of new treatment options. The exception to this was a small cadre of patients with hemophilia who seemed to have the same level of access to care as their adult counterparts.

While clearly no policy existed that encouraged equal access to treatment protocols for adolescents, the confusion over how to deal with adolescents as a group was further typified by the lack of a consistent definition for who qualifies to be thought of as an adolescent. The Centers for Disease Control, the government agency responsible for maintaining surveillance of the growing number of AIDS cases, classifies *adolescents* as individuals who are between ages 13-20. While one government agency is using this definition for record keeping, however, another is using a different definition to determine who is eligible for clinical trials. The National Institute of Allergy and Infectious Diseases (NIAID) defines *adolescence* as the period spanning ages 13-18. The upper limit is established to coincide with the legal definition of *adulthood*, the "age of majority," when an adolescent would be allowed to consent to participate in clinical research. Finally, the issue of an age definition is further complicated by a nongovernmental organization that is focused on providing health care for all adolescents. The American Academy of Pediatrics is rather low-key in its approach to establish acceptable guidelines for practice. In doing so, however, it directly states that patients are appropriately cared for by pediatricians until their 21st birthday. While this is not a true "definition" of adolescence, it is an operational definition in that pediatricians traditionally are thought of as the primary physicians for the care of children and adolescents. While a "practice issue," the ramifications of this are tremendous in terms of getting adolescent patients appropriate treatment and of making treatment protocols available to them.

If the inconsistencies of the policies that address the question of access to research-based care were of concern to some, the policies of the two largest "consumers" of youth manpower—the United States armed forces and the Job Corps—while unambiguous, were clearly not beneficial to youth. Mandatory testing without the provision of follow-up care poses a unique dilemma for adolescents. Although this approach has not been adopted by other federal agencies or state or local jurisdictions, its success in documenting a widespread level of HIV infection certainly will increase the pressure for "policies," one of which might be for universal testing. Few if any believe that such testing would be appropriate for all teens (Hein, 1991). In patients for which predicting the risk of infection is difficult (D'Angelo, Getson, Luban, & Gayle, 1991), however, more specific criteria for who should be tested, what sort of consent is appropriate for such testing, how confidentiality will be maintained, and how patients will have access to clinical care are questions that must be answered.

Public Policy and HIV: The Role of Federal Agencies

Part of the confusion surrounding the policies that do exist with regard to HIV infection in teenagers has been the lack of a mandate to any federal agency to champion the concerns of adolescents. While a number of agencies have programs that *relate* to adolescents, few are involved in direct research or service provision for adolescents. Some of those that do and the programs they support are the following:

1. Centers for Disease Control
   a. Division of Adolescent and School Health (DASH): Unique in that it is one of the few federal activities to have the word *adolescent* in its title, DASH has taken the lead in many areas primarily concerned with prevention through the fostering of educational initiatives on a local and state level, monitoring risk behaviors in teens, and implementing programs to reduce these risk behaviors.
   b. Division of STD/HIV Prevention (DSTD/HIVP): Although many prevention programs initiated by DSTD/HIVP do not specify that they are aimed at adolescents, they clearly have an effect on teenagers, as well as adults. One project that is aimed primarily at adolescents is the Hemophilia Behavioral Intervention Research Project, which the division supports, along with the Bureau of Maternal and Child Health and the National Hemophilia Foundation. In many ways, this program, although focused on a special population, provides a model for other HIV-prevention programs.
   c. Division of HIV/AIDS: Through many of the surveillance projects that are ongoing, the Division of HIV/AIDS is responsible for monitoring the prevalence of HIV infection and AIDS. Special

concerns surrounding adolescents have been expressed, and a number of studies directed toward this age group have been initiated. The Seroepidemiology Branch carefully monitors the two largest studies of HIV-infected adolescents—the Job Corps and the U.S. military.

2. Health Resources and Services Administration (HRSA)

   a. Bureau of Maternal and Child Health: Traditionally active in the support of adolescent health issues, this bureau has maintained a high level of interest and activity surrounding the question of HIV among adolescents. Current undertakings include a series of pediatric demonstration projects that are focused primarily on adolescents. These projects have served as a model for how primary and specialty services could be provided for HIV-infected or at-risk youth.

   b. Bureau of Health Care Delivery and Assistance (BHCD): This bureau funds the provision of primary care services in impoverished areas, including several homeless shelters for adolescents. BHCD also funds drug treatment programs, many of which reach adolescent clients.

3. Alcohol, Drug Abuse and Mental Health Administration (ADAMHA)

   a. National Institute of Drug Abuse (NIDA): Along with its ADAMHA sister organization, the National Institute of Mental Health (NIMH), NIDA funds a program addressing homeless and runaway youth. AIDS prevention and education services are addressed in this program. Additionally an ongoing research program announcement on the role of drug use in the transmission of HIV infection targets this same group of runaway youth.

   b. National Institute of Mental Health (NIMH): Almost half of the research projects funded by NIMH that deal with interventions to change risk behaviors target adolescents. Included are projects on cognitive and behavioral antecedents of HIV infection, and behavioral strategies to prevent spread of HIV infection in minority youth.

4. National Institutes of Health (NIH)

   a. National Institute of Allergy and Infectious Disease (NIAID): The administrative site of the AIDS Clinical Trials Group (ACTG), the institute recently made the first meaningful step toward providing adequate access to clinical trials for adolescents. With the support of a congressionally funded mandate, the Division of AIDS (DAIDS) established nine programs specifically aimed at recruiting adolescents for clinical trials. Epidemiologic projects conducted by the division include adolescents, but these are not directed solely at this age group.

b. National Institute of Child Health and Human Development (NICHD): This institute is the traditional home of research projects that involve the exploration of scientific issues surrounding adolescents. Funding limitations, however, have hindered it from initiating projects dealing with a host of issues, including psychologic, pharmacologic, and neurologic aspects of HIV infection in adolescents.

While a number of other agencies are involved in some aspect of HIV infection and adolescents, the above represent those that have actual ongoing programs targeted toward adolescents or have had a previous mandate to work with research or service programs for adolescents. The list represents surprisingly little substance, however, and what is clearly missing is any semblance of coordination of these programs with the sort of clearly articulated objectives that underlie successful program development. At a federal level, this coordination is definitely a desirable next step.

Local Policy-Making and Adolescents: What Is It, and Who Does It?

If federal agencies have been less than successful in establishing a coherent approach to policy development concerning HIV infection and adolescents, their lack of success certainly has been echoed by the equally ineffective efforts of state and local governments. For most of these, policy-making has been confined to producing and attempting to implement educational policies and debating the legal status of adolescents with regard to the HIV epidemic. With the notable exception of places like San Francisco, no concerted effort has been made to ensure the availability of appropriate medical services, nor pressure exerted on academic medical centers linked to the AIDS clinical trials network to incorporate adolescents into these trials. While many jurisdictions have focused on education and legal issues, even articulated policies often have failed to be operationalized at the local school and community level.

Because both of these topics are reviewed elsewhere in this volume, I will comment only on the role of state and local governments in the provision of care for HIV-positive or at-risk youth. It is not surprising that few communities have thought about formulating policy concerning medical issues and HIV infection in teens. The same inattention fostered by an established policy of determining resource allocation by "counting cases" of AIDS that has plagued national policy has similarly confounded the creation of local policies sympathetic to the needs of adolescents. This in itself has been an extension of the long-standing apathy that most communities have displayed toward the development of health services for adolescents. This is evident in the lack of adolescent-specific services, in inadequate training of most of the health care providers who see teenagers, and in a lack of adequate financing for services that do exist. A notable exception to this trend has been the growth of school-based or -linked health services established in many urban areas to provide accessible health services for teens. Unfortunately the economic problems being felt by many school districts have necessitated a curtailing of many of these services. Even where they did or do exist, however, the constraints on the nature of services provided (limiting information on sexuality and contraception and not allowing condom distribution) often have limited these clinics' usefulness in combating HIV infection.

Where local jurisdictions have had an opportunity to focus clinical services for HIV treatment and prevention, they have often unknowingly excluded adolescents. An excellent example of this is the treatment adolescents and their advocates have received under the Ryan White Comprehensive AIDS Resources Emergency (CARE) Act. This legislation, divided into four "Titles" or separately funded sections, does not make specific reference to the needs of adolescents. Title I provides "emergency" funding to metropolitan areas with more than 2,000 cases of AIDS or with a per capita incidence of 2.5 cases per 1,000. Grants for the 1991 fiscal year went to 16 cities. Although the application requirements call for "appropriate allocations for services for women, children, women, and families with HIV disease," advocates for adolescents generally have found that carving out any services for adolescents has been difficult at best. The Health Care Services Planning Councils, whose role is to establish priorities for the organization and delivery of health services, have frequently resisted attempts to have those concerned with adolescents included in the planning process. When this political "jockeying" is combined with the fact that only $87.8 million of the authorized $275 million has been appropriated, services for adolescents have rarely been part of local allocations. The irony, which apparently has escaped many, is that Ryan White, who gave his life to AIDS and his name to the act, was an adolescent.

Adolescents have fared no better under the other titles of this grant. Title II grants call for the establishment of local "consortia" to allocate funding for a variety of health care and support services for individuals and their families with HIV disease. While the requirements for Title II grants include targeting services for the needs of "infants, children, women, and families," adolescents are not specifically mentioned, and their advocates have in many locales been omitted from the established consortia. In some places, services for adolescents have become available when they have been linked to services for HIV-infected individuals represented by larger, better recognized interest groups, such as those concerned with neonatal infection and those that advocate for the health needs of gay men. Both of these avenues, while often successful in the short run, distort the overall approach to the provision of clinical services for HIV-infected or at-risk youth. Adolescents find themselves having access to care because they are pregnant or because they are gay, rather than because they are adolescents, at risk for HIV infection, or infected by HIV and in need of age-appropriate services.

Title III, which meant to provide outpatient "early intervention services," would appear to be the portion of the act most supportive of the needs of the growing number of asymptomatic HIV-infected adolescents. Unfortunately it has been poorly funded, with many of the appropriated funds going to replace services for other groups whose funding previously was interrupted. Title IV, for which no funds were appropriated in 1991, has provisions for the establishment of pediatric demonstration projects for clinical services and research. While a potential source of support for teens needing services, even when funded, adolescent advocates will need to convince local authorities, as well as the federal agencies that will administer the grants, of the specific needs of adolescents.

In summary, although potential mechanisms for establishing policies with regard to the care, education, and legal status of adolescents exist, most state and local jurisdictions have done little, outside of the irregular establishment of educational policies that may or may not be implemented, to address the needs of teenagers. At this time, the mandate is still not clear to develop new programs or to ensure that the old ones are undertaken.

What Needs to Be Done?

Unfortunately the almost complete lack of established public policy on either a federal or state/local level has served to amplify the problem of HIV infection in adolescents. Preoccupation with counting AIDS cases while ignoring the problem of a large number of asymptomatically infected adolescents has given a false sense of security to youth, putting them at still greater risk of infection. Education efforts stymied by local politics or reticent school systems have served to leave ignorant or even to mislead teens about their own risk of acquiring HIV infection. An unclear set of legal and ethical guidelines with regard to adolescents has compounded the dilemma of getting teens who are at risk appropriately counselled and tested for the presence of HIV. Finally, the lack of age-specific services for care or access to treatment research protocols has left adolescents without a place to turn that will provide for their needs and increase our knowledge of the natural history of HIV infection in teenagers.

Although much needs to be accomplished, relatively few policy directives from critical federal and state/local authorities could rapidly clear the way for a systematic approach to prevention and treatment services. Suggestions for such policies include the following:

1. *Create a federal government standing task force/working group to deal with questions of prevention, care, and research concerning HIV infection in adolescents.* Although other committees have addressed these concerns, the lack of a standing committee identified with the needs of adolescents has hindered severely the development of an adolescent-specific policy agenda. This committee should have representatives from all agencies directly involved in care or research questions dealing with adolescents, as well as substantial representation from those who advocate for adolescents, with particular emphasis on those who have been involved in care or research questions specific to HIV infection in adolescents. Part of the charge of this committee would be to assist in coordinating the

activities of government agencies as they relate to HIV infection and adolescents. In addition, this committee would be expected to advise state and local jurisdictions and to assist them in developing responsible policies for education, prevention, and care of adolescents with regard to HIV infection.

2. *Mandate the implementation of appropriate HIV-educational programs for all children and adolescents.* While guidelines for such programs have been proposed (Centers for Disease Control, 1988), each local jurisdiction has had the responsibility for developing programs for such educational efforts and for assuring that they are implemented. While the individual content of these programs could be determined by state and local school boards, federal funding to support education should be linked to the demonstration that each school district has such a program and that it meets "federal standards."

3. *Establish a national consensus that HIV is a sexually transmitted disease.* Although this would appear to be obvious, many states have not clearly recognized HIV disease as a sexually transmitted disease. Until this is done, adolescents with concerns about their risk and health status will not be afforded the protection they have under the law for evaluation and treatment of other STDs. Also by making HIV reportable nationally, we may get a much more accurate picture of the impact of this infection in adolescents.

4. *Require that services for adolescents be part of any federally or state funded programs for the evaluation or treatment of HIV infection.* It should be understood that programs cannot exclude adolescents from care or bar them from access to research protocols. All programs should consider the unique needs of adolescents and not allow the assumption that these needs will be met in the process of serving other groups.

5. *Establish a coordinated research effort to define specific risk factors for adolescent infection, to determine the natural history of HIV infection in adolescents, and to develop treatment protocols appropriate for adolescents.* To date, little research has been done to define how HIV infection may differ in adolescents as compared with children and adults. Comparatively few adolescents have been enrolled in

clinical trials, and little has been done to define what risk behaviors have had the greatest impact on the growing number of teenagers infected with HIV. Because many different aspects of HIV disease are represented in this research recommendation, the establishment of priority research areas should rest with the working group outlined in recommendation #1.

6. *Develop national standards for HIV counseling and testing of adolescents.* Although no national policy with regard to counseling and testing of adolescents exists, the programs of the military and Job Corps actually may be misused to establish standards for other groups of adolescents and young adults. To avoid this misuse, national standards for counseling and testing of adolescents should be established. These guidelines should ensure that whenever testing is undertaken, it is done for the benefit of the adolescent; that safeguards, including an interim court-appointed guardian (if necessary), are in place to avoid coercion; that appropriate steps are taken to ensure confidentiality; and that appropriate support systems are in place for posttest counseling of "positive" and "negative" adolescents.

While the existence of policies that are directed toward the unique needs of adolescents will help establish on national, state, and local levels the appropriate framework for preventing and treating HIV infection in adolescents, only systematic implementation of these policies can hope to reverse the growing trend of the steady increase in HIV infection in adolescents. This is the work that all involved with adolescents will need to dedicate themselves to in the years ahead.

References

American Medical Association. (1990). *Healthy youth 2000: National health promotion and disease prevention objectives for adolescents* (pp. 1-50). Chicago, IL: Author.
Centers for Disease Control. (1988). Guidelines for school health to prevent the spread of AIDS. *MMWR, 37*(Suppl. S-2), 1-13.
D'Angelo, L. J., Getson, P. R., Luban, N. L. C., & Gayle, H. D. (1991). Human immunodeficiency virus infection in urban adolescents: Can we predict who is at risk? *Pediatrics, 88,* 982-986.

DiClemente, R. J. (1990). Adolescents and AIDS: Current research, prevention strategies and public policy. In L. Temoshok & A. Baum (Eds.), *Psychosocial perspectives on AIDS: Etiology, prevention, and treatment* (pp. 52-64). Hillsdale, NJ: Lawrence Erlbaum.

Ginzburg, H. M. (1991). Limitations to an adolescent's access to medical care, Part II. Medical confidentiality. *Pediatric AIDS and HIV Infection, 2,* 290-295.

Hein, K. (1987). AIDS in adolescents: A rationale for concern. *New York State Journal of Medicine, 87,* 290-295.

Hein, K. (1991). Risky business: Adolescents and human immunodeficiency virus. *Pediatrics, 88,* 1052-1054.

Kegeles, S. M., Adler, N. E., & Irwin, C. E. (1988). Sexually active adolescents and condoms: Changes over the year in knowledge, attitudes, and use. *American Journal of Public Health, 78,* 460-461.

Steiner, J. D., Sorokin, G., Schiedmayer, D. L., & Van Susteren, T. J. (1990). Are adolescents getting smarter about acquired immunodeficiency syndrome? *American Journal of Diseases of Children, 144,* 302-306.

Strunin, L., & Hingson, R. (1987). Acquired immunodeficiency syndrome and adolescents: Knowledge, beliefs, attitudes, and behaviors. *Pediatrics, 79,* 825-828.

Vermund, S. H., Hein, K., Gayle, H. D., Cary, J. M., Thomas, P. A., & Drucker, E. (1989). Acquired immunodeficiency syndrome among adolescents: Case surveillance profiles in New York City and the rest of the United States. *American Journal of Diseases of Children, 143,* 1220-1225.

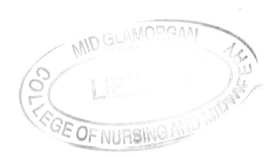

15

Expanding Access to HIV Services for Adolescents: Legal and Ethical Issues

ABIGAIL ENGLISH

Introduction

Design and implementation of interventions and research related to the prevention, diagnosis, and treatment of HIV infection in adolescents involve a wide array of legal and ethical concerns. Resolution of these concerns requires consideration of the developmental issues of adolescence and cannot simply rely on the perspectives that are appropriate either for adults or for young children. Moreover, as a result of their psychosocial circumstances and legal status, adolescents experience serious barriers in gaining access to essential health

AUTHOR'S NOTE: This chapter was supported by the Maternal and Child Health Bureau, Health Resources and Services Administration, Department of Health and Human Services (Grant No. BRH PH0908-01-0), the Public Health Service Panel on Women, Adolescents and Children with HIV Infection and AIDS, and the Working Group on Legal and Ethical Issues Related to HIV of the Public Health Services Task Force on AIDS. The views expressed herein do not necessarily reflect those of the funding entities.

care and related services. The development of HIV-related interventions and research for this age group must take these barriers into account and include strategies for overcoming them.

Legal and Ethical Issues
in Intervention and Research

The legal issues involved in providing HIV-related services and conducting HIV research with adolescents include consent for testing and treatment, confidentiality and disclosure of HIV-related information, financing of care and services, participation in clinical trials and other research, and discrimination. Significant ethical issues include the importance of establishing a linkage between testing and treatment, the tensions that may exist between the basic ethical principles of avoiding harming and maximizing benefits, the need for counseling and informed consent that is appropriate for adolescents, and the potential conflicts that may occur between the importance of enrolling adolescents in clinical trials or other research studies and the mandate to protect them from harm.

Linkage Between Testing and Treatment

One of the most critical ethical issues that must be considered in providing HIV-related services to adolescents is the linkage between HIV testing and treatment (English, 1991b). This issue has both broad ramifications for many aspects of HIV service delivery to this age group and very specific implications for the counseling and informed consent procedures associated with HIV testing.

Early therapeutic intervention with the potential for delaying the onset of symptoms and/or prolonging life recently has become available for individuals who are infected with HIV but are asymptomatic (National Institutes of Health, 1990). This development has had a profound effect on attitudes toward HIV testing among health care professionals and service providers, AIDS advocacy organizations, and the general public. Despite the continued social and psychological risks that may be associated with HIV testing, it is now widely viewed as an important gateway to early intervention services and treatment (Altman, 1989).

It cannot be assumed, however, that this model works equally effectively for all groups of infected individuals. Adolescents, for example, often encounter more obstacles than adults and younger children do in establishing access to essential health care (U.S. Congress, 1991a); and those who are in high-risk situations—and may be at highest risk for HIV infection—experience especially great difficulty in meeting their needs for both health care and basic survival services (English, 1991b; Hein, 1991). These general difficulties, together with the limited availability of HIV-specific services for adolescents, suggest that HIV testing will not automatically result in linking infected adolescents with treatment.

From an ethical perspective, unless access to treatment can be reasonably assured for adolescents who test positive, the balance of benefits and risks associated with HIV testing shifts dramatically.[1] This has several important implications for HIV testing of adolescents. First, at minimum, the issue of adolescents' access to treatment must be reflected in the informed consent and counseling procedures for HIV testing. Second, communities should not implement HIV testing for adolescents apart from a context in which linkage to services can be established. Third, increased efforts to expand adolescents' access to health care and HIV-specific services are more important than ever.

Consent for Testing and Treatment

For some adolescents, an essential element of accessible health care is the ability to obtain services on an independent basis. Thus one major concern in providing services to adolescents in high-risk situations is whether they are able to give their own consent for HIV testing and treatment. This question raises issues that involve both the HIV-specific laws enacted during the past few years and the broader legal context in which health care services are provided to adolescents. In addition, to the extent that adolescents are legally authorized to consent to HIV testing and/or treatment, serious ethical considerations arise with respect to counseling and informed consent, as well as to the balance of risks and benefits, that must be incorporated into the framework of providing services to this age group.

Laws Authorizing Minors to Consent

Some adolescents are legally adults (age 18 or older in almost every state) and therefore are able to give consent for their own medical care. Many adolescents are younger than age 18, however, and in the eyes of the law are "minor children" (throughout this discussion of consent, the term *minors* will be used to refer to adolescents who are under age 18). Although the law generally requires parental consent when health care is provided to minor children, this basic requirement has numerous exceptions, based on the minor's status or the specific services sought (English, 1990; Gittler, Quigley-Rick, & Saks, 1990). Many of these exceptions are relevant in determining the extent to which adolescents who are minors can consent to their own HIV testing and treatment. Both the HIV-specific laws and the other provisions for minors to consent to their own care vary among different states (English, 1990). Although this variety makes the development of consistent national policy difficult, a sufficient number of different bases exist for minors to consent to their own care to facilitate access for many adolescents in high-risk situations.

HIV-Specific Consent Laws

Beginning in the mid-1980s, states have enacted numerous HIV-specific laws, including statutes that govern consent for HIV testing and treatment. At least 11 states have statutes that explicitly authorize minors to consent to HIV testing.[2] Only three of these states also explicitly authorize minors to consent to treatment for AIDS or HIV infection.[3] This does not mean that minors in other states are unable to consent to HIV testing or treatment, however; they may be able to do so based on laws that pertain to specific services—STDs, contagious or communicable disease, pregnancy, or family planning services—or that authorize minors to consent based on their status (English, 1990; North, 1990).

Consent Laws Based on STDs and Contagious or Communicable Disease

While every state has a law that enables minors to consent to diagnosis and treatment of sexually transmitted disease (STD) or venereal disease (VD), not every state has classified HIV infection or AIDS as an STD or VD (English, 1990; North, 1990). At least 13 states do, however, and in these states minors would be able to consent to testing and treatment of HIV on that basis.[4] Moreover, in at least seven states in which minors are authorized to consent to diagnosis and treatment of communicable, contagious, or infectious disease, HIV infection is classified as one of these conditions.[5] In addition, in at least two states that permit minors to consent to diagnosis and treatment of reportable diseases, they may be able to consent to HIV care on the basis that AIDS cases are reportable even if HIV infection is not.[6]

Consent Laws Based on Other Specific Services or Conditions

In addition to the laws that are specific to HIV, STDs, and other communicable, contagious, or infectious diseases, laws in most states enable minors to consent to treatment for other conditions, including mental health problems, drug or alcohol problems, rape or sexual assault, and pregnancy (English, 1990; Gittler et al., 1990). In particular, minors' independent access to family planning services is protected by the constitutional right of privacy, and minors have a right to obtain family planning services without parental consent in federally funded Title X family planning programs and by specific provisions of state law in approximately half the states (English, 1990; Gittler et al., 1990; Paul & Klassel, 1987). As a result of the increasing frequency with which HIV testing is being offered as an integral part of family planning services, some of these laws may enable minors to consent to HIV testing.

Consent Laws Based on Status of Minor

In addition to the consent laws that are oriented to specific services, many states have laws that enable minors to consent to their own medical care based on their living situation or legal status. For example, by statute in varying numbers of states, the following groups of minors may give consent for their own care: (a) those who are living apart from their parents, such as runaways and homeless youth (at least 11 states), (b) emancipated minors (at least 16 states),[7] (c) mature minors (at least 5 states),[8] (d) high school graduates (at least 3 states), and (e) married minors (at least 25 states) or minor parents (at least 13 states) (Gittler et al., 1990).

Counseling and Informed Consent

The foregoing discussion demonstrates that numerous circumstances exist in which minors are legally authorized to consent to HIV testing and treatment, as well as related health care services, and that minors may be receiving HIV testing and treatment in a wide variety of settings. In addition to the settings mentioned above, adolescents are also sometimes tested for HIV when they seek other health care services—surgical care in a hospital setting, for example.

Regardless of the setting in which HIV testing and/or treatment is provided to adolescents, it is essential that in implementing these services, procedures are in place to ensure that appropriate counseling is provided and informed consent is obtained (English, 1989). Research studies have suggested that, compared with adults, adolescents (particularly those who are older than about 14) do have the capacity to make health care decisions (Gittler et al., 1990). Clinicians have found also that most adolescents are capable of understanding the risks and benefits of medical treatment and therefore of giving informed consent (Morrissey, Hofmann, & Thrope, 1986). In situations in which an adolescent lacks capacity to give informed consent, it must be sought from a parent, guardian, or court (Holder, 1985).

Significant attention has been paid to the question of pretest and posttest counseling and informed consent for HIV testing. In certain settings, counseling and informed consent have been incorporated as an integral part of the testing process (Larkin Street Youth Center, 1990). In other settings, however, individuals are tested without their consent and/or without adequate counseling. Recent federal legislation—the Ryan White Comprehensive AIDS Resources Emergency (CARE) Act—requires counseling and informed consent for HIV testing performed in any facility receiving Ryan White funds whether or not the testing is paid for with federal monies (Ryan White CARE Act, 1990).

A multidisciplinary group of experts has recommended that all adolescents who are tested for HIV should receive pretest and posttest counseling that is age appropriate, developmentally appropriate, and in a language they can understand (English, 1989). In addition, informed consent procedures, including both the protocols for dialogue between patient and health care professional and any written consent forms, should be reviewed to ensure that they are designed to be meaningful to adolescents (Larkin Street Youth Center, 1990). Some programs have involved adolescents themselves in developing the protocols and forms. In order to ensure that adolescents are making a voluntary decision about whether to undergo a test, the counseling and informed consent procedures should incorporate sufficient information about the accessibility of treatment services if they test positive.

Participation in Clinical Trials and Research Studies

One important mechanism for expanding adolescents' access to treatment for HIV is to enable them to participate in clinical trials. Until very recently, adolescents have been largely excluded from clinical trials[9] (Hein, 1991) that have been limited to the pediatric (0-13) and the adult age groups, although under a recent initiative of the National Institute of Allergy and Infectious Disease (NIAID), their access to pediatric HIV trials is being expanded (National Pediatric HIV Resource Center, 1991). Adolescent participation in other HIV research studies can also indirectly help expand adolescents' access to services by providing important information to be used in designing appropriate prevention and treatment strategies for this age group and in advocating for increased services (Hein, 1991; English, 1989). From an ethical perspective, the goal with respect to HIV research involving adolescents should be twofold: first, to facilitate the research when it will benefit adolescents either individually or as a group; and second, to protect them from undue risk.

The participation of adolescents as subjects of research raises a number of legal and ethical questions (Leikin, 1989; Melton, 1989). Specifically, such participation must occur, if at all, in conformity with the federal research regulations (Protection of Human Subjects, 1989). These regulations establish requirements for the protection of human subjects of research funded by the Department of Health and Human Services, although they are widely regarded as establishing the basic ethical requirements for research funded by other sources as well. The regulations include special provisions applicable to children, establish a hierarchy of acceptable levels of risk, and set forth requirements for parental consent (Additional Protections for Children, 1989). The basic regulations apply to research studies and clinical trials that involve adolescents of any age, and the Additional Protections for Children (1989) also apply when the adolescent subjects of the research would be considered children under the regulations.[10]

Hierarchy of Risk

The Additional Protections for Children establish criteria for determining the circumstances under which research involving varying levels of risk is acceptable. These criteria would be particularly relevant in evaluating research that involves HIV testing of subjects, or clinical trials of drugs with significant side effects. Research involving no greater than minimal risk or greater than minimal risk but also a possibility of direct benefit to the individual research subjects is acceptable under the regulations. Research involving greater than minimal risk but no prospect of direct benefit may also be acceptable under more limited circumstances if it is likely to yield generalizable knowledge of vital importance.

Parental Permission and Waiver

One of the basic requirements of the regulations is that participation in research must be based on informed consent of either the subject of the research or, in certain circumstances, the parent or guardian of a child. In the case of adolescents who meet the definition of *children* under the regulations, both parental permission and the assent of the adolescents ordinarily are required for their participation. The regulations also provide for the requirement of parental permission to be waived if the research is "designed for conditions or for a subject population for which parental or guardian permission is not a reasonable requirement" (Additional Protections for Children, 1989).

The body of law that permits minors to consent to their own medical care is highly relevant in determining the circumstances in which a requirement of parental permission might not be reasonable. For example, the National Commission for the Protection of Human Subjects of Biomedical and Behavioral Research (1977) suggested that it would be appropriate to waive parental permission for research related to conditions for which minors legally may consent to their own treatment or research in which the subjects are "mature minors" and the research entails no more than minimal risk that they might "reasonably assume on their own." The Commission (1977) also suggested that the requirement might not be reasonable for abused or neglected children, and data suggest that a high percentage of adolescents have been physically or sexually abused.

Thus for research related to HIV, if under state law minors may consent to HIV testing and/or treatment or if the adolescent research subjects are capable of giving informed consent—and may therefore be considered "mature minors"—and the research does not entail more than minimal risk, the requirement of parental permission may be waived. Determining the level of risk to adolescents associated with a particular research study should include consideration not only of the risks specifically associated with any medical intervention that is involved but also of the overall impact on the adolescents in the social and psychological circumstances of their lives.

Special Protections

The regulations explicitly require that when parental permission is waived, an alternative mechanism for protecting the children (or adolescents) must be substituted. The specific mechanism must be designed around the particular risks involved in the research, as well as the maturity and other characteristics of the adolescents who are the research subjects. Moreover, if the subjects of research are wards of the state or any agency or institution and the research involves greater than minimal risk and no prospect of direct benefit, an advocate (in addition to anyone else acting as guardian or in loco parentis) must be appointed to protect the best interests of each child or adolescent who is a research subject.

Despite the legal and ethical complexities involved in the participation of adolescents in HIV clinical trials and research studies, such participation can be one important avenue to the care they need. In order for adolescents to benefit from their participation, however, research protocols must be designed carefully to ensure that adolescents' participation is voluntary and that a mechanism is in place to ensure that those who choose to be involved are linked with services they need. Some efforts of this nature are already underway. For example, funding recently made available by NIAID is designed to support ancillary services for adolescents who enroll in clinical trials (National Pediatric HIV Resource Center, 1991).

Access to Health Care and Related Services

Although clinical trials are an important element in a comprehensive system of HIV treatment and related services for adolescents, adolescents' access depends on numerous other factors as well. For adolescents, access to health care and related services is dependent not only on their ability to give independent consent but also on the existence of a source of funding for the services (U.S. Congress, 1991b). In addition, programs with funding that enables them to serve an adolescent population must be accessible in other ways as well. Many adolescents are reluctant to utilize health care services that are geographically distant or difficult to identify or that do not take adolescents' psychosocial characteristics into account in the program's design. Moreover, unless a program that funds services for adolescents includes both a mechanism for adolescents to establish eligibility, independently of their families if necessary, and the range of services that are important in meeting adolescents' needs, adolescents will not be able to benefit fully from the program.

Funding Sources

Numerous sources of public funding exist for services to address the prevention, diagnosis, and treatment of HIV (Winkenwerder, Kessler, & Stolec, 1989). The most recent source of federal funding, which is designed to fund comprehensive services, is the Ryan White Comprehensive AIDS Resources Emergency (CARE) Act (1990). Medicaid has been the major source of public funding for treatment of indigent AIDS patients (Winkenwerder et al., 1989).

The Pediatric AIDS Demonstration Projects have been a critically important source of care for the pediatric population and are beginning to focus greater attention on the needs of adolescents (Hemophilia and AIDS Program Branch, 1991). Finally, some states have implemented specialized funding programs to provide HIV services that have been or could be utilized to meet the needs of adolescents.

Ryan White CARE Act. The Ryan White CARE Act (1990) authorizes funding for a system of comprehensive HIV care for individuals and families to be provided by cities, states, and other public and private entities (English, 1991a). For the first year of this ambitious program, FY 1991, Congress authorized a total of $875 million but appropriated only a quarter of that—$225 million. Nevertheless, each of the three major programs included in the act—the Emergency Relief Grant Program, the Care Grant Program, and Early Intervention Services—could support HIV services that are essential for adolescents, particularly if advocates for this population work hard to ensure that an adequate portion of the funding is used for this purpose.

For example, under the Emergency Relief Grant Program, which funds comprehensive treatment and case management services in geographic areas hardest hit by the epidemic, one half of the funds is awarded as supplemental grants to areas that provide assurances that their use of funds will include appropriate allocations for infants, children, women, and families. To ensure that adolescents receive some of the benefits of these allocations, however, advocates for adolescents must participate actively in the HIV Health Services Planning Council, which establishes priorities for the allocation of funds. Similarly under the Care Grant Program, which supports a broad range of health services, support services, and home- and community-based services, at least 15% of the funds must be used for services to infants, children, women, and families, but targeted advocacy may be needed to ensure that programs serving adolescents receive funds so that adolescents actually benefit. The Early Intervention Services program also has the potential to support services, including counseling, testing, referrals, clinical and diagnostic services, periodic medical evaluations, and therapeutic services, that are needed urgently by adolescents with or at high risk for HIV infection, but adolescents will benefit only if programs receiving Ryan White Early Intervention funds—such as STD clinics and substance abuse treatment programs—ensure that their services are accessible to and appropriate for this age group.

Pediatric AIDS Demonstration Projects. For the past few years, the Maternal and Child Health Bureau in the Health Resources and Services Administration has provided funding for Pediatric AIDS Demonstration Projects (Hemophilia and AIDS Program Branch, 1991). These projects have been mandated to provide comprehensive, coordinated, community-based, family-centered care for children and families affected by HIV. The funding for these projects offers them broad flexibility in designing services that are responsive to the needs of their target population, and for this reason they could be critically important in meeting the needs of adolescents. Until very recently, only a few of these projects have been specifically targeted at adolescents, although within the last 2 years the ability to serve adolescents has been an important criterion in selecting projects for funding.

Medicaid. Medicaid has paid for the HIV-related health care of an estimated 40% of all patients with AIDS (Winkenwerder et al., 1989). For adolescents, Medicaid has both advantages and disadvantages as a funding source (U.S. Congress, 1991b).

The primary advantage of Medicaid is that, to the extent that adolescents can establish eligibility, they are entitled to receive whatever services Medicaid covers in their state, in contrast to other programs that provide services but do not create any enforceable individual entitlement for program beneficiaries. An additional advantage is that state and local governments can extend scarce resources by utilizing Medicaid because of the guaranteed federal match of at least 50%.

Two major disadvantages of Medicaid are that (a) it is difficult for many adolescents to qualify and (b) the covered benefits often do not include some of the services that are critically important for adolescents. For the most part, eligibility requirements restrict Medicaid eligibility for adolescents to those who are dependent children in AFDC families, who are pregnant or parenting a child, who are eligible for SSI or federal foster care or adoption assistance, or who qualify, in some states, as "medically needy." Many adolescents who are poor are nevertheless unable to qualify for Medicaid. Moreover, because of limitations in services under many state Medicaid plans, even those adolescents who qualify may be unable to receive many of the nonmedical health care services they need.

Two recent developments in the Medicaid program at the federal level, however, may make the program a more accessible resource for adolescents, including those at risk for HIV (Perkins & Melden, 1991). First, in addition to recent expansions of Medicaid eligibility for infants and pregnant women, in 1990 Congress mandated that states begin including children over age 6 who are poor according to federal guidelines on a phased-in basis, 1 year at a time, until all poor children are covered up to age 18. Second, in 1989 Congress enacted major reforms in the Early and Periodic Screening, Diagnosis and Treatment (EPSDT) program (Johnson, 1990; Perkins & Melden, 1991). One provision that could be critically important in expanding the scope of services available to Medicaid-eligible adolescents is a requirement that states must provide any federally reimbursable service that is necessary to diagnose or treat a problem identified in an EPSDT screen of a Medicaid-eligible child whether or not that service is ordinarily included in the state's Medicaid plan.

Medicaid Waivers and Other Specialized State Programs. Several states have adopted specialized programs to fund diagnosis and treatment and other health-related services for individuals with HIV. These programs include both the Medicaid "AIDS Waiver" programs and special programs developed under other authority, such as the California Children's Services HIV Children Program.

Beginning in 1981, Congress granted states authority to seek waivers of basic federal Medicaid requirements in order to allow them to meet the needs of certain populations more effectively (English, Jameson, & Warboys, 1989; Fox, 1990). Under this authority, several states have established "AIDS Waiver" programs to provide a broader range of home- and community-based services to individuals with AIDS than would ordinarily be available under the state's Medicaid plan. The eligibility criteria and services provided for in AIDS waivers are determined by the waiver application filed by the state and approved by the Health Care Financing Administration. Thus the effectiveness of these AIDS waivers in meeting the needs of adolescents depends on the specific provisions of each state's program. For example, depending on the level of diagnosis—of HIV infection or AIDS—that is required to establish eligibility for the program, many adolescents who are infected with HIV but asymptomatic may not be able to qualify.

Adolescents may be able to establish access to essential health care and related services through other special programs at the state level. California, for example, has established the HIV Children Program under the auspices of California Children's Services (CCS) (California State Department of Health Services, 1989). For any child or adolescent up to age 21, the HIV Children Program pays for any diagnostic procedures necessary to establish the presence or absence of HIV infection. If HIV infection is definitively diagnosed, children or adolescents who meet financial eligibility requirements (which are more generous than the eligibility requirements for Medi-Cal, California's Medicaid program) are eligible for treatment under the regular CCS program. It is advantageous for adolescents to establish eligibility for CCS because it provides more comprehensive benefits than the Medi-Cal program.[11]

Confidentiality of HIV-Related Information

For many adolescents, in addition to a source of funding for the care and the option of giving independent consent, protection of confidentiality is a critical element in their willingness to seek health care for sensitive issues (Hofmann, 1980), including HIV. The importance of confidentiality is also underscored by the continuing risks of discrimination that individuals with HIV or AIDS experience, despite extensive statutory and judicial protections against discrimination. The legal requirements of confidentiality that apply to HIV-related information derive from a complex body of law. Moreover, numerous ethical issues arise with respect to the circumstances under which disclosure of HIV-related information by health care professionals and others serving adolescents may be necessary or appropriate.

Sources of the Confidentiality Obligation

Mandates to protect the confidentiality of HIV-related information are found both in the confidentiality requirements that apply to medical information in general and in specific requirements recently enacted to protect the confidentiality of HIV tests result and other HIV information (English, 1990, 1991b). These mandates are contained in HIV-specific statutes, medical records laws, licensing laws for professionals and facilities, tort law, social services and child welfare statutes, education and vocational rehabilitation laws, laws related to drug and alcohol treatment, developmental disabilities statutes, and a broad range of statutes governing the provision of health care (Rennert, 1991). Some of the strictest nondisclosure requirements are contained in the HIV-specific statutes of several states. In addition, the Ryan White CARE Act (1990) now requires, as a condition of federal funding, that states have in place adequate protections of confidentiality.

Disclosure

Disclosure of HIV-related information is nevertheless required under a variety of circumstances. The critical issues involve determining when and to whom disclosure is appropriate and what if any authorization is required. At minimum, mechanisms must be in place to ensure that information necessary to the provision of appropriate care can be communicated among those who are providing direct services to an adolescent. Although the law sometimes authorizes such communication among direct providers of health care without specific authorization from the patient or a legal representative, obtaining authorization in writing is preferred in most circumstances even if it is not legally required. It is also important for adolescents to understand clearly what the limits are with respect to confidentiality.

Authority to Disclose

For adolescents, one of the critical questions is whether the adolescent has the right to authorize—or refuse to authorize—disclosure of HIV-related information or whether authorization must be obtained from a parent or other decisionmaker. As a general matter, the person (or court) with legal authority to make health care decisions for the adolescent will be the one from whom authorization to release information concerning HIV should be obtained (Rennert, 1991). Thus in the absence of a specific contrary legal requirement, adolescents who are legally authorized to consent to HIV testing or treatment would usually have the right to control disclosure of related information (English, 1990, 1991b; Rennert, 1991).

In certain circumstances, disclosure is either permitted within the discretion of the health care professional or service provider or is mandated by law. For example, in a few states, physicians have statutory discretion to decide whether to notify the partner of a patient who is infected with HIV; and in all states, confidentiality is overridden by the mandatory reporting requirements of child abuse reporting laws and by the necessity for taking preventive measures when a patient is suicidal (English, 1990). While these latter circumstances would require breaking confidentiality, they would not necessarily require disclosure of the adolescent's HIV status.

Partner Notification

One of the most controversial issues with respect to confidentiality of HIV-related information is the question of whether partner notification is required or is appropriate. At the present time, no HIV-specific statute or court decision requires physicians or other youth-serving professionals or agencies to notify the partners of adolescents who are infected with HIV (Rennert, 1991). Some states explicitly permit, but do not require, physicians to do so. In addition, many states require psychotherapists (and possibly physicians) to warn individuals against whom their patients have made specific threats of serious harm, although whether this "duty to warn" will be applied in the HIV context remains unclear at this time (Rennert, 1991). The preferred approach would be to work with infected adolescents themselves to assist them in disclosing their HIV status to their partners and in avoiding behaviors with a risk of transmitting the virus.

Disclosure to Residential Care Providers

Residential care providers, including foster parents and group home or institutional staff, frequently are concerned about the HIV status of adolescents under their care (Child Welfare League of America, 1989). These concerns generally stem from a desire to protect other residents and staff from transmission and from a concern about the provider's potential liability if transmission occurs from one resident or foster child to another. While concerns about transmission and liability are understandable, disclosure of an adolescent's HIV status to foster parents, residential care staff, and other foster children or residents does not necessarily address those concerns.

Reliance on the "knowledge" of an adolescent's HIV status can be misleading and can provide a false sense of security. Because a window period exists between infection and seroconversion, and because adolescents may continue to engage in high-risk behaviors and become infected after testing negative for HIV, residential care providers cannot rely on a negative test result to assume that a risk of transmission does not exist. By implementing universal precautions, making condoms available, and providing all adolescents in residential care with effective prevention education, agencies can more appropriately reduce the risk of both transmission and liability[12] (CWLA, 1989; Hein, 1991). Moreover, even if the HIV status of youth in residential care were known, it would be difficult to use the information to prevent transmission effectively without serious infringement of the adolescent's rights—either by forced isolation or exclusion from the program.

Protection From Discrimination

To the extent that the desire to know an adolescent's HIV status is motivated by the intention to exclude that young person from a program, a high likelihood exists that to do so would violate one or more of the many prohibitions against discrimination on the basis of AIDS or HIV status. These protections include Section 504 of the Rehabilitation Act, the Americans with Disabilities Act, and numerous other federal, state, and local antidiscrimination laws (Rennert, Parry, & Horowitz, 1989). One of the greatest problems for adolescents, however, is that they simply do not have either the detailed knowledge necessary to use these laws to protect themselves against discrimination or sufficient access to lawyers and other advocates to represent them. Often the very adolescents who are at greatest risk of the kind of discrimination that can result from disclosure that they are infected with HIV are also the ones least likely to be able to obtain help from attorneys or other advocates (English, 1988).

Conclusion

HIV infection in adolescents presents a major challenge to policymakers, service providers, and advocates to resolve the many legal and ethical issues that may present barriers to providing this vulnerable population with the services they need. To meet the ultimate goal of preventing HIV infection in adolescents and providing appropriate health care and related services to those who are infected, important concerns with respect to (a) consent for HIV testing and treatment, (b) confidentiality of information, and (c) funding for services must be addressed. One of the most critical issues is the necessity for establishing a linkage between testing and treatment in order to encourage adolescents who are at high risk for infection to learn their HIV status, while providing a benefit to justify the increased risks of loss of confidentiality and discrimination that may occur as a result of identification. In order to establish this linkage effectively, the available sources of funding for HIV treatment and related services, including clinical trials, must be fully utilized and if necessary adapted to make them accessible to the adolescent population.

Notes

1. Moreover, the efficacy of treatment for adolescents with HIV infection has not yet been established, so the degree of benefit associated with early intervention is not clear.

2. **Arizona** (Ariz. Rev. Stat. Ann. §§ 36-661(2) and 36-663 (Supp. 1990) [written informed consent required for an HIV test; capacity to consent determined without regard to age]); **California** (Cal. Health & Safety Code §§ 199.22 and 199.27(a) (West 1990) [written consent of competent subject of HIV antibody test required; minors under age 12 deemed incompetent to consent to test]); **Colorado** (Colo. Rev. Stat. Ann. § 25-4-1405(6) (1990) [minor may be examined and treated for HIV infection without consent of parent]); **Delaware** (Del. Code Ann. tit. 16, § 1202(f) (Supp. 1988) [minors age 12 and older may give informed consent for HIV testing and counseling]); **Iowa** (Iowa Code Ann. § 144.22 (West Supp. 1991) [minor may apply and give consent for screening or treatment for AIDS]); **Michigan** (Mich. Comp. Laws Ann. § 333.5127 (West Supp. 1991) [minor may consent to medical or surgical care, treatment, or services for HIV]); **Montana** (Mont. Code Ann. § 50-16-1007 (1989) [minors may consent for HIV related test]); **New Mexico** (N.M. Stat. Ann. § 24-2B-3 (Supp. 1990) [minor has capacity to give informed consent for HIV test]); **New York** (N.Y. Pub. Health Law §§ 2780(5) and 2781(1) (McKinney Supp. 1991)[written informed consent required for an HIV related test; capacity to consent is

determined without regard to age]); **Ohio** (Ohio Rev. Code Ann. § 3701.242(B) (Page Supp. 1990) [minor may give consent for an HIV test]); and **Wisconsin** (Wis. Stat. Ann. § 146.025(2)(a)(4) (West Supp. 1990) [consent of a competent minor age 14 or older is required for an HIV test]).

3. **Colorado** (Colo. Rev. Stat. Ann. § 25-4-1405(6) (1990) [minor may be examined and treated for HIV infection without consent of a parent]); **Iowa** (Iowa Code Ann. § 144.22 (West Supp. 1991) [minor may apply and give consent for screening or treatment for AIDS]); **Michigan** (Mich. Comp. Laws Ann. § 333.5127 (West Supp. 1991) [minor may consent to medical or surgical care, treatment, or services for HIV]).

4. **Alabama** (Rules of State Bd. of Health, Division of Disease Control § 420-4-1-03 (1987) [HIV classified as STD]; Ala. Code § 22-11A-19 (Supp. 1989) [minors may consent to STD care]); **Florida** (Fla. Stat. Ann. § 384.23 (West Supp. 1991) [Department of Health shall consider HIV in designating STDs]; Fla. Stat. Ann. § 384.30 [minors may consent to confidential treatment for STDs]); **Illinois** (Ill. Ann. Stat. ch. 111 1/2, para. 7403(3) (Smith-Hurd Supp. 1991) [HIV is classified as STD]; Ill. Ann. Stat. ch. 111, paras. 4504 and 4505 (Smith-Hurd Supp. 1988) [minors age 12 or older may consent to VD diagnosis and treatment]; **Kentucky** (Ky. Rev. Stat. Ann. § 214.410 (Baldwin 1991) [STD defined to include AIDS and HIV]; Ky. Rev. Stat. Ann. § 214.185 (Baldwin 1982) [minors may consent to diagnosis and treatment of VD]); **Mississippi** (Miss. State Dept. Health 1990 List of Reportable Diseases [HIV classified as STD]; Miss. Code An.. § 41-41-13 (1981) [minors may obtain treatment for VD without parental consent]); **Montana** (Mont. Code Ann. § 50-18-101 (1989) [AIDS is defined as STD]; Mont. Admin. R. 16.28.204 (1987) [HIV is reportable]; Mont. Code Ann. § 41-1-402 (1989) [minors may consent to care for reportable STDs]); **Nevada** (P. Albert, R. Eisenberg, D. A. Hansell, J. K. Marcus (Eds.). (1991). *AIDS practice manual: A legal and educational guide* (3rd ed.). (App. A). San Francisco: National Lawyers Guild AIDS Network. [HIV is classified as STD]; Nev. Rev. Stat. Ann. § 129.060 (Michie 1986) [minors may consent to examination and treatment for VD]; **South Carolina** (S.C. Dept. Health 1990 List of Reportable Diseases and S.C. Code Ann. § 44-29-10, -70 (Law Co-op. Supp. 1989) [HIV is reportable STD]; S.C. Code Ann. § 20-7-280 (Law Co-op 1985) [minors 16 or older may consent to any health services except operations]; S.C. Code Ann. § 20-7-290 (Law Co-op 1985) [minors of any age may receive without parental consent health services deemed by the provider necessary to maintain the well-being of the child]); **Tennessee** (*AIDS practice manual* (App. A) [HIV classified as STD]; Tenn. Code Ann. § 68-10-104 (1987) [minors may be examined, diagnosed, and treated for VD without parental consent]); **Vermont** (Vt. Stat. Ann. tit. 18, § 1091 (1968) and *AIDS practice manual* (App. A) [HIV classified as STD]; Vt. Stat. Ann. tit. 18, § 4226 (1982) [minors age 12 and older may consent to VD treatment]); **Washington** (Wash. Rev. Code Ann. § 70.24.017 (Supp. 1991) [STD defined to include HIV and AIDS]; Wash. Rev. Code Ann. § 70.24.110 [minors age 14 and older may consent to diagnosis and treatment of STDs]; and **Wyoming** (Wyo. Stat. § 35-4-130(b) (Supp. 1990) [AIDS defined as reportable STD]; Wyo. Stat. § 35-4-131 (1988) [minors may consent to examination and treatment for VD]. (Although the classification of HIV—as STD or VD—does not exactly match the designation of conditions—STD or VD—for which minors are authorized to consent to treatment in each of these states, it is likely that a

court would construe broadly the minor consent statute to facilitate access to HIV-related care.)

5. **Alabama** (Ala. Code § 22-11A-14 (1984) [HIV is reportable disease]; Ala. Code § 22-8-6 (1984) [minors of any age may consent to diagnosis and treatment of reportable diseases]; **Idaho** (Idaho Code § 39-601 (1990) [AIDS, ARC and HIV classified as contagious, infectious, and communicable]; Idaho Code § 39-3801 (Supp. 1988) [minors age 14 or older may consent to diagnosis and treatment of reportable infectious, contagious, or communicable diseases]); **Montana** (Mont. Admin. R. 16.28.204 (1987) [HIV is reportable]; Mont. Code Ann. § 41-1-402 (1989) [minors may consent to care for reportable communicable diseases]); **North Carolina** (N.C. Gen. Stat. § 130A-135 (1989) [HIV is a reportable communicable condition]; N.C. Gen. Stat. § 90-21.5 (1985) [minors may consent to medical services to prevent, diagnose, and treat reportable diseases]); **Oklahoma** (Okla. State Board of Health, Regulations for Reporting Cases of Disease, § 100 *et seq.* [HIV is reportable communicable disease]; Okla. Stat. Ann. tit. 63, § 2602 (1984) [minors may consent to treatment of reportable communicable diseases]); **Texas** (Tex. Health & Safety Code Ann. § 81.041(e) (Vernon 1991) [HIV and AIDS are reportable diseases]; Tex. Fam. Code Ann. § 35.03 (Vernon 1986) [minors may consent to treatment of reportable, infectious, contagious, or communicable diseases]); and **Virginia** (Va. Code Ann. § 32.1-116.3 (Supp. 1990) [HIV is defined as communicable disease for certain purposes]; Va. Code Ann. § 54.1-2969(D)(1) (1988) [minors may consent to diagnosis and treatment of any reportable infectious or contagious disease]).

6. **California** (17 Cal. Code Reg. 17, § 2500 (4-1-90) [AIDS is reportable communicable disease]; Cal. Civ. Code § 34.7 (West 1982) [minors age 12 or older may consent to diagnosis and treatment of reportable infectious, contagious, or communicable diseases]; and **Pennsylvania** (Pa. Stat. Ann. tit. 35, § 7607(9) (Purdon Supp. 1991) [HIV reporting to state permitted]; Pa. Stat. Ann. tit. 35, § 10103 (Purdon 1977) [minors may consent to treatment of reportable diseases]).

7. It is also likely that in the other 10 states that have enacted emancipation statutes, and in situations in which minors meet the common law criteria for emancipation—marriage, service in the armed forces, or living apart from parents and managing their own financial affairs—courts would consider emancipated minors as being able to consent to their own medical care.

8. Even in the absence of an explicit state statute, courts have found that minors meeting certain criteria of maturity may give their own consent.

9. In addition, adolescents in foster care would likely experience additional barriers in establishing access to clinical trials, because few states have established mechanisms to enable foster children to obtain HIV treatment in this way. (Martin & Sacks, 1990).

10. The regulations define *children* as persons who do not have the legal authority to consent to the treatments or procedures involved in the research under the law that applies in the jurisdiction in which the research is to be conducted.

11. It is not entirely clear to what extent adolescents—such as runaway and street youth—who are separated from their parents are able to qualify for the CCS program independently of consideration of their families' income. In contrast, the Medi-Cal Minor Consent program clearly permits adolescents to establish eligibility based on their own incomes for services to which they are legally able to give

their own consent, although it is not clear to what extent treatment for HIV infection would be covered under this program.

12. Limited circumstances may exist in which an agency might have a legal responsibility to inform other residents of the status of an adolescent with HIV infection or to take other protective measures—when, for example, that adolescent is unable or unwilling to practice safer behaviors and the partners or potential partners of the adolescent are also clients or wards of the agency and are unable to protect themselves. (Rennert, 1991).

References

Additional Protections for Children Involved as Subjects of Research, 45 C.F.R. Part 46, Subpart D (1989).

Altman, L. K. (1989, April 24). Experts on AIDS, citing new data push for testing. *New York Times*, pp. A1, A12.

California State Department of Health Services. (1989). *California Children's Services: HIV Children Program guidelines*. Sacramento: Author.

Child Welfare League of America (CWLA). (1989). *Serving HIV-infected children, youth and their families*. Washington, DC: Author.

English, A. (1988). Adolescents and AIDS: Legal and ethical questions multiply. In M. Quackenbush & M. Nelson (Eds.), *The AIDS challenge: Prevention education for young people* (pp. 255-268). Santa Cruz, CA: Network Publicatons.

English, A. (1989). Work group recommendations: AIDS testing and epidemiology for youth. *Journal of Adolescent Health Care, 10*(3), 52S-57S.

English, A. (1990). Treating adolescents: Legal and ethical considerations. *Medical Clinics of North America, 74*(5), 1097-1112.

English, A. (1991a). New federal law may help children and adolescents with HIV. *Youth Law News, 12*(2), 1-5.

English, A. (1991b). Runaway and street youth at risk for HIV infection: Legal and ethical issues in access to care. *Journal of Adolescent Health, 12*(7), 504-510.

English, A., Jameson, E., & Warboys, L. (1989). Legal issues in pediatric and adolescent AIDS. In C. Hockenberry (Ed.), *AIDS law* (pp. 4.3-4.15). San Francisco, CA: AIDS Legal Referral Panel.

Fox, D. M. (1990). Financing health care for persons with HIV infection. *American Journal of Law & Medicine, 16*(1&2), 223-247.

Gittler, J., Quigley-Rick, M., & Saks, M. J. (1990). *Adolescent health care decision making: The law and public policy*. Washington, DC: Carnegie Council on Adolescent Development.

Hein, K. (1991). Fighting AIDS in adolescents. *Issues in Science and Technology*, Spring, 67-73.

Hemophilia and AIDS Program Branch, Division of Services for Children with Special Health Care Needs, MCHB, HRSA, PHS, DHHS. (1991). *Pediatric AIDS/HIV Demonstration Program agenda*. Washington, DC: Author.

Hofmann, A. D. (1980). Toward a rational policy for consent and confidentiality. *Journal of Adolescent Health Care, 1*(1), 1-9.

Holder, A. R. (1985). *Legal issues in pediatrics and adolescent medicine* (2d ed.). New Haven, CT: Yale University Press.

Johnson, K. (1990). Improving health care programs for teens. *Adolescent Pregnancy Prevention Clearinghouse Reports.* Washington, DC: Children's Defense Fund.

Larkin Street Youth Center. (1990). *HIV and homeless youth: Meeting the challenge.* San Francisco: Author.

Leikin, S. L. (1989). Immunodeficiency virus infection, adolescents, and the institutional review board. *Journal of Adolescent Health Care, 10*(6), 500-505.

Martin, J. M., & Sacks, H. S. (1990). Do HIV-infected children in foster care have access to clinical trials of new treatments? *AIDS & Public Policy Journal, 5*(1), 1-7.

Melton, G. B. (1989). Ethical and legal issues in research and intervention. *Journal of Adolescent Health Care, 10*(3 Supp.) 36S-44S.

Morrissey, J. M., Hofmann, A. D., & Thrope, J. C. (1986). *Consent and confidentiality in the health care of children and adolescents: A legal guide.* New York: The Free Press.

National Commission for Protection of Human Subjects of Biomedical and Behavioral Research. (1977). *Research involving children: Report and recommendations* (DHEW Publication No. OS77-0004). Washington, DC: Government Printing Office.

National Institutes of Health. (1990). Recommendations for Zidovudine: Early treatment. *Journal of the American Medical Association, 263,* 1606.

National Pediatric HIV Resource Center. (1991, June 27). *Funding Alert.* Washington, DC: Author.

North, R. L. (1990). Legal authority for HIV testing of adolescents. *Journal of Adolescent Health Care, 11*(2), 176-187.

Paul, E. W., & Klassel, D. (1987). Minors' right to confidential contraceptive services: The limits of state power. *Women's Rights Law Reporter, 10*(1), 45-63.

Perkins, J., & Melden, M. (1991). *An advocate's guide to the Medicaid program.* Los Angeles: National Health Law Program.

Protection of Human Subjects, 45 C.F.R. Part 46 (1989).

Rennert, S. (1991). *AIDS/HIV and confidentiality: Model policies and procedures.* Washington, DC: American Bar Association.

Rennert, S., Parry, J., & Horowitz, R. (1989). *AIDS and persons with developmental disabilities: The legal perspective.* Washington, DC: American Bar Association.

Ryan White Comprehensive AIDS Resources Emergency (CARE) Act, Pub. L. No. 101-381, 104 Stat. 576 (1990); 42 U.S.C.A. § 300ff *et seq.* (West Supp. 1991).

U.S. Congress, Office of Technology Assessment. (1991a). *Adolescent health—Volume I: Summary and policy options.* Washington, DC: Government Printing Office.

U.S. Congress, Office of Technology Assessment. (1991b). *Adolescent health—Volume III: Crosscutting issues in the delivery of health and related services.* Washington, DC: Government Printing Office.

Winkenwerder, W., Kessler, A. R., & Stolec, R. M. (1989). Federal spending for illness caused by the human immunodeficiency virus. *New England Journal of Medicine, 320*(24), 1598-1603.

Name Index

Subject Index

Aaron Diamond Foundation, 243
Additional Protections for Children, 269
Adolescence, definitions of, 195, 234
Adolescents:
    access to health care, 271-275
    African-American, 181, 205, 209
    AIDS as cause of death in, 4
    anal intercourse by, 6, 57
    bisexual, 226
    in clinical trials and research studies, 268-271
    community-based   HIV-prevention programs for, 194-210, 237
    demographics of, 4
    emotional response of HIV-positive, 65-66
    endorsement of teenage sexuality by, 215
    factors affecting HIV infection rate in, 4-6
    Hispanic-American, 181
    HIV infection in, 195-196, 251-253
    HIV-positive, 212
        modifying HIV-prevention programs for, 221-226, 227
        secondary prevention for, 213, 226
        suicidal ideation by, 222
    HIV-risk behaviors
        primary prevention programs, 217-221
    HIV services
        expanding access to, 262-279
        funding for, 271-272, 279
    homosexual, 8, 12, 196, 219, 226
    and knowledge of AIDS, 18-19, 20, 28, 173
    local policymaking and, 255-258

About the Contributors

Charles J. Baker, M.D., is Medical Director, Los Angeles County Department of Health Services/Juvenile Court Health Services Division where they are responsible for providing medical care to juveniles in two Los Angeles County Juvenile Halls and 16 Residential Treatment Facilities. Delivery of health care is also provided to the Department of Children's Services shelter care facility, MacLaren Children's Center. He received his B.S. degree from the School of Pharmacy, Purdue University and his M.D. from the Indiana School of Medicine, Indiana University. His rotating internship was completed at Good Samaritan Hospital, Los Angeles, and he was a pediatrician resident at Children's Hospital, Los Angeles. He is also a Colonel in the U.S. Army Reserves.

Albert Bandura, Ph.D., is David Starr Jordan Professor of Social Sciences in Psychology at Stanford University. He received his bachelor's degree from the University of British Columbia in 1949 and his Ph.D. degree in 1952 from the University of Iowa. After completing his doctorate, he joined the faculty at Stanford University, where he has remained to pursue his career. He served as Chairman of the Department of Psychology and was honored by Stanford by being awarded an endowed chair.

Bandura is a proponent of social cognitive theory. He has authored countless articles and seven books on a wide range of issues in psychology. He has been elected to the American Academy of Arts and Sciences and to the Institute of Medicine of the National Academy of Sciences. He was elected to the Presidency of the American Psychological Association and the Western Psychological Association. Awards he has received include the Distinguished Scientific Contributions Award of the American Psychological Association, the Distinguished Scientist Award, Division 12 (APA), the William James Award of the American Psychological Society for outstanding achievements in psychological science, the Distinguished Contribution Award from the International Society for Research in Aggression and a Guggenheim Fellowship. He is the recipient of a number of honorary degrees.

Benjamin P. Bowser, Ph.D., is currently Associate Professor of Sociology and Social Services at California State University at Hayward. He is a former Research Director for the Bayview-Hunter's Point Foundation in San Francisco and has held research and administrative appointments at Stanford, Santa Clara, and Cornell Universities. He also is Associate Editor of *Sage Race Relations Abstracts* (London), editor of *Black Male Adolescents* (University Press America, 1991) and co-editor of *Impacts of Racism on White Americans* (Sage, 1981), and has written articles for *Youth and Society*, *Urban Anthropology*, and *Journal of the National Medical Association*. His research has focused on race relations, community studies, and community-based AIDS prevention. He received his Ph.D. from Cornell University in 1976.

Thomas J. Coates, Ph.D., is Professor of Medicine (with joint appointments in the Departments of Psychiatry and Epidemiology and Biostatistics), Director of the Behavioral Medicine Unit in the Division of General Internal Medicine, and Director of the Center for AIDS Prevention Studies (CAPS) at University of California, San Francisco (UCSF). Dr. Coates came to UCSF from Johns

Hopkins in 1982. Prior to that time he was on the faculty of the Stanford Heart Disease Prevention Program. His interests and experience have focused on the study of disease-related behavior, with an emphasis on interventions to modify high risk behaviors in adolescents and adults. He is the author of many recent publications on theoretical underpinnings of AIDS prevention programs, the effects of antibody testing on high risk behavior, reducing high risk behavior among seropositive men, and AIDS risk reduction among minority gay men. Dr. Coates is a member of the Committee on AIDS and the Statistical, Social, and Behavioral Sciences of the National Research Council/National Academy of Sciences. He is Chairman of the Steering Committee for the Social and Behavioral Studies Unit at the Global Programme on AIDS at the World Health Organization, and a consultant to USAID-funded AIDS prevention programs in developing countries.

Lawrence J. D'Angelo, M.D., M.P.H., is Chairman of the Department of Adolescent and Young Adult Medicine at Children's National Medical Center, Washington, DC and Professor of Pediatrics, Medicine, and Health Care Sciences at George Washington University. He is a graduate of Harvard College, Duke University Medical School, the Harvard University School of Public Health, and he trained in internal medicine at Georgetown University Hospital. He completed a medical chief residency at the Veterans Administration Hospital in Washington, then he joined the U.S. Public Health Service and was stationed as an Epidemic Intelligence Service Officer at the Centers for Disease Control in Atlanta, Georgia. He returned to Washington, DC to help found the Division of General Medicine at Georgetown University in 1979 and in 1982 accepted his current position at Children's.

D'Angelo is the author of more than 50 articles and book chapters. His particular area of interest is the epidemiology of a variety of acute and chronic diseases in adolescents and young adults. Under the sponsorship of the Centers for Disease Control, he has conducted an annual seroprevalence study to track the rate of infection with the human immunodeficiency virus in Washington, DC adolescents and has shown a 500% increase in seroprevalence rate in teenaged patients coming to CNMC for care during the past 5 years. In addition, he is also interested in the participation of HIV-infected adolescents in AIDS clinical trials. As a visiting scientist at the National Institute of Allergy and Infectious Diseases' Division of AIDS, he worked to incorporate adolescents into the clinical trials network. He is the recipient of a special NIAID award recognizing these efforts.

Ralph J. DiClemente, Ph.D., is a Research Psychologist at the Center for AIDS Prevention Studies and the Institute for Health Policy Studies, University of California San Francisco School of Medicine. He is also a Senior Research Scientist at the Bayview-Hunter's Point Foundation, a community-based organization engaged in HIV-prevention research focused on the African-American community. He received his B.A. from the City University of New York (CCNY), an M.S. from the Harvard School of Public Health in Behavioral Sciences and Epidemiology, and earned his Ph.D. from the University of California San Francisco in Health Psychology. He was also an American Cancer Society Fellow at the University of California San Francisco from 1984-1986.

Abigail English, J.D., is an attorney at the National Center for Youth Law in San Francisco and is Project Director of the Center's Adolescent Health Care Project. She is a recognized expert on legal issues in adolescent health care. She has litigated major cases affecting adolescents' rights in the health care system, lectured frequently, authored numerous publications, and served as a consultant to professional organizations on legal issues in the health care of children and adolescents.

Her current work includes a special focus on problems in pediatric and adolescent AIDS. She was honored by the Society for Adolescent Medicine in 1987 as a Gallagher Lecturer on legal and ethical aspects of sexually transmitted diseases and AIDS in adolescents. Her article, "The HIV-AIDS epidemic and the child welfare system: Protecting the rights of infants, young children, and adolescents," will appear in a special symposium issue of the *Iowa Law Review* in 1992.

Jeffrey D. Fisher, Ph.D., is Professor of Psychology at the University of Connecticut. He is co-principal investigator of a large 5-year NIMH-sponsored AIDS risk-reduction grant and has written extensively on HIV prevention. His articles on HIV prevention have appeared in *American Psychologist, Psychological Bulletin,* and in several edited volumes. He was a member of the Psychobiological, Biological, and Neurosciences Subcommittee, Mental Health Acquired Immunodeficiency Syndrome Research Review Committee of the National Institutes of Mental Health from 1989-1991 and was Chair of the Social Psychology Program at the University of Connecticut from 1989-1990. Before focusing his research on HIV prevention, he did extensive research on factors that affect recipient reactions to help.

William A. Fisher, Ph.D., is Professor in the Department of Psychology and is cross-appointed to the Department of Obstetrics and Gynecology at the University of Western Ontario in London, Canada. He was educated at Tel Aviv University (B.A.) and Purdue University (M.S., Ph.D.), and is well know for his work on the prevention of adolescent pregnancy (*Adolescents, sex, and contraception,* 1983, co-edited with Donn Byrne) and on the prevention of STD/HIV infection (*Psychological Bulletin,* 1992, co-authored with Jeffrey D. Fisher). He is a Fellow of the Society for the Scientific Study of Sex, a Director of the Planned Parenthood Federation of Canada, and is on the editorial board of *The Journal of Sex Research.* Dr. Fisher has published more than 50 scientific papers and chapters in the area of sexual health promotion, and he has received departmental, university, and provincial awards for excellence in teaching. He is co-directing a major AIDS risk reduction education project for the National Institute of Mental Health.

Adam N. Gordon, D.S.W., is Senior Associate Director of Mental Health Services at Elmhurst Hospital Center in New York. Formerly he was a Senior Research Associate at Columbia University School of Social Work where he managed the organization and evaluation of field trials in such areas as drug abuse prevention and treatment, AIDS risk reduction, and HIV risk assessment. He was also the Project Director for the AIDS Prevention Research Center at Columbia University School of Social Work.

His current research interests include the development and testing of culturally relevant social learning and cognitive behavior models of treatment to a variety of human service problems.

Karen Hein, M.D., is currently Professor of Pediatrics and Associate Professor of Epidemiology and Social Medicine at Albert Einstein

College of Medicine in New York. In July 1987, she founded and is the Director of the Adolescent AIDS Program at Montefiore Medical Center in the Bronx. She is the President of the Society for Adolescent Medicine. She attended the University of Wisconsin for undergraduate training, attended Dartmouth Medical School from 1966-1968, and in 1970 graduated with an M.D. degree from Columbia University's College of Physicians and Surgeons. Between 1970-1973, she completed three years of Pediatric residency at the Bronx Municipal Hospital Center and then did an additional year of postdoctoral fellowship training in Adolescent Medicine (1973-1974) at Montefiore Hospital. She was Director of the Division of Adolescent Medicine at Columbia University, College of Physicians and Surgeons Babies Hospital from 1980-1984. Before and after, she has been on the faculty of Albert Einstein College of Medicine involved in program development, clinical research, teaching, and patient care related to adolescents.

Hein has written more than 100 articles, chapters, and abstracts related to adolescent health, particularly focusing on high-risk youth. She has been the Principal Investigator of 20 grants, 16 of the most recent awards from foundations and federal agencies related to HIV/AIDS in adolescents. She serves as a consultant to many federal and health organizations, including the New York City Department of Health, Board of Education, Girls Clubs, and the American Medical Association. She is a manuscript and abstract reviewer for many medical journals and medical societies. She co-authored the book *AIDS: Trading Fears for Facts*, a guide for young people published by Consumer Reports Books in 1989.

Ralph Hingson, Sc.D., is Professor of Public Health and Chair of the Social and Behavioral Sciences Department at Boston University School of Medicine, School of Public Health. He received his Sc.D. in Behavioral Sciences and Public Health from Johns Hopkins University. He has published extensively on alcohol and substance abuse. His recent publications include articles in *American Journal of Public Health, JAMA, New England Journal of Medicine, Pediatrics, Journal of Studies on Alcohol, The International Journal of the Addictions* and *Alcohol, Drugs and Driving.*

His research includes evaluations of maternal drinking; marijuana and cocaine use on fetal development; drunk driving laws and other traffic safety interventions; studies of alcoholism treatment in occupational settings, and research on adolescent and adult knowledge, and attitudinal and behavioral changes in response to the AIDS epidemic.

Robert C. Hornik, Ph.D., is Professor in the Annenberg School for Communication at the University of Pennsylvania and is the Director of the Center for International, Health, and Development Communication. He is the author of *Development Communication: Information, Agriculture and Nutrition in the Third World.* He has been a frequent consultant to the World Health Organization, Global Programme on AIDS.

Susan Huscroft, M.D., is the Chief Physician for the Los Angeles County Department of Health Services/Juvenile Court Health Services division, which is responsible for providing medical care to the juveniles in two Los Angeles County Juvenile Halls, 16 Residential Treatment Facilities, and the Maclaren Children's Center (the Los Angeles County shelter care facility). She received her B.S. and M.D. degrees from the University of California San Francisco Medical Center; and her Pediatric Internship and Residency at Los Angeles County/University of Southern California Medical Center.

Douglas Kirby, Ph.D., is Director of Research at ETR Associates. Formerly he was Director of Research for the Center for Population Options. He has directed nationwide studies of adolescent sexual behavior, sexuality education programs, direct mailings of STD/AIDS pamphlets to adolescent males, and schoolbased clinics. He has authored or co-authored numerous volumes, articles, and chapters both on these programs and on methods of evaluating them. Currently he is evaluating programs for teenage mothers, is directing statewide surveys of adolescent risk-taking behaviors, and is helping design and evaluate comprehensive school-wide programs to reduce unprotected sexual behavior.

Cheryl Koopman, Ph.D., is Assistant Professor of Clinical Psychology in the Department of Child Psychiatry, Columbia University and Research Associate in the Department of Psychiatry, Stanford University. Her previous positions include research scientist in the HIV Center for Clinical and Behavioral Studies at the New York State

Psychiatric Institute, visiting scholar in the Columbia University School of International and Public Affairs, and postdoctoral fellow at Columbia Teachers College and Harvard Medical School. She was co-principal investigator on Dr. Rotheram-Borus's study targeting runaway and gay adolescents for HIV/AIDS prevention.

Her publications include articles in the *American Psychologist, JAMA, Journal of AIDS Education and Prevention,* and *Journal of Social Issues.* Her primary area of research interest is risk assessment and high risk behavior. Currently she is continuing to work with Drs. Rotheram-Borus and Rosario on HIV/AIDS prevention research targeting adolescents. Her other research examines the psychological effects of a disaster (the Berkley/Oakland firestorm), and she is evaluating the effectiveness of hypnosis to help people stop smoking cigarettes.

Stephen J. Misovich, is a doctoral student in Psychology at the University of Connecticut. His work on AIDS risk reduction among college students, health care workers, and other groups has been published in *AIDS Education and Prevention* and in edited volumes. He has also published work on the initiation and maintenance of personal change. His current research involves studying the effects of reference group norms on personal change.

Robert E. Morris, M.D., is a senior physician for Los Angeles County and Assistant Clinical Professor of Pediatrics at the University of California Los Angeles. He coordinates the UCLA medicine and pediatric residents during the adolescent rotation at Los Angeles Central Juvenile Hall. Before his UCLA position, he was Associate Director of the Emergency Department at Children's Hospital of Los Angeles. He has had articles published in *Annals of Emergency Medicine, Pediatric Emergency Care,* and *Journal of Adolescent Health Care,* as well as chapters in several books. During the past 4 years, he has been involved in research regarding sexually transmitted diseases, especially in the area of AIDS. He has contributed abstracts to the past three International AIDS meetings and has lectured to national organizations concerning AIDS and the detained juvenile.

Daniel Romer, Ph.D., is a Research Director in the Center for International, Health, and Development Communication at the Annenberg

School for Communication at the University of Pennsylvania. His research interests are in the social psychology of persuasive communication, the use of mass media for social change, and the design of AIDS education.

Margaret Rosario, Ph.D., is Assistant Professor of Clinical Psychology, Department of Psychiatry, College of Physicians and Surgeons, Columbia University; Assistant Professor of Clinical Public Health, Social Medical Sciences, School of Public Health, Columbia University; and Research Scientist III, Division of Child Psychiatry, New York State Psychiatric Institute. She received her M.A. and Ph.D. in Psychology from New York University. Her publications include articles in the *Journal of Personality and Social Psychology*, *The Community Psychologist*, and *Journal of Community Psychology*. Currently she is working with Drs. Rotheram-Borus and Koopman on HIV/AIDS prevention research targeting adolescents.

Mary Jane Rotheram-Borus, Ph.D., is Clinical Professor of Medical Psychology, Division of Child Psychiatry, Columbia University College of Physicians and Surgeons, and a Research Scientist at the New York State Psychiatric Institute. She received her B.A. at the University of California, Irvine and her Ph.D. in clinical psychology at the University of Southern California. Her research interests include assessment and modification of children's social skills, ethnic identity, group processes, and cross-ethnic interactions. Her work on assertiveness training was selected as an exemplary model of primary prevention by the American Psychological Association and her work on suicide prevention was selected the Outstanding Child and Adolescent Mental Health Project in New York State, 1986. She currently is conducting a five-year study evaluating the effectiveness of an intensive AIDS prevention program with runaway and gay youths in New York City, which was chosen as an exemplary model of primary prevention by the American Medical Association. Her research has been funded by the National Science Foundation, National Institute of Mental Health, Society for Research in Child Development, and W. T. Grant Foundation.

Steven P. Schinke, Ph.D., received his doctoral degree in Social Welfare from the University of Wisconsin at Madison in 1975.

Subsequently he served on the faculty of the University of Washington School of Social Work in Seattle. He joined the faculty at Columbia University in 1986 and is currently a Professor in the School of Social Work. His research interests center on prevention training, with a special focus on substance abuse and minority culture adolescents. Currently he is Head of an AIDS Minority Research Center. He presently serves as a consulting editor for a number of journals, including *Addictive Behaviors, Behavioral Medicine Abstracts,* and *Children and Youth Services Review,* and has published more than 150 articles dealing with preventive interventions and skills training for adolescents.

Diane L. Sondheimer is currently Chief, Research Demonstration Program, Child and Family Support Branch, Division of Applied and Services Research Branch, National Institute of Mental Health. In this capacity, she directs a national program that seeks to expand the research base on the effectiveness of new models of organizing, delivering, and financing mental health services to children and adolescents with or at risk for serious emotional or mental disorders and their families. Prior to this, she was the Coordinator of Adolescent HIV Research at the National Institute of Child Health and Human Development, National Institutes of Health. She is a doctoral student in Medical Anthropology at the Catholic University of America and holds a master's degree in Public Health from the Johns Hopkins School of Hygiene and Public Health. She has published articles, editorials, and book chapters on the subject of adolescents and HIV and has presented posters and abstracts at major meetings, including the IV, V, and VI International AIDS Conferences.

Lee Strunin, Ph.D., is Assistant Professor of Public Health in the Social and Behavioral Sciences Department of Boston University School of Medicine, School of Public Health. She received her Ph.D. in Anthropology from Brandeis University. Her recent publications include articles in *Social Science and Medicine, American Journal of Public Health, Pediatrics,* and *The International Journal of the Addictions.*

Her research interests include adolescent sexuality; substance use and AIDS-related risk behaviors among adolescents; ethnic and cultural differences in health beliefs and behaviors; sociocultural issues in health and health care, and medical students' socialization.

James A. Wells, Ph.D., a medical sociologist and epidemiologist, is Senior Research Associate with the Center for Health Policy Studies in Columbia, Maryland. He formerly has held the positions of Senior Policy Analyst at the Project HOPE Center for Health Affairs and Associate Research Scientist in Pediatrics, Yale University School of Medicine. He has published the monograph *Learning AIDS: A Special Report on Readability, Literacy and the HIV Epidemic* and has published in several journals, including *Health Affairs, Journal of the American Medical Association,* and *Health and Social Behavior.* He recently has been involved in research into the role of literacy in health education, the impact of health insurance reform on coverage of AIDS therapies, and a survey of AIDS educational messages and behavior change in the United States, Great Britain, and France. He has served as a consultant to the American Foundation for AIDS Research, the National AIDS Clearinghouse, and the World Health Organization's Global Program on AIDS. He currently is a member of the National Institutes of Health Study Section on Aging and Human Development. He received his Ph.D. in Sociology from Duke University and was a Fellow in Epidemiology at the Yale University School of Medicine.

Gina M. Wingood, M.P.H., is a doctoral candidate at Harvard University School of Public Health in the department of Health and Social Behavior. She received her M.P.H. in Maternal and Child Health from the University of California, Berkeley. Formerly she served as a data analyst and a community educator at the Bayview Hunter's Point Foundation in San Francisco. She has co-authored articles in *Multicultural Inquiry and Research on AIDS, AIDS Education and Prevention,* and the *Journal of Ethnicity and Disease.* She also co-authored a chapter with B. Bowser in *AIDS and Adolescents: Emerging Issues.* Currently she is conducting research on social/behavioral predictors of HIV infection among African Americans and designing HIV/AIDS intervention/prevention programs tailored toward African American female adoescents and women.